Radiographic and Imaging Techniques for Radiology Residents and Technologists

Rajesh Gothi

Radiographic and Imaging Techniques for Radiology Residents and Technologists

Springer

Rajesh Gothi
Department of Imaging
Holy Family Hospital
New Delhi, India

ISBN 978-981-96-4815-3 ISBN 978-981-96-4816-0 (eBook)
https://doi.org/10.1007/978-981-96-4816-0

This Springer imprint is published by the registered company Springer Nature Singapore Pte Ltd.
The registered company address is: 152 Beach Road, #21-01/04 Gateway East, Singapore 189721, Singapore

This book is dedicated with love and gratitude to my wife, Swarna, whose patience and unwavering support allowed me to immerse myself fully in writing. Her patience, understanding and encouragement have been my guiding light and source of strength throughout this journey.

To my wonderful children—Nikita, Priyanka, Gaurav and Ankit—and my beloved grandchildren—Anika, Siddharth, Radhika and Madhav—your boundless energy, mischief and love have filled my life with joy and inspiration.

I also extend a special dedication to my esteemed teachers at AIIMS, particularly Prof. Sneh Bhargava, whose excellence as an educator left an indelible mark on me, and my revered mentor, the late Dr. R.K. Goulatia, whose guidance shaped my career. I am deeply grateful to Prof. Sima Mukherjee, a brilliant teacher, and to Dr. Manorama Berry, Dr. Mira Rajani, Dr. Ratni Gujral and Dr. S. Satyanath, all of whom have played significant roles in my professional growth.

Foreword

Navigating the vast and complex world of medical imaging can be an intimidating challenge for a beginner. The sheer volume of technical jargon and intricate procedures often overwhelms new students, residents, and technologists alike. This is where Dr. Rajesh Gothi's book *Radiographic and Imaging Techniques for Radiology Residents and Technologists* plays a valuable role, providing a much-needed, concise, and lucid guide to the fundamentals of the field. The author with his vast experience in the field successfully delivers a book that simplifies complex topics without sacrificing accuracy, making it an indispensable companion for anyone starting their career in radiology.

The book's well-defined structure is one of its greatest strengths. Divided into thirty well-organized chapters, the content flows logically, building knowledge from one section to the next. The author places appropriate emphasis on essential topics, starting with a thorough exploration of chest radiographs—covering both technique and interpretation—before moving on to barium studies for the gastrointestinal tract and the intricacies of bone radiography.

The book also effectively demystifies modern imaging modalities. It provides an introduction to basic **CT** and **MR techniques**, defining key terminology in a way that is accessible and easy to grasp. Another crucial topic, **radiation protection**, is given suitable coverage, highlighting its importance in clinical practice.

As the title suggests, this book is specifically tailored for **radiology residents** and **technologists**, and is the perfect beginner's guide. It doesn't aim to replace the comprehensive, multi-volume radiology textbooks but rather to serve as a practical, easy-to-read primer that makes the learning process smoother. Students of imaging technology will also find this book useful for its straightforward explanations and practical focus.

I thoroughly enjoyed reading this book and was particularly impressed by the author's clarity of thought. I recommend this guide to all beginners in radiology and imaging technology. It is a useful resource that will undoubtedly make the initial stages of their professional journey comfortable and less daunting. Dr. Gothi's passion for the subject is suitably reflected in the book.

Department of Radiodiagnosis &
Interventional Radiology
All India Institute of Medical Sciences
New Delhi, India
2 August 2025

Raju Sharma

Preface

A Gentle Introduction to Radiology for Beginners

Starting a journey in radiology can be both exhilarating and overwhelming. The field is filled with technical depth and precision, but for newcomers, this complexity can be daunting. There are numerous renowned textbooks, written by leading experts, which offer in-depth knowledge and advanced insights. However, for those just stepping into the world of radiology, these classics may seem like a mountain to climb—immense, detailed and often beyond the immediate grasp of a beginner.

For students, whether aspiring radiologists or medical technologists, the most frequent question is: "Where do I begin?"

The ideal starting point, in my view, is a resource that eases you into the discipline. A book that simplifies the basics and serves as a companion throughout your early training, providing practical, hands-on guidance. This book is designed to do just that. It walks you through the foundational concepts of radiology in an approachable and clear manner, offering step-by-step discussions of key techniques and core principles essential for anyone new to the field.

Over the years, the world of radiology—now integrated within the broader domain of medical imaging—has advanced dramatically. Technologies like CT, ultrasound, PET scans and MRI have not only revolutionized diagnostics but also enhanced the precision and quality of patient care. With each advancement, departments continually adapt and update their protocols to stay ahead and maintain high standards. Yet, despite these technological leaps, every radiologist's journey begins in the same place: the beginning, where one sets on the process of developing a solid understanding of the basics.

This book aims to guide you through that crucial beginning, laying a strong foundation without attempting to replace the more comprehensive, specialized texts you will soon encounter in your training. Instead, it serves as a stepping stone—a resource to ground you in the field before you explore its deeper and more complex aspects.

Inside, you will find key areas of radiology and imaging presented in a structured, digestible format, making it an ideal guide for students in their early training. The content is straightforward, with minimal jargon, focusing instead on practical knowledge that you can apply immediately in the department. My goal is to help you build a confident, reliable foundation in radiology, preparing you to approach more advanced topics with ease as you continue your learning journey.

This book is written not just for the classroom, but as a resource you will return to throughout your education. I welcome your feedback, suggestions and corrections, as learning is a lifelong process, and your input will help improve this work for the future readers.

As you begin this exciting journey, I want to leave you with a thought: "When people leave this world, an entire library of knowledge leaves with them". In writing this book, I hope to share what I have learned—and continue to learn—with the coming generation of radiologists and medical technologists.

New Delhi, India Rajesh Gothi

Acknowledgements

I am deeply indebted to the students of the Department of Imaging at Holy Family Hospital, New Delhi. Their passion for radiology, both its theoretical and practical aspect, served as the primary inspiration for this book. The curiosity they brought to their studies, coupled with their willingness to confront challenges and self-doubt, has left a profound and lasting impact on me. Their enthusiasm, be it through volunteering as models, contributing images or fulfilling my various requests—no matter how trivial—without hesitation, has been invaluable in shaping this work.

I extend my sincere gratitude to our esteemed medical technology educators: Rajshree, Saroj Thakur, Sunil (Baba), Dinesh and Bhupinder. Your dedication to teaching and your steadfast support throughout this journey have been pivotal.

A special acknowledgement goes to our exceptional technologists: Santosh, Dinesh, Sylvester, Sarita, Vandana, Bandana, Sagar and Tanupriya. Your expertise, collaboration and willingness to contribute have greatly enriched this book.

I would also like to express my heartfelt thanks to our models, Mr. Yash and Mr. Harsh, for their patience, cooperation and essential contributions.

To our respected faculty—Drs. Renee Kulkarni, P.S. Uppal, Amit Kumar, Syed Rehan, Charu Ghai, Neeti Purkait and Neha Nischal, Mr. Muein, Mr. Bhuvan and the extraordinary, Mrs. Huma—your unwavering support and encouragement have been instrumental throughout this process, and I am truly grateful.

Lastly, I owe a special debt of gratitude to Dr. Amit Sahu, Dr. Diwan Chand Aggarwal Imaging Centre, South Delhi Ultrasound and X-ray Clinic, and the Department of Imaging at Holy Family Hospital, New Delhi, for providing the images that form an integral part of this book.

Contents

Part I Radiography

1 Introduction to the Basics of Radiology, Physical Principles, Safety Issues and Terminologies 3

2 Positioning in Chest X-Rays 11

3 The Normal Chest X-Ray 21

4 Systematic Interpretation of Chest X-Ray 31

5 Interpretation of Lung Lesions 39

6 Pleural Pathology 55

7 Evaluation of the Heart 63

8 The Intrathoracic Vasculature 71

9 The Mediastinum and Its Normal Structures 77

10 Plain X-Ray of the Abdomen 85

11 Evaluation of the Pharynx and Oesophagus 95

12 Stomach and Duodenum 107

13 The Small Bowel 111

14 The Large Bowel 121

15 The Urinary Tract 131

16 Bones and Joints 145

17 The Peritoneal Spaces 161

18 X-Rays of the Skull 167

Part II CT Scans

19 CT Scans: Basics of CT Scanning 173

20 Types of CT Scanners 179

21 Meaning of Commonly Used Acronyms and Words in CT: A Beginner's Guide 187

22 Artefacts in CT and How to Deal with Them 199

23 CT Protocols 207

24 Guide to Patient Safety in the Radiology Department 237

Part III MRI (Magnetic Resonance Imaging)

25 MRI: Some Basic Facts 245

26 Acronyms and Artefacts in MRI: A Beginners Guide 251

27 Commonly Used MRI Sequences 277

28 Contrast Studies in CT and MRI 293

29 Image Gently: Patient Safety in the Radiology Department . . . 297

Part IV PET Scans

30 Introduction to PET Scan 303

Part I

Radiography

1 Introduction to the Basics of Radiology, Physical Principles, Safety Issues and Terminologies

Abstract

The history of medical radiology is short. X-rays were discovered by Wilhelm Conrad Roentgen on the 8th of November 1895. Since that accidental discovery, we have come a long way. Conventional radiography has progressed to digital radiography, dark field radiography and CT scans. Image quality has improved considerably, so much so, that radiology has become an all-important part of medical diagnostics and treatment. In this chapter, the student will be given a brief introduction to the subject. There are several terms used in radiology, which need to be known to the students. Also, while there has been increased use of radiation, there is a growing fear of side effects of radiation exposure. We will briefly touch upon some of the topics which are essential for learning.

Keywords

X-rays · Radiation · Terminology · Side effects

Radiology is a highly technical subject. There is plenty of physics and chemistry involved in the process of generating an X-ray, something which needs to be understood.

Briefly speaking, X-rays are electromagnetic radiation, having an extremely short wavelength but a high frequency.

An X-ray beam is produced inside a vacuum tube, also called a "Cathode ray tube", by passing a current and heating the cathode, which is a negative electrode. The cathode consists of a tungsten filament/coil. High-energy unbound electrons [1] are emitted by thermionic emission from the heated cathode. The electrons being negatively charged are repelled by the cathode and driven towards the positively charged tungsten anode. The speed at which the electrons travel in the vacuum X-ray tube is determined by the potential difference between the cathode and anode. Upon hitting the anode, the electron energy is converted into heat (99%) and X-ray photons (1%). The X-ray photons unlike electrons, neither have a charge nor a mass. The X-ray photons are electromagnetic energy similar to gamma rays but differ from it in several aspects, such as how they are produced, the wavelength and frequency as well as in their application in medical practice. They are let out as a beam or spectrum having photons of different strengths which can pass through soft tissues and low-density structures but do not get easy passage through structures having high density. Since the photons have variable strength, some of them get absorbed by the high-density tissue while the rest penetrate the exposed region. The ability to penetrate tissues, therefore depends on the strength of the X-ray photons and

R. Gothi, *Radiographic and Imaging Techniques for Radiology Residents and Technologists*,
https://doi.org/10.1007/978-981-96-4816-0_1

the density of the obstacle in the path of the X-ray beam as it converges towards the receiving device, such as the X-ray film, an imaging plate or a digital receiver. Air allows free passage. Fat, water and soft tissues hinder their passage to a variable extent. Calcium, bone, heavy metal, barium and iodinated contrast medium block the X-ray beam significantly. Consequently, when the X-rays penetrate the patient and reach the film or any other device, they show an image having various shades of gray ranging from a completely black area (representing the region in the patient's body which it could easily pass through, such as an air-containing regions) to completely white regions (corresponding to bone or any other high-density objects). All other tissues produce intermittent shades of gray, depending upon the extent to which they can obstruct the X-ray beam penetration.

Having understood why an X-ray film has that typical look, we will proceed with areas which are frequently examined by X-rays. But before we do that, let us talk briefly about radiation safety.

1.1 Radiation Safety

Radiation exposure has increased substantially over the years, especially with the extensive deployment of CT scans as a potent medical imaging tool [2].

Radiation exposure is potentially harmful to the patient and should be used judiciously. Minimally needed radiation dose **(As Low As Reasonably Achievable—ALARA)**, and avoidance of repeating X-rays unnecessarily, should be the aim of the radiation technologist and radiologist.

1.2 Radiation Exposure in Childhood

Paediatric patients, on account of their size, are more sensitive to radiation than adults. As a consequence, they are at an increased risk of developing radiation-related complications, including cancers. X-rays and CT scans must be done only when necessary and by using paediatric protocols. Care should be taken to obtain images appropriate for interpretation and by using the lowest possible radiation parameters. An experienced technician should preferably do the x-ray to avoid unnecessary repeats. Fortunately, with the availability of digital radiography, most X-rays of both children and adults are of good quality and need no retakes unless there is an issue with positioning or artefacts degrading the image.

We can still try some more, by doing the following to further limit radiation exposure:

1. By taking X-rays without an anti-scatter grid in small and thin patients. The radiation dose is reduced when the grid is not used. A minor improvement in image quality by using the grid, in this category of patients, is insufficient to justify its use [2].
2. By reducing exposure time.
3. When films are being used, by using a fast film-screen combination.
4. The body parts not required to be exposed should be shielded by a lead shield.
5. If there is a recently performed X-ray, it should be reviewed first and further X-rays of the same region, be considered only, if necessary.
6. Collimate the beam so that only the required area is exposed.
7. It is always useful to talk to the referring physician before performing any radiation-related investigation [3].

1.3 Radiation Exposure in Pregnancy

The importance of recognizing the additional risk of radiation in pregnancy is because radiation may have an adverse effect on the embryo and foetus.

During an entire pregnancy, a cumulative effective dose to the foetus below 5.0 mSv can be taken as the cut-off limit. Foetal radiation dose below 50 mGy is considered safe in the first trimester. During the second and third trimesters, a dose above 150 mGy may probably be the trigger for adverse foetal side effects. Most of the diagnostic studies performed during the pregnancy are below the threshold level [4] and can be considered as safe. A single X-ray chest PA delivers a dose of 0.01 mSv. This radiation dose does not threaten the foetus.

The effect of radiation also depends on the foetal age. The embryo/foetus is most susceptible to radiation during organogenesis (2 to 7 weeks gestational age) in the first trimester. The 10–17 weeks is a sensitive time as it is linked with foetal CNS development. Later, the effect of diagnostic radiation is unlikely to cause any significant effect. However, if the foetus is exposed to more than 100 mGy, there may be some untoward effects including miscarriage, growth reduction, IQ reduction and severe mental retardation. This level of dose is probably administered during radiation therapy but not in a diagnostic procedure. However, "stochastic" effects which are due to DNA damage are carcinogenic and increase with increasing doses. Unfortunately, there is no threshold below which there is no risk from the stochastic effect. Therefore, clinicians and radiologists should counsel pregnant patients regardless of the gestational age and avoid unnecessary and repeated exposures.

Considering all factors, if it is clinically possible, delay or avoid X-rays unless considered necessary and keep it below 100 mGy [5]. It is also worth knowing that radiation to parts of the body other than the pregnant abdomen is unlikely to affect the foetus and foetal or gonadal shielding is no longer recommended in diagnostic radiology [6]. It should also be remembered that if a diagnostic radiological investigation is vital, it should not be withheld out of fear of harmful side effects of radiation [6].

1.4 Radiation Dose in CT

The advent of CT has ushered in a revolution in diagnostic imaging. However, this revolution has also increased radiation exposure to patients.

The effective radiation dose varies from patient to patient, from procedure to procedure and from area to area of the body being examined. It can range anywhere from 1 mSv to 10 or more mSv.

The radiation dose can be kept to a minimum by employing the following manoeuvres.

1. Use the automatic exposure control (AEC). This automatically changes the tube current by taking into consideration the patient's anatomy.
2. Adequate collimation of the area to be scanned, so that the coverage is limited to the area of interest and does not expose areas of no particular interest.
3. Using a low kV or a low mAs technique.

Radiation dose for the head, paranasal sinuses, chest and bones can be kept low because there is adequate contrast between bones, air and soft tissues. Children should be examined using child-specific protocols. All CT scans should be planned based on the clinical situation and requirement and only then the scanning be done. Wherever possible, if another investigation such as ultrasonography or MRI is likely to give similar or even better information, that imaging modality must be preferred. It is therefore important to discuss this with the referring physician before performing the CT.

1.5 Radiation Dose in PET-CT

The radiation dose given to a patient undergoing PET-CT is a summation of both CT and PET-related radiation. Almost every patient gets a whole-body CT which can give an effective radiation dose from 7 to 30 mSv. To this is added the radiation dose given by 18F-FDG PET scan which can be as much as 8 mSv [7]. Hence, the risk-benefit ratio must be weighed first before referring the patient for a PET-CT [8]. An earnest attempt should be made to ensure that the total effective radiation dose received from PET-CT does not climb up beyond 32 mSv in addition to the background radiation dose, the patient will anyway receive [8].

1.6 How Much Radiation Is Generally Given in an Imaging Study

This is one of the most frequently asked questions. There are several charts and tables available which discuss this issue.

Listed in this table is some information about the radiation doses with radiological procedures.

Radiation dose to foetus while examining the pregnant patient:

Plain film	Radiation dose to foetus (mSv)	Threshold for safe radiation (mSv)
Lumbar spine	1–3, maximum 10	50
Abdomen	1–3	50
Chest X-ray	0.01	50
CT head	0.01–0.1	50
CT chest	0.2	50
CT abdomen and pelvis	10–13	50
CT KUB	10	50

Radiation dose to adults	Typical case
LS spine	1.4 mSv
NCCT brain	1.6 mSv
NCCT spine	8.8 mSv
CT abdomen	10 mSv
NCCT head and neck	1.2
CECT chest	3–5 mSv
Low-dose CT	1–1.5 mSv
Chest X-ray	0.01 mSv

1.7 Dose-Related Radiation Risk [9]

Doses below 0.02 mSv are considered as low doses with radiation risk below 1:1,000,000.

Doses under 2 mSv are considered medium doses with a radiation risk between 1:1,000,000 and 1:10,000.

Dose above 2 mSv are high doses, equivalent to one CT scan of the head. The radiation risk is between 1:10,000 and less.

For further information on radiation exposure to adults, the reader is encouraged to visit one of the many authoritative sites [9, 10] on this subject.

1.8 Some Common Terms Used in Radiation [11]

Absorbed Dose The amount of energy which radiation deposits in a mass or tissue is called the "absorbed dose". The unit used for measuring this absorbed dose is expressed as gray (Gy). This term can be used for all types of radiation but does not describe the biological effect of radiation on tissues.

ALARA Principle ALARA stands for "As low as reasonably achievable". In other words, it means exposing the patient to the minimum possible radiation dose. Required to produce a satisfactory radiological examination. This can be done by adjusting factors to reduce the exposure dose, increasing the distance between the source of radiation and the part being examined as well as by using protective shielding, wherever possible.

Anode The positive-end of the X-ray tube from where X-ray photons are generated.

Anode Cooling When the electrons emitted from the cathode are focused on the anode, the focal spot on the gets heated. This heat is transferred by the molybdenum stem of the anode to the oil which surrounds the stem. The heat from the oil is then transferred by convection currents to the x-ray tube housing, from where it gets dissipated into the atmosphere.

Background Radiation This is the radiation present in the atmosphere and freely available from natural sources.

BEIR The abbreviation stands for "Biological Effects of Radiation".

Collimation This is a process by which the projection of the x-ray beam can be limited to the area of interest. The device which does this is called the collimator device.

Compton Effect This is a phenomenon which happens when an X-ray photon interacts with an outer electron of a valence shell. It results in a change in direction (scattering) and transference of energy to the electron. This results in a decrease in energy or an increase in the wavelength of an X-ray photon.

Computed Radiography The system consists of a phosphor imaging plate (IP). On being exposed to X-rays, by use of digitizing processing, a latent image of the irradiated object is created and embedded on this plate. Subsequently, on being exposed to a laser beam, the latent image is released and captured by a computer which converts it into a pixelated form. This is subsequently printed on an imaging film, where it appears as a radiograph of the irradiated object.

Contrast In imaging, it stands for the ability to distinguish between closely approximated densities.

Cumulative Dose This is the total sum of doses exposed to the body.

Deterministic Effects These effects due to radiation occur after a threshold of radiation dose is crossed. It has primarily a somatic effect on the skin, hair, nails and lenses.

Digital Radiography In this system, instead of a phosphor imaging plate (IP), there is a digital detector array or a flat panel detector, which directly captures and immediately displays the image. The intermediate steps are omitted. The radiation dose is less and the time to display the image is also shortened.

DLP "Dose Length Product" is a product of CTDI vol multiplied by the scan length. It is used as a surrogate marker for the amount of radiation received by a body part during the CT scan study.

Equivalent Dose It is the radiation dose given to particular organs and is measured in millisievert (mSv). The source of radiation could be X-rays, gamma rays or any other source of radiation.

Effective Dose This term is used to describe the radiation dose to the whole body from any source. It is the addition of an equivalent dose to all organs. It is measured in Sievert, or mSvs, where 1 Sv is equal to 1 J/kg of tissue.

Electromagnetic Radiation (EMR) Waves of energy (photons) that have both electric and magnetic fields and travel through space at the speed of light are called electromagnetic radiation. These waves of energy can be natural or man-made. X-Ray is electromagnetic radiation emitted by an X-ray tube. Gamma-ray is also electromagnetic radiation but is generated by radioactive nuclei. Similarly, there are radio waves and light which are also electromagnetic radiation.

Exposure This word refers to the concentration of X-rays at a particular point. It is also a measure of ionization of air caused by X-rays. Exposure is measured in Roentgen.

Focal Film Distance (FFD) This is the distance between the focal spot of the x-ray anode and the x-ray film/image plate. Increasing the FFD reduces the radiation dose to the patient because the radiation is distributed over a larger area as compared to a smaller FFD.

Focal Spot A focal spot is a small area on the X-ray anode, which is bombarded by electrons, resulting in the production of X-ray photons. The smaller the focal spot the sharper the images. Small focal spots tend to get heated by high radiation doses, hence are reserved for areas needing less radiation, for example, the hands.

Grid A grid is a device meant to reduce scattered radiation. It does this by allowing the straight or primary X-ray beam to pass through but absorbing the obliquely directed radiation emerging from the X-ray beam. It is made of lead strips with gaps in between the strips. A grid could be focused, non-focused, criss-cross and tapered. A grid could be stationary or moving. A stationary grid casts shows of the lead strips, on the image. A mobile grid, also called "Potter-

Bucky grid", blurs the lines cast by the lead strips in the grid which renders them invisible in the X-ray image.

Image Intensifier This is a device used in fluoroscopy. It converts the X-ray image into a light image which can then be displayed on an image monitor.

Intensifying Screens These are a pair of plates present inside the conventional X-ray cassette. The X-ray film is placed between these plates. When the X-ray photons fall on the screens, they emit light photons. Since the X-ray film is coated with silver halide emulsion on both sides, the light photons produce the imprint of the exposed area on the X-ray film.

Ionization It is either the addition or subtraction of electrons from an atom, thus creating an ion.

Ionizing Radiation Any radiation which can result in the production of ions by displacing electrons from atoms is called ionizing radiation.

Isotope It is a variant of an element which has the same number of protons (atomic number) and electrons but different numbers of neutrons, hence having different mass numbers (sum of protons and neutrons).

Kilovoltage Peak (kVp) [12] The difference in the electrical charge between the cathode and anode is called the potential difference. Potential difference is measured by a unit called kilovolt peak (kVp), which is the maximum/peak difference in the electrical charge (potential difference) between the cathode and anode during exposure. The higher the kVp, the higher the speed gained by the electrons as they travel from the cathode to the anode. This increases the penetrating power of the X-ray beam which reduces the need for generating additional quantum of radiation to produce an image.

Milliampere (mA) mA represents the quantity of electric current needed to expose the X-ray film/image plate and is produced by changing the potential difference between the cathode and anode. The quantity of current produced depends upon the time, in seconds, needed for generating an image. The mAs can be adjusted as per the requirement of that study.

Non-stochastic Effect (Deterministic Effect) It is the effect on the body caused by exposure to radiation dose above a threshold level. For example, loss of hair, effects on nails and skin burns.

Nucleons Within the atom, there is a nucleus which consists of protons and neutrons. Together, these are called nucleons and they are denoted by the alphabet "A". The protons are denoted by the alphabet "Z", which also determines the atomic number of the element.

Noise Noise is the presence of randomly deposited gray-black mottled images, thereby compromising the image quality.

PACS System The abbreviation stands for a "picture archiving and display system". In this system, images can be stored as well as immediately retrieved from any site, where access to the PACs is available.

Photon This is a particle or unit of electromagnetic energy such as X-rays, visible light and microwaves. It has no mass and travels at the speed of light. X-rays and gamma rays are photons.

Rad It is an abbreviation for "Radiation Absorbed Dose". It is a unit of the radiation given by any source which is absorbed by the tissue. The term "Rad" is now replaced by the unit "Gray". One unit of gray is equal to 100 Rads [13].

Radiation Sources In the X-ray room, radiation sources include the main X-ray beam, leakage from the equipment and scattered radiation from the patient's body as well as from the collimation device.

Roentgen It is the unit of exposure to X-rays.

Rotating Anode For the target (anode) to be uniformly bombarded by an X-ray beam and not being pitted at one point, the anode is made to rotate at high speeds. This results in even pitting of the anode. The exposure, hence pitting, is not confined to a single spot as it happens in a stationary anode used in portable low mAs as well as fluoroscopic units, used for many procedures, including pacemaker insertion.

Spatial Resolution The ability to resolve different details, approximated closely in a tissue, is called spatial resolution.

Shielding It is for protecting a person or a part from being exposed to radiation.

Sievert This is a unit which is related to the absorbed dose. However since absorbed doses from different sources do not have a similar effect, it is called a dose equivalent and measured in sieverts, which is equivalent to 100 Rem.

Stochastic Effect It is the effect of radiation on the body which is neither determined by dose nor by the duration of radiation exposure, but whose probability of occurrence increases both with an increase in radiation dose and duration of radiation exposure. Stochastic effects are like development of radiation-induced cancers or genetic mutation.

Thermoluminescent Dosimetry Badge (TLD Badges) This is a badge which is used to measure radiation exposure. It is worn over the clothes or under the lead apron, by the radiation worker. The process by which the radiation exposure is determined is called "Thermoluminescent dosimetry". The material used in these badges is in the form of three discs made of crystalline material such as lithium fluoride which has an atomic number similar to the exposed surface. Beneath the discs are filters, made of aluminium and copper on the top and Perspex in the centre. The lowest disc does not have a filter beneath it. Upon exposure to radiation, the dosimeter stores the energy within its latticework. This stored energy is released by heating the material, resulting in the emission of light by a process called "thermoluminescence". The amount of light emitted enables determining the quantum of radiation received by its wearer [14].

References

1. McCollough CH. The AAPM/RSNA physics tutorial for residents. X-ray production. RadioGraphics. 1997;17(4):967–84.
2. http://www.sprmn.pt/pdf/EuropeanGuidelinesEur16261.pdf
3. https://www.fda.gov/radiation-emitting-products/medical-imaging/pediatric-x-ray-imaging
4. Yoon I, Slesinger TL. Radiation exposure in pregnancy. [Updated 2023 May 1]. In: StatPearls. Treasure Island, FL: StatPearls Publishing; 2024. https://www.ncbi.nlm.nih.gov/books/NBK551690/.
5. Applegate KE, et al. Radiation exposures in pregnancy, health effects and risks to the embryo/foetus—information to inform the medical management of the pregnant patient. J Radiol Prot. 2021;41(4):S522.
6. Mainprize JG, Yaffe MJ, Chawla T, et al. Effects of ionizing radiation exposure during pregnancy. Abdom Radiol. 2023;48:1564–78. https://doi.org/10.1007/s00261-023-03861-w.
7. https://www.iaea.org/resources/rpop/health-professionals/nuclear-medicine/pet-ct/patients
8. Huang B, Law MW-M, Khong P-L. Whole-body PET/CT scanning: estimation of radiation dose and cancer. Risk Radiol. 2009;251(1):166–74.
9. Allisy-Roberts P, Williams J. Farr, physics for medical imaging. 2nd ed. Saunders; 2008.
10. https://www.radiologyinfo.org/en/info/safety-xray
11. https://www.cdc.gov/nceh/radiation/emergencies/glossary.htm#:~:text=Rad%20(radiation%20absorbed%20dose)%3A,is%20equivalent%20to%20100%20rad
12. Sy E, Samboju V, Mukhdomi T. X-ray image production procedures. [Updated 2022 Oct 17]. In: StatPearls. Treasure Island, FL: StatPearls Publishing; 2024. https://www.ncbi.nlm.nih.gov/books/NBK564352/.
13. https://www.cdc.gov/nceh/radiation/emergencies/measurement.htm#:~:text=The%20rad%2C%20which%20stands%20for,is%20equal%20to%20100%20rad
14. Goel A, Chieng R, Kasáč Z, et al. Intensifying screen. Radiopaedia.org. https://doi.org/10.53347/rID-30319.

Further Reading

http://icrpaedia.org/Main_Page
http://icrpaedia.org/ICRP_Glossary
Goel A, Chieng R, Kasáč Z, et al. Intensifying screen. Radiopaedia.org. https://doi.org/10.53347/rID-30319

2 Positioning in Chest X-Rays

Abstract

Amongst all X-ray requests, the most common request is for a chest X-ray. A good quality chest X-ray is a must to detect chest diseases. A proper X-ray is correctly centred and taken with the correct exposure factors while the patient holds breath in deep inspiration. It is essential for both the radiologic technologist and radiologist to be familiar with what a good quality X-ray looks like and the various positions in which a chest X-ray can be performed.

Keywords

X-ray quality · Exposure factors · Positioning · Chest X-ray

There are various positions and views in chest radiography. Listed below, are the multiple views and how to do them.

2.1 Erect PA Chest X-Ray

A posteroanterior view (PA) X-ray of the chest, is amongst the commonest X-ray asked for in medical practice.

The X-ray is performed in either standing or sitting position with the legs slightly apart (to ensure stability). The patient's back is towards the X-ray tube which is approximately 180 cm away from the image receiver (which can be a cassette (holding the X-ray film) or the imaging plate) (Fig. 2.1a, b). The front of the chest touches the image receiver with the neck extended to allow the chin to rest on the top edge of the image plate. The X-ray beam is centred below the inferior angle of the scapula at the level of the T7 spinous process. If the patient has problems in standing, the X-ray can be obtained in a sitting position. In a sick patient, the X-ray will have to be done in either a supine or recumbent position. In a child, it is easier to do the X-ray in the supine position with the hands above the chest, held against the head. This helps in keeping the head straight and not tilted sideways. The lower limbs are held down against the X-ray table by placing the palm over the knee joints. The reasons for preferring an erect film over a film done in the supine position include (a) more accurate evaluation of the heart size, which is magnified in the supine X-ray, (b) easy delineation of pathologies of the pleural space, (c) achievement of the lower position of the diaphragms, hence clearer view of the lung bases. The film obtained with the patient standing and taking a deep inhalation allows better chest expansion and evaluation of the lower lobes. Pleural effusion and pneumothorax are easy to evaluate in the erect position, the latter seen better in an expiratory phase film. In the supine position, the free

R. Gothi, *Radiographic and Imaging Techniques for Radiology Residents and Technologists*,
https://doi.org/10.1007/978-981-96-4816-0_2

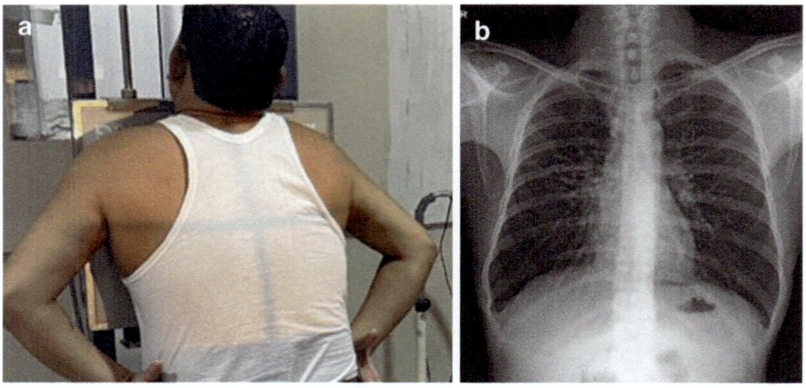

Fig. 2.1 (**a, b**) Positioning for an erect chest x-ray. The film should be properly centred so that the medial end of both clavicles are equidistant from the spinous process of the dorsal vertebra. The film should include the entire rib cage and soft tissues of the chest wall, part of the scapula, the lower neck and a portion of the upper abdomen

Fig. 2.2 (**a, b**) Positioning for AP view of the chest (**a**). Note the scapula (arrow) overlapping on the lung fields (**b**)

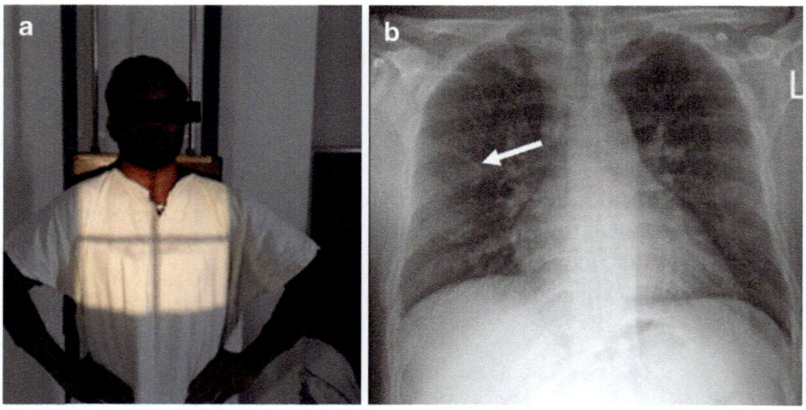

pleural fluid spreads out and envelops the surface of the lung, giving a hazy appearance to the lung parenchyma (Fig. 2.2).

The normal hila is of soft tissue density, tapers down smoothly and does not appear prominent or lobular in the erect position unless there is a hilar or perihilar pathology. Another advantage of the erect view is improved evaluation of the pulmonary vessels. Normally, in the erect view, the upper lobe pulmonary veins are smaller in calibre as compared to the lower lobe veins. This is not only the effect of gravity but also the result of increased blood supply to the lower lobes. It is a helpful observation because, if in the erect film, the upper lobe vessels are prominent, (cephalization of pulmonary veins), it indicates raised pulmonary venous pressure. In the supine view, pulmonary veins have a similar size as the effect of gravity is neutralized by the supine position of the patient. This, unfortunately, hampers interpretation of raised pulmonary venous pressure in patients with increased left atrial pressure (normal value of LA pressure is 5–10 ml/Hg and raised pressure is 10–15 ml/Hg). Therefore, erect views are better for the evaluation of dilatation of pulmonary veins. An erect view also shows fluid levels in cavities, abscesses, dilated bronchi (bronchiectatic cavities) in a dilated oesophagus (as seen in cases of achalasia cardia) and in the gastric fundus. Hence, for all these reasons, the erect view of the chest is the preferred view.

2.2 Supine Chest X-Ray

In the supine AP view, the diaphragms are high in position, resulting in the crowding of pulmonary vessels in the lung bases. The cardiac shadow appears more prominent due to magnification as well as due to slight rotation caused by the elevated left diaphragm. The shadows of the scapula overlies the lung shadows (Fig. 2.2).

Free pleural fluid can float upwards behind the lung tissue, in the supine position, thereby falsely increasing the density of the lung parenchyma. In cases of pneumothorax, the air in the pleural cavity migrates forwards beneath the anterior chest wall, and downwards into the anterolateral pleural sulcus. The anteriorly located air is somewhat difficult to appreciate. The air in the anterolateral sulcus can be appreciated if large in quantity.

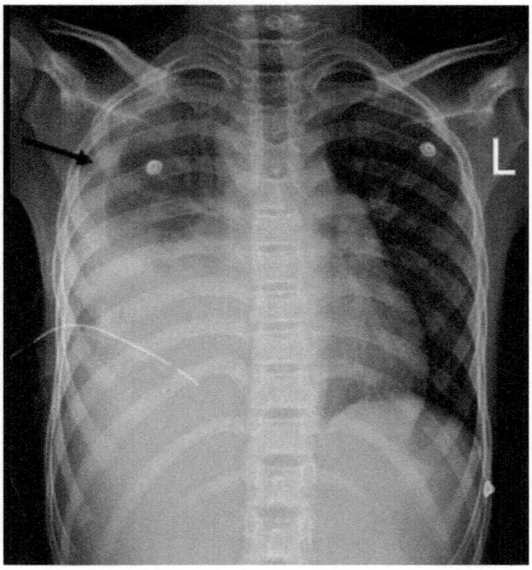

Fig. 2.3 Supine chest AP view. Note the large right pleural effusion resulting in a hazy appearance of the right lung parenchyma as compared to the left

2.3 Other Views

These include an AP erect view, a lateral view, a penetrated chest AP view, an apical lordotic view and a decubitus view.

- **AP Erect View**
  A chest X-ray can also be obtained with the patient's front facing the X-ray tube, the back being against the image receiver (plate or cassette). This position is used in patients who are unable to stand. The X-ray tube should be a minimum of 120 cm from the image plate. The arms are kept by the side. In this position, the heart size is magnified. Therefore, no comment can be made on the cardiac size and shape, unless it is obviously abnormal.
- **The Lateral View** is performed by turning the patient sideways, either to the right or left, depending upon the area of interest (Fig. 2.3a, b). The patient bends slightly forwards with the arm raised above the head. The image should include both the lung apices and diaphragms, the sternum as well as the dorsal vertebral column. The film is centred at the T7 level. The lateral view helps in evaluating the retrocardiac area, the dorsal spine, the pleural fissures, the posterior costophrenic sulcus, the anterior superior mediastinum and the posterior segments of the lung lobes. It is, therefore, an additional help in correctly assigning the exact position of a lung lesion to it's appropriate lung lobe/segment.
- In the lateral view, the hila can also be evaluated in greater detail (Fig. 2.4a, b). The position of the right and left pulmonary arteries can be made out by relating them with their corresponding bronchi (Fig. 2.5). The right pulmonary artery projects anterior to the bronchus while the left pulmonary artery projects above and posterior to the bronchus.
- When performing the lateral view, the arms should be raised and folded above the head, so that the shadow of the soft tissues of the upper arm and the humerus does not obscure the lung apices (Figs. 2.6 and 2.7).
- The lateral view of the chest is infrequently used these days because of the easy availability of CT scans. There are, however, many things a lateral chest X-ray shows, which may not be evident in a chest PA view. These include the sternum, retrosternal space, pathological soft tissues overlapping the vertebral bodies, hilar masses and cardiac enlargement, especially of the right ventricle. Often a com-

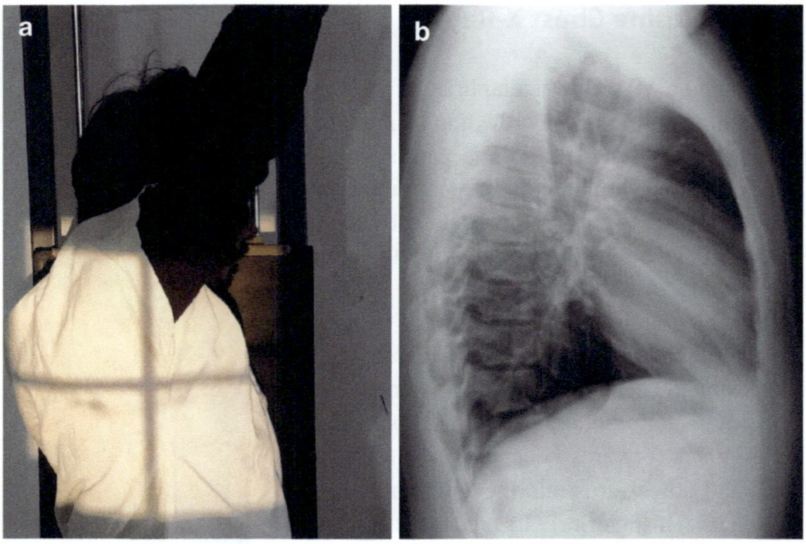

Fig. 2.4 (**a, b**) Chest X-ray positioning (**a**) for lateral view (**b**)

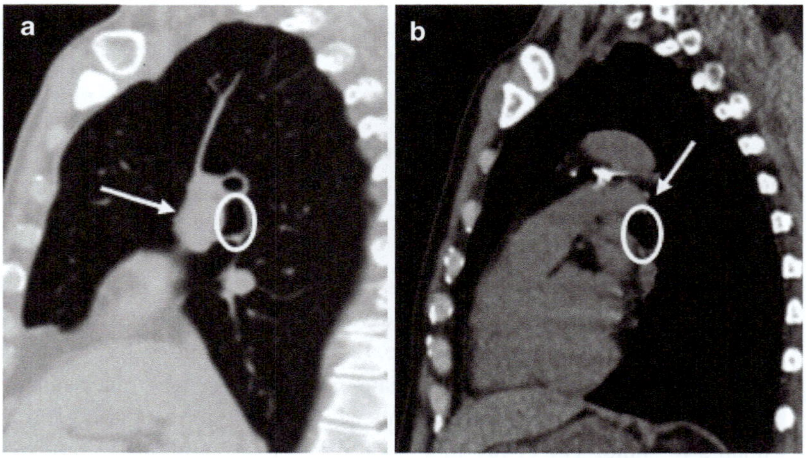

Fig. 2.5 (**a, b**) CT scan, sagittal view of the right and left chest (resembling lateral view of the chest X-ray), showing the relationship of the right and left pulmonary arteries (arrows) with their respective bronchi (circles). The right pulmonary artery in (**a**) is anterior to the right upper lobe and intermediate bronchus. The left pulmonary artery in (**b**) is above the left main bronchus

bination of PA and lateral view give a good idea about the presence and exact location of a chest lesion.

- **Supine Penetrated AP View**. This is an AP projection of the chest done in the supine position using a high kV technique for penetrating the mediastinal soft tissues. It is obtained using a moving grid (a bucky)and by greater penetrating power of the X-ray beam, which allows better visualization of the mediastinal structures, especially the tracheal bifurcation and retrocardiac densities. The patient lies supine with the arms raised above the head or by the side but away from the chest wall. The X-ray tube is kept 120 cm away from the image receiver. This view also enables better delineation of the dorsal spine, paraspinal soft tissues and posterior end of the ribs. The pulmonary air spaces appear dark with obscured vascular markings caused by the greater penetration of the X-ray beam. In this view, it might also be difficult to appreciate pneumothorax against the dark lung background. In such a situation, "the deep sulcus sign" should be looked for which is a sharp inferior extension of the pneumothorax into the anterior costophrenic angle (Fig. 2.8).
- **The Apical Lordotic (Apicogram).** This view is used to evaluate the apices of the lungs, the middle lobe and the inferior end of

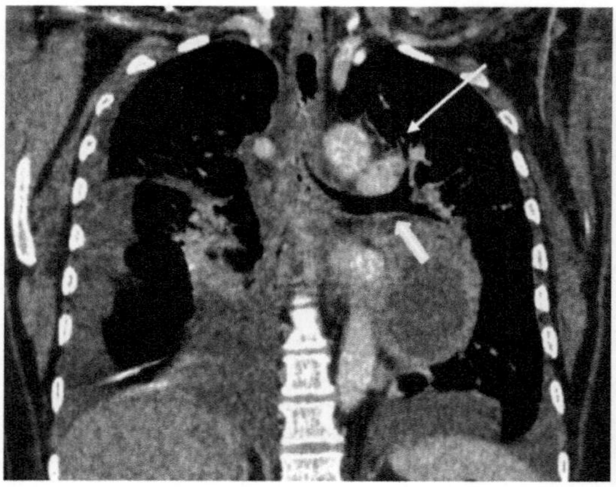

Fig. 2.6 Coronal view of CT scan of the chest (corresponding to PA/AP view of a chest X-ray). Note the position of the left pulmonary artery (thin arrow), which is above the left main bronchus (thick arrow)

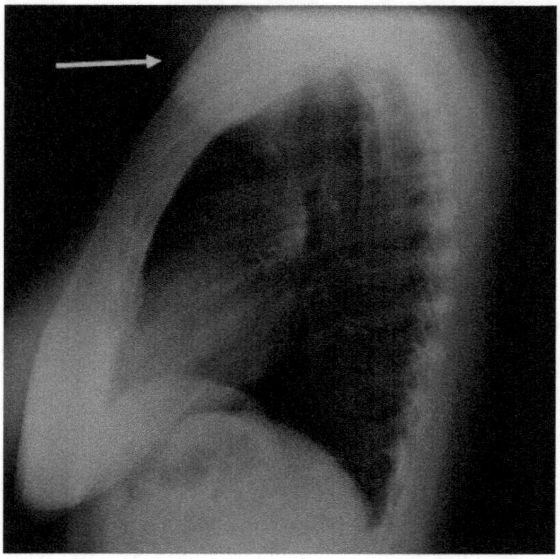

Fig. 2.7 X-ray obtained with the elbows kept above the head in the flexed position. Note the linear soft tissue shadow of the raised upper limbs, crossing the anterior chest (arrow) which is difficult to avoid, but is penetrable, hence does not give much of a problem. Sometimes, the patient is unable to raise the arms well above the head, in which case, the shadow of the humeri will overlap the lung apices

the oblique fissure. In this view, while still facing the X-ray tube, the patient bends backwards with his arched back touching the imaging plate/cassette. The arms are kept by the side. The patient holds the breath in deep inspiration. The diverging X-ray beam lifts the clavicle off the pulmonary apices, thereby per-

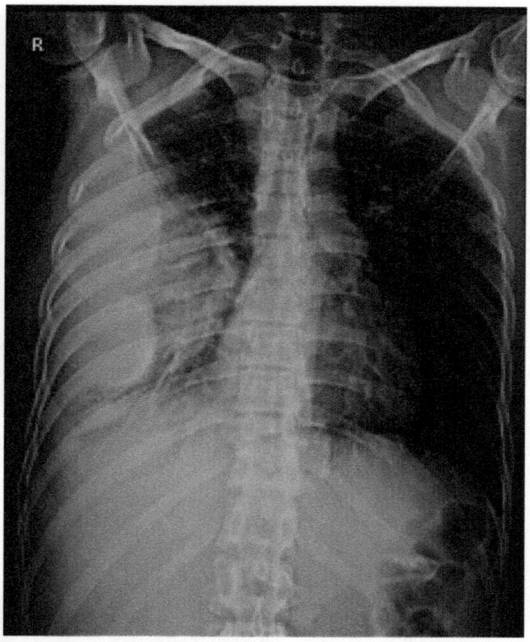

Fig. 2.8 Penetrated view of the chest. The high kV penetrating beam highlights the mediastinal structures and the right-sided loculated pleural fluid collection. Greater penetration comes at a price, which is increased blackening of the surrounding lung parenchyma

mitting a clearer view of the lung apices. The middle lobe and inferior end of the oblique fissure are also better seen in this view (Fig. 2.9).

- **A Decubitus View** is obtained to ascertain the presence of small quantities of free pleural fluid. The patient lies on the side with the affected hemithorax being in the dependent position. The arms are raised above the head. The knees and hips are flexed. If necessary, the torso is lifted off the table with the help of a non-opaque sponge sheet or even a pillow, which is kept beneath the chest. This allows proper coverage of the dependent lung without being obscured by the edge of the X-ray table. The X-ray beam is centred on the sternum. A cross-table view is obtained in expiration, with the X-ray beam passing through the front of the chest and exposing the film kept against the back. The presence of fluid in the dependent part of the hemithorax results in the formation of a linear soft tissue opacity in this region. The dependent lung is also less expanded as compared to the non-dependent lung. Its diaphragm is therefore at

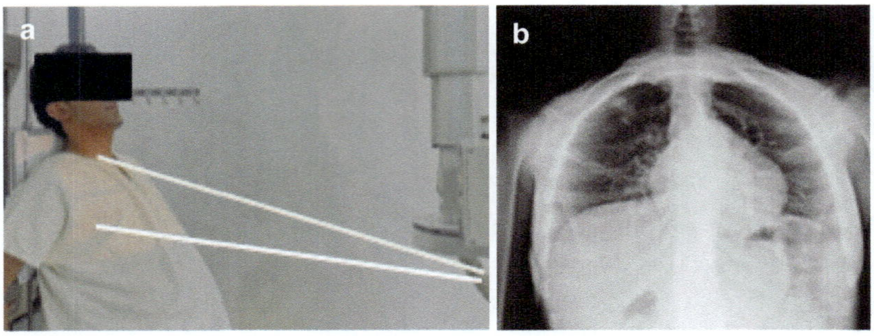

Fig. 2.9 (**a, b**) Positioning for apicogram. Note how the top line falls on the chest. It lifts off the clavicle, thereby exposing the lung apices clearly (**a**). Note the presence of an opacity (**b**) in the right apex, which is well demonstrated in the apical lordotic view, but was masked by the overlapping shadows of the clavicles and ribs in the standard chest X-ray

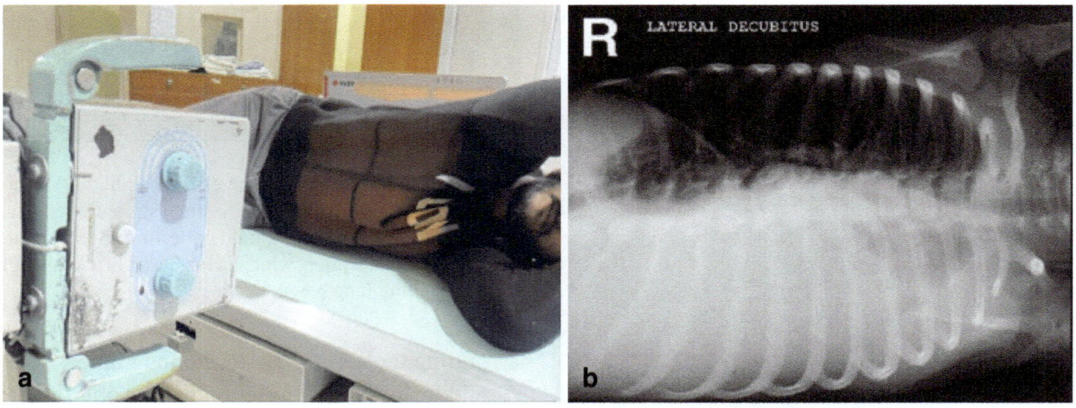

Fig. 2.10 (**a**) Decubitus view, showing position of the patient and (**b**) the decubitus X-ray demonstrating presence of pleural fluid. Note the well aerated non dependant lung

a higher level as compared to the well expanded non-dependent lung (Fig. 2.10).

- **Oblique and Tangential Projections**
  Oblique views are performed to evaluate the ribs for any fracture or destruction.

  The tangential views are acquired under fluoroscopy to determine the relationship of a soft tissue shadow in the chest wall with the underlying rib.

  These X-rays can be obtained in both lying down and standing positions with 15–20-degree rotation to either side.
- **Chest X-Ray of Paediatric Patients**
  While it is ideal to obtain a chest X-ray in an upright position, often it is difficult, especially if the child is restless or very sick. In such cases, a supine X-ray can be performed. The child is restrained by either using a restrainer or, by holding firmly but gently, taking care to protect gonads from radiation, by using a lead apron. The arms are held against the head, (which keeps the baby straight) and the knees are held together against the X-ray table. The exposure is timed to coincide with the apnoeic phase which occurs during crying. This moment of apnea, is the one which provides a deep inspiratory film (Fig. 2.11).

2.3.1 A Good Quality X-Ray

A word about good quality X-rays!

The interpretation of a chest X-ray should always be preceded by first ensuring its quality. The technical quality should be such that it carries the correct information and does not mislead the interpreter.

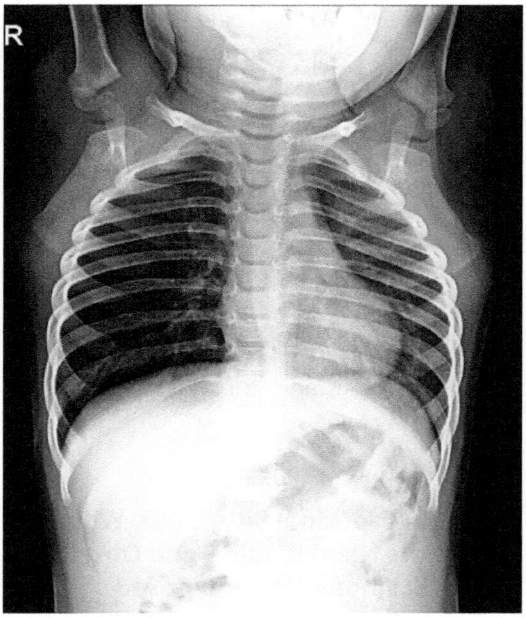

Fig. 2.11 The arms are held against the head, which results in the neck remaining straight. The feet are held together with one hand and the knee, restrained with the other. Note that in a small child, some parts of the upper abdomen often get included in the chest x-ray

What, then, is a good quality chest X-ray?

A well-performed X-ray should have the following qualities.

1. First, the film should be well-centred and not rotated towards any side. This means that the sternoclavicular joints should be equidistant from the spinous process of the upper dorsal vertebral body. If the spinous process is not visible, then the sternoclavicular joint should be equidistant from the lateral vertebral margins.
2. A good X-ray includes all parts of the chest including the soft tissues of the chest wall. The lungs appear gray, not black or white.
3. When the spine and intervening discs just start to be seen and when there are no extraneous marks on the image, then the X-ray is of good quality.
4. The X-ray chest should have been taken in deep inspiration and not during expiration (exception: an expiratory film is obtained to look for pneumothorax. It also helps when looking for foreign bodies blocking a bronchus which traps air in the lobe distal to the obstructed bronchus. This happens because, during expiration, the patent airway permits the exit of the intrapulmonary air, from the unaffected side while a blocked airway does not. This makes the obstructed lung/lobe/segment look larger and more lucent as compared to the remaining lung parenchyma).
5. A good inspiratory film shows up to 6–9 ribs anteriorly and 10–11 ribs posteriorly.
6. The right diaphragm is approximately 1 intercostal space above the left.
7. The pulmonary vessels should be visible and not be obscured by a penetrating exposure which darkens the film. A good X-ray, therefore, has a good contrast, which means that one can distinguish various soft tissue and bony structures. Most X-rays are routinely obtained using a low-kilovoltage technique. The kilovoltage (kV) ranges from 46 for children to 86 for heavy adults.
8. An X-ray of the chest, taken using a vertical bucky or grid needs a higher kV to penetrate through the grid. It appears better and sharper as the scattered radiation, which adds to the "noise", is cut off, leaving the useful X-ray photons in the beam to do their job of producing a good film. The use of a bucky to cut off the scatter is particularly recommended in large patients where the quantum of radiation needed to produce the film is greater than average. In thin patients and children as well as in pregnant patients, lower radiation should be used. In these patients, a film can be obtained without the use of bucky/grid. A high kV technique using a bucky enables better visualization of soft tissues of the mediastinum, spine and ribs. Hence it is the preferred way to perform an X-ray of the chest (Fig. 2.12).

2.3.2 Suboptimal X-Rays

Occasionally it might not be possible to obtain a good quality film.

1. A breathless patient, a patient who is unable to stand, an uncooperative child and the use of poor technical factors, may result in a poor-quality film.

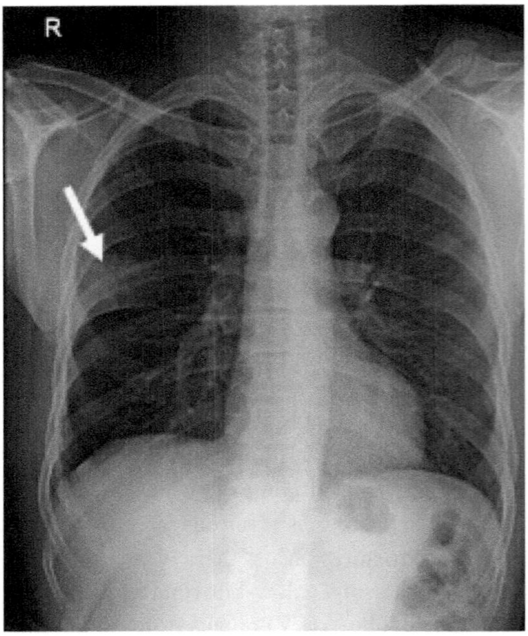

Fig. 2.12 Example of an over-exposed film. Compared to a pathology (arrow), the rest of the normal lungs looks black. It should look gray because a normal lung is composed of soft tissue structures, such as bronchi, blood vessels, interstitium and walls of air spaces. If the lung is dark on a normal exposure, it is indicative of air trapping, presence of air filled cystic spaces or paucity of overlying soft tissues such as muscles and fat. Pulmonary parenchymal diseases and pleural pathologies appear white. Interstitial lung disease, give a streaky pattern

2. When interpreting an X-ray, make sure that the X-ray is interpretable.
3. If not, then repeat it.

2.3.3 What Should Be Done to Improve the Quality?

1. Technical factors can be adjusted. The exposure time can be shortened in a breathless patient.
2. Faster film-screen combinations, fresh and chemicals digital X-rays should be used for processing X-ray films, if the conventional darkroom technique is still being used.
3. The X-ray films should be properly stored and handled to avoid the development of artefacts which are unwanted distortions of the image. Several types of artefacts were seen in a conventional X-ray. These included nail marks, static electricity marks, dust-related artefacts, partially exposed film and many more. In the CR system, also, several types of artefacts can be seen [1]. Amongst them, the common ones are unerased previous images which superimpose on the new image, imaging from the wrong side of the cassette, exposure-related factors, light bulb artefacts and many more.
4. The screen or image plate should not be aged or scratched.
5. If a patient is restless or unable to stand comfortably, it would be better to do the X-ray in the supine position. Rarely sedation is also needed to obtain X-rays.

2.3.4 Exceptional Situations, Where the Need Would Be to Obtain Either an Underexposed (White) or an Overexposed (Dark) X-Ray

2.3.4.1 Underexposed X-Rays

There are situations where one would ask for a whitish X-ray (soft/underexposed/under-penetrated film). This is when soft tissue lesions (Fig. 2.13), smaller peripheral pulmonary vessels, pneumothorax (air in the pleural cavity) and rib lesions in thin patients need to be seen.

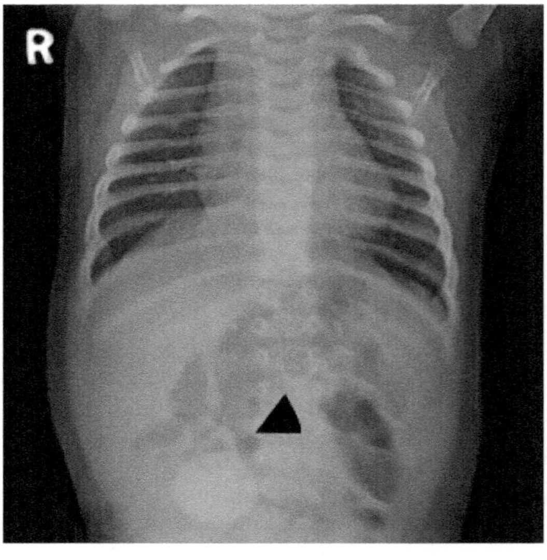

Fig. 2.13 An underexposed film. Note how the gray-shaded subcutaneous fat is visible between the skin and soft tissues of the chest and upper abdomen. Note also the arrowhead pointing towards the soft tissue shadow cast by the umbilical hernia (black arrowhead)

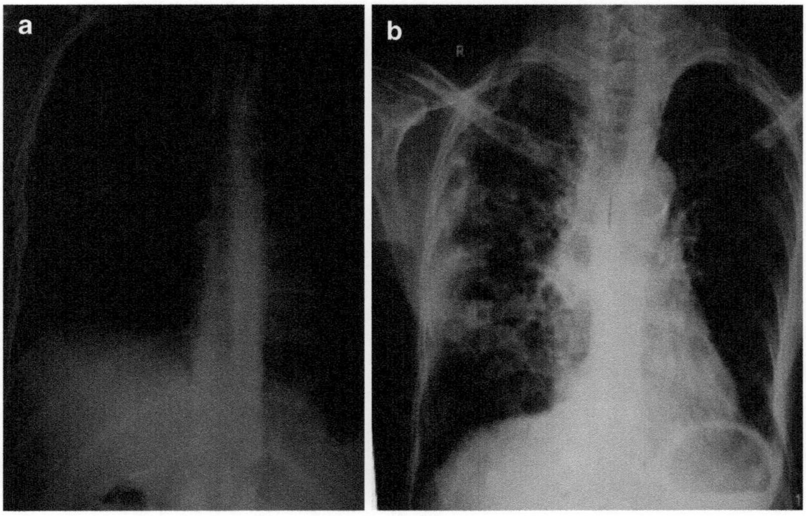

Fig. 2.14 (**a**) An over-penetrated X-ray film. No lung markings are seen in this image. The shadow of the carina and spine are visible. However, an overinflated lung field (**b**) as seen in patients of chronic obstructive pulmonary disease (COPD), may also appear dark, despite using normal exposure factors

2.3.4.2 Overexposed X-Rays

An overexposed film is a dark X-ray due to a high influx of photons on the film. This results in the obscuration of soft tissue density pulmonary shadows (Fig. 2.14).

The chest X-ray is of profound importance in daily practice. One needs a thorough knowledge of the technical aspects to provide high-quality imaging to the referring clinicians. This chapter is meant to introduce beginners to the fine art of chest radiography. They are encouraged to read excellent books on this subject [2, 3].

References

1. Shetty CM, Barthur A, Kambadakone A, Narayanan N, Rajagopal KV. Computed radiography image artifacts revisited. Am J Roentgenol. 2011;196(1):W37–47.
2. Swallow RA, Naylor E. Clark's positioning in radiography. 11th ed. New Delhi: CBS Publisher; 1989.
3. Sloane C, Holmes K, Anderson C, Whitely AS. Clakk's pocket handbook for radiographers. London: CRC Press; 2014.

3 The Normal Chest X-Ray

Abstract

Interpretation of a chest X-ray in the early days of training must be through a systematic assessment of all four corners and the centre of an X-ray film. X-rays are a two-dimensional study of a three-dimensional structure. The first step in interpretation is to know what a normal X-ray looks like. Only then can we proceed to recognize abnormalities. The process of interpreting an X-ray is not easy and even the most experienced radiologists stumble and make mistakes. It is also essential to know, that a normal-looking X-ray may still be harbouring abnormality. Hence, it is fair to say that no abnormal finding is visible in the X-ray rather than stating that the X-ray chest is normal, which might be mistaken for the absence of any abnormality in the chest. In this chapter, we will learn how to analyze a chest X-ray.

Keywords

Normal chest X-ray · Chest X-ray interpretation

Once the X-ray is in your hand and you are satisfied with its quality, then proceed with the interpretation.

Let's follow a search pattern.

3.1 Look at the Following Structures

1. **Lung Apices:** These are seen extending symmetrically above the level of the clavicles in a PA View (Fig. 3.1)

   The pulmonary apex is surrounded by a combined layer of extrapleural fat and pleura, which together form the "apical pleural cap (Fig. 3.2)". Its thickness should be bilaterally symmetrical. Any thickening more than 5 mms or having a convex/lobular appearance should be viewed with suspicion and investigated further.
2. **Pulmonary Vessels**: The vessels visible in the lung parenchyma are pulmonary arteries and veins (Fig. 3.3). The arteries are seen tapering towards the periphery. The veins are seen converging towards the left atrium. Bronchial arteries are small in calibre and not seen in a normal chest X-ray. The pulmonary vessels should appear bilaterally symmetrical. The upper lobe vessels are smaller in size as compared to the lower lobe vessels in an erect X-ray.
3. **Lung Expansion**: The lung may be considered adequately expanded if, at least, the anterior end of the 6–9th ribs or posterior 10th rib is visible (Fig. 3.4).
4. **The Diaphragms:** These should be inverted cup-shaped (Fig. 3.5). The right diaphragm should be at the most one and a half intercos-

R. Gothi, *Radiographic and Imaging Techniques for Radiology Residents and Technologists*,
https://doi.org/10.1007/978-981-96-4816-0_3

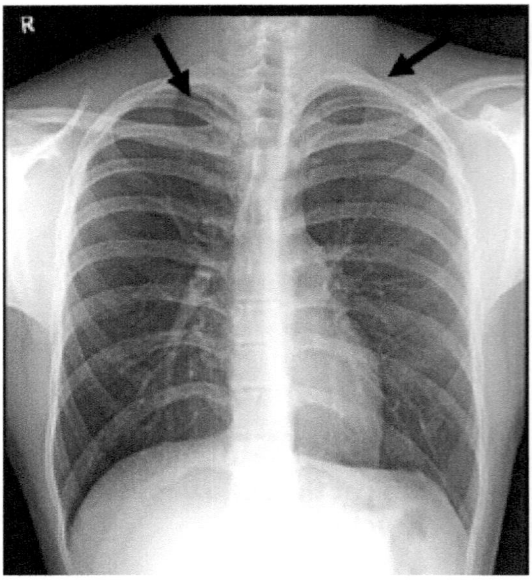

Fig. 3.1 The lung apices (arrows) should have identical density on both sides. Any asymmetry in the density will appear white against the gray background of the underlying air-filled lung. The reasons for the difference in density could be parenchymal fibrosis, calcification, nodule, mass, or a pleural or bony lesion

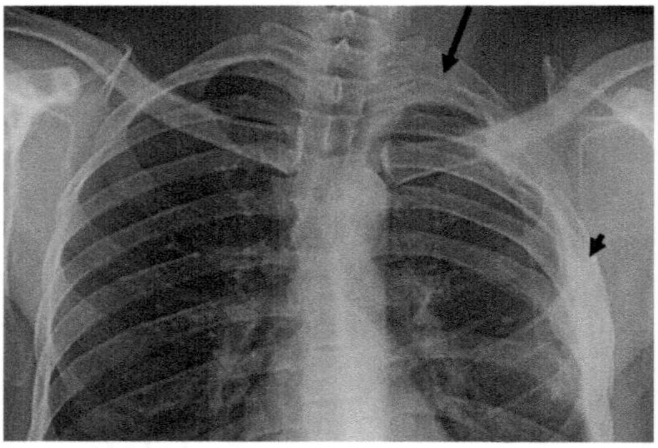

Fig. 3.2 In this case, there is an asymmetry in the apices due to left pleural fibrosis (long arrow) which has resulted in crowding of the left-sided ribs (short arrow)

tal space higher than the left. It can also be at the same level. If it projects below the left diaphragm, it should be considered abnormal and the reason identified.

Reasons for the low position of the right diaphragm include compensatory overexpansion of the right lung, elevation of the left diaphragm due to a distended stomach or colon (Fig. 3.6), eventration or phrenic nerve palsy.

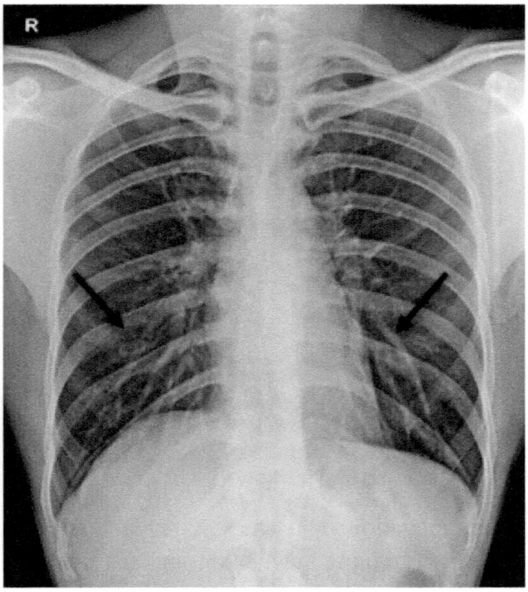

Fig. 3.3 The lower lobe vessels (arrows), in particular the inferior pulmonary veins, are more prominent in the erect position due to the effect of gravity. In the supine position, the blood flow is redistributed uniformly and both upper and lower lobe veins appear similar in size

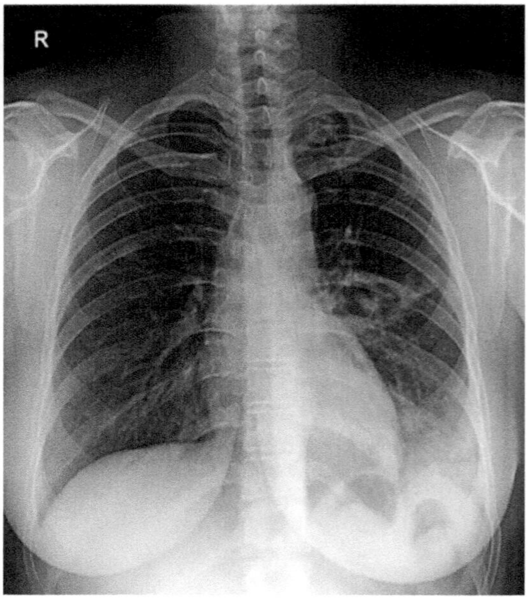

Fig. 3.4 Adequately expanded lung fields. Note that, despite pathology in the left lung, the lung expansion is adequate

If the right diaphragm is significantly higher than the left (Fig. 3.7), it could be due to a subdiaphragmatic pathology such as

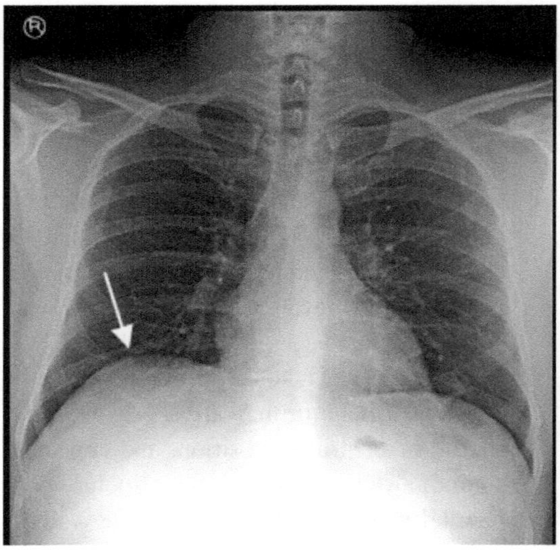

Fig. 3.5 Note the normal position of the diaphragms. The peak of the cupola of the right diaphragm (arrow) is central. If it is more to the periphery, consider the possibility of subpulmonic effusion. In a normal situation, there should be no evidence of tenting, flattening or obscuration of the diaphragms by any intrathoracic pathology. However, sometimes, mediastinal fat deposition can cast a faint shadow in the pericardial region, through which the normal pulmonary vasculature will be visible

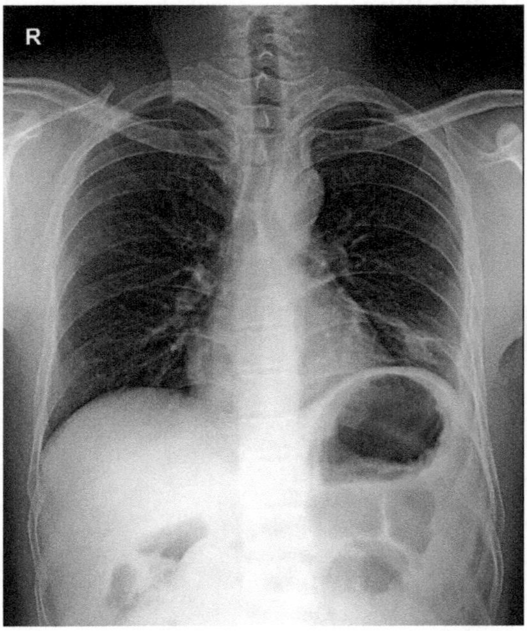

Fig. 3.6 The left diaphragm is elevated by a distended gas-filled stomach

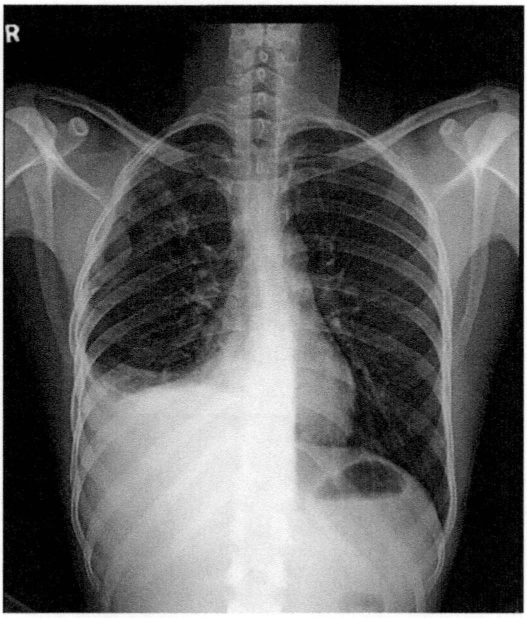

Fig. 3.7 A case of hepatomegaly caused by an amoebic liver abscess, elevating the right dome of the diaphragm. Note that the diaphragm is still visible along with the pleural shadow

subphrenic abscess or liver enlargement. Make sure that what you are seeing is the diaphragm and not a pathology mimicking the diaphragm. A large subpulmonic fluid collection can be mistaken for a raised diaphragm. In doubtful cases, do an ultrasound of the chest or obtain a right lateral decubitus film to rule out subpulmonic effusion.

5. **The Cardiac Shadow** should be in the mid-chest, with one-third protruding to the right of the midline (Fig. 3.8). Its transverse diameter should not be more than 15.5 cm. The cardiothoracic ratio (CT ratio) is the ratio of the width of the cardiac shadow compared with the maximum width of the chest. It should not be more than 50–55% of the maximum width of the chest. The exception is infants where up to 60% is acceptable as normal.
6. **The Aortic Knuckle** is typically located to the left of the midline. Its maximum diameter is not more than 3.5 cm (Fig. 3.9).

7. **Both Costophrenic** (CP) angles should be sharp and acutely angled.
8. **The Mediastinum and Hila**: The centre of the chest, called the mediastinum, contains the trachea, carina, blood vessels, cardiac shadow, esophagus, mediastinal fat and lymph nodes (Fig. 3.10). Nodes, unless enlarged or calcified, are normally not visible in a chest X-ray. Large nodes may cast a lobular bulge, enlarge hilar shadows or result in superior mediastinal widening.

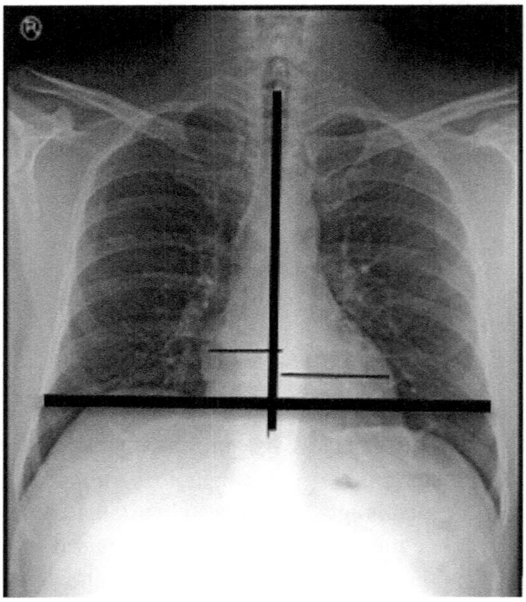

Fig. 3.8 Measurement of the cardiothoracic ratio

9. **Elderly people** may have aortic knuckle calcification, tortuous aorta and probably an enlarged heart with a left ventricular configuration. Any deviation from the normal contours of the heart and aorta must be due to some cardiovascular abnormality, such as aortic dilatation, aortic aneurysm, cardiac chamber enlargement or pericardial disease. Hence, careful evaluation of the cardiovascular outline is necessary (Fig. 3.11).
10. **The Trachea** extends from the level of the cricoid cartilage to the carina (Fig. 3.12). It should be central in position, and appear as smooth air containing tubular structure with parallel walls. The thickness of the walls is 3 mm on average and the dimensions are 2.3 cm and 1.8 cm, respectively in coronal and sagittal planes [1]. There may be an impression on its wall on the left side, caused by the aortic knuckle. The walls may show calcification in part or in the entire "C"-shaped cartilage ring which surrounds it. The muscular posterior part is formed by the trachealis muscle and does not calcify.
11. **The Hilar Shadows** should be symmetrical in thickness, shape and density. The hila are composed of pulmonary arteries, the main right and left bronchi, central lobar bronchi, pulmonary veins, bronchial arteries and veins, lymph nodes, nerves and areolar tissue. The pulmonary arteries are the predominant residents of the hila and give form to the

Fig. 3.9 The aortic knuckle is seen as a round shadow indenting the left tracheal border

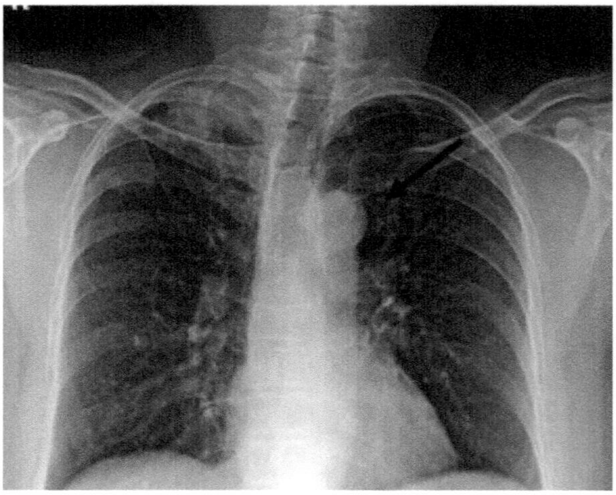

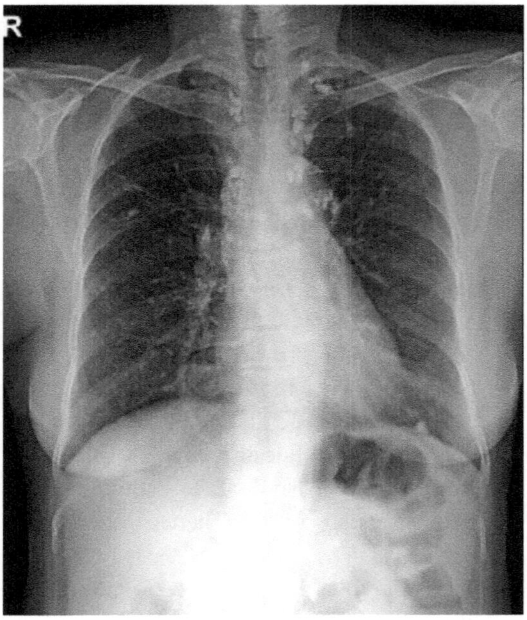

Fig. 3.10 Calcified neck and mediastinal nodes are seen in this view

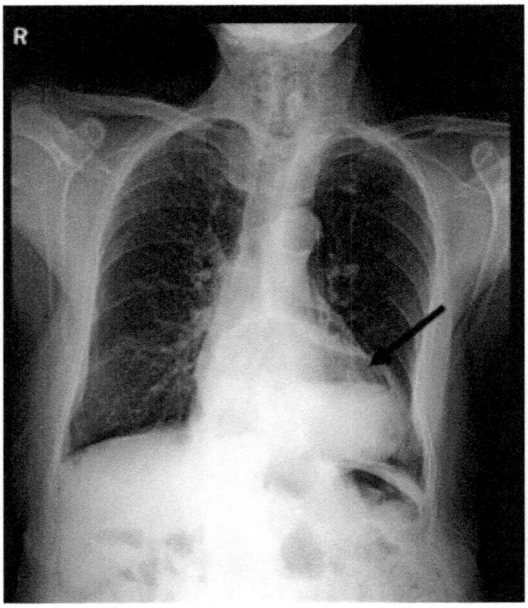

Fig. 3.11 In this patient, there is a soft tissue shadow within the cardiac borders. It shows a fluid level. While it could be due to hydropneumopericardium or a mediastinal gas-containing abscess, note that the normal gastric fundus shadow is not seen below the left diaphragm. This shadow is due to a hiatus hernia with an intrathoracic stomach

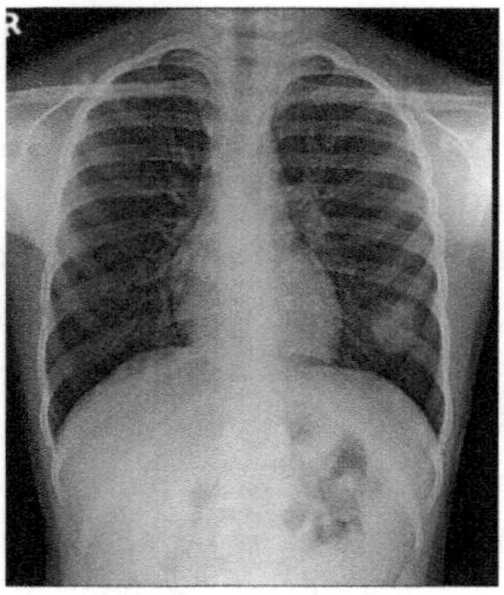

Fig. 3.12 A chest x-ray showing the normal appearance of the trachea in the midline. Observe the shape of the air column. The shape changes from round in children to ovoid in adults. The tracheal walls may show calcification, especially in older patients. Distortion of the trachea can be caused by adjoining fibrosis which exerts traction on the tracheal wall. Alternatively, a mass, such as an enlarged thyroid, or middle mediastinal mass may also cause an extrinsic impression on its walls. The tracheal lumen becomes narrow in the coronal plane due to the thinning and softening of the cartilage-containing walls caused by chronic lung disease in chronic smokers. As a result, it acquires a sabre-shaped deformity

hilar shadow. They taper smoothly from the centre downwards. Hence the hila looks like drooping moustaches, having soft tissue density. They are neither lobular in outline nor very dense. The tapering is caused by the inferior pulmonary arteries, as they descend from the centre to the periphery of the lower lobes. The right hilum will be at a lower level as compared to the left, because of the lower position of the right main pulmonary artery as compared to the left pulmonary artery (Fig. 3.13). The right upper lobe bronchus lies above the right main pulmonary artery and is called the eparterial bronchus (Fig. 3.14).

The left upper lobe bronchus lies below the left main pulmonary artery and is called the hyparterial bronchus (Fig. 3.15).

If one of the hilar shadows appears larger than the other, make sure that the film has been taken properly without rotation of the patient to the right or left. If there is rotation, the lung parenchyma towards the side of rotation is closer to the imaging plate or cassette. This makes the hila of this lung look more prominent and better visible. The opposite hilar shadow falls on the spinal/cardiac shadow and is therefore obscured.

The hilar shadow can be masked by an enlarged tortuous atherosclerotic aorta (Fig. 3.16), superior vena cava (Fig. 3.17), an enlarged heart or by any pathological lesions overlying the hila. Middle lobe lesions or lesions in the apical segment of the lower lobe can also mask the hila.

12. **The Bony Cage** should be looked at carefully. The ribs should be bilaterally symmetrical, and equally spaced out on both sides. They should be traceable in their entirety. The widening of intercostal space could be either due to a missing rib or the fusion of two closely approximated ribs, resulting in the widening of the adjoining intercostal spaces. Differences in the densities of the ribs could be due to lysis (destruction) or sclerosis. Irregularity in the outlines of the ribs is seen mostly along their inferior border, where the bronchial arteries and intercostal nerves are located. Enlarged bronchial arteries or neurogenic tumours can cause rib notching or focal destruction. So, look at the ribs carefully. Also don't forget to count the number of pairs of ribs. There can be 11 pairs of ribs, as in trisomy 21.
13. The spine should be examined for any altered curvature. Scoliosis will result in an asymmetrical right and left chest. Kyphosis will result in a symmetrical reduction in the posterior intercostal spaces. A gibbus will result in localized crowding of the posterior end of the rib shadows at the site of the gibbus. It may be difficult to detect vertebral destruction in a routine chest X-ray unless carefully looked for. A penetrated AP view and a lateral view (obtained with a long exposure, without holding breath) may, by blurring of the superimposed pulmonary shadows, show the lateral projection of the

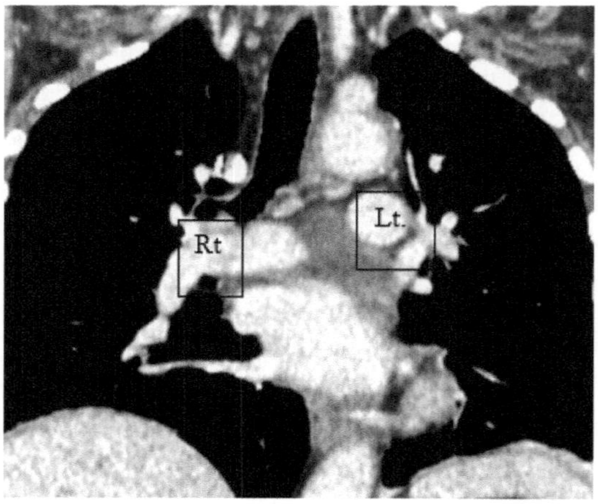

Fig. 3.13 Coronal image of CT scan of the chest: Note the slightly lower position of the right pulmonary artery as compared to the left

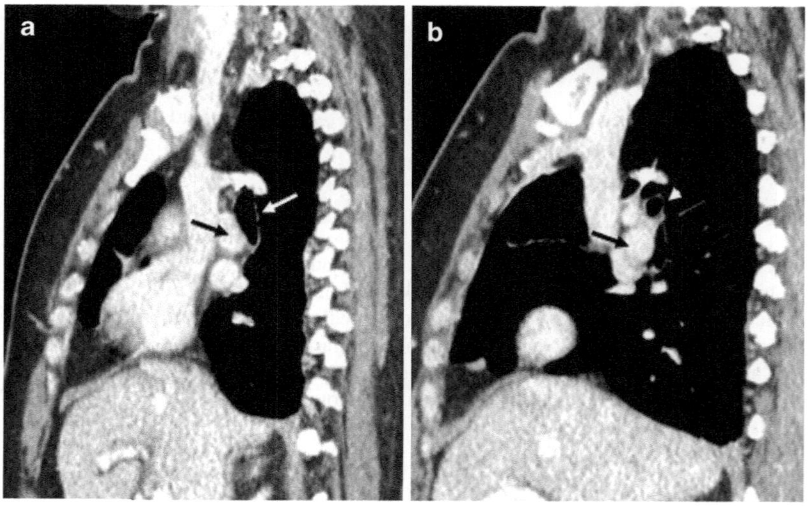

Fig. 3.14 (**a, b**) Sagittal images from a CT scan of the chest:- Figure shows the right pulmonary artery (black arrow) located anterior and slightly inferior to the right main bronchus (white arrow)

dorsal spine clearly. It will be noticed that in a lateral view, the lower dorsal vertebra appears relatively darker as compared to the upper dorsal vertebral bodies. This is because they are overlapped by the larger air containing lower lobes. Any increase in the soft tissue density in this region should be viewed with suspicion. It could be due to lower lobe consolidation, a mass in the lower lobe, pleural effusion, elevation of the diaphragm or the presence of a paraspinal abscess.

14. The right posterior costophrenic recess extends behind the liver shadow. The lucency of the posterior lobes should, therefore, be visible below the level of the diaphragms (Fig. 3.18).
15. **X-Ray Chest in the Elderly Patient**

    Elderly patients may occasionally show evidence of fibrosis in the periphery and especially in the lung bases. This is to be expected because, with age, the interstitium thickens due to several causes and becomes visible. Chest expansion is also reduced as compared to the younger persons. The diaphragms may be raised, especially in an obese patient. The heart shadow enlarges and the aorta unfolds and calcifies. The patient also may be unable to hold his breath or take deep inspiration due to hearing impairment or weakness. The spine may show a kyphotic deformity in the lateral radiograph. These factors may affect the quality of the X-rays and may be mistaken for a pathology (Fig. 3.19).
16. **The Pendulous Breast Shadows** often overlap on the lung bases in the erect PA position and cast a haze in the lower zones (Fig. 3.20).

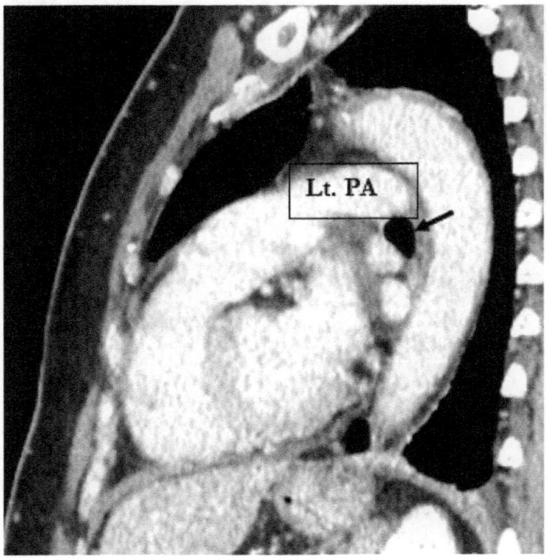

Fig. 3.15 Note the left main bronchus (arrow) located below the left main pulmonary artery

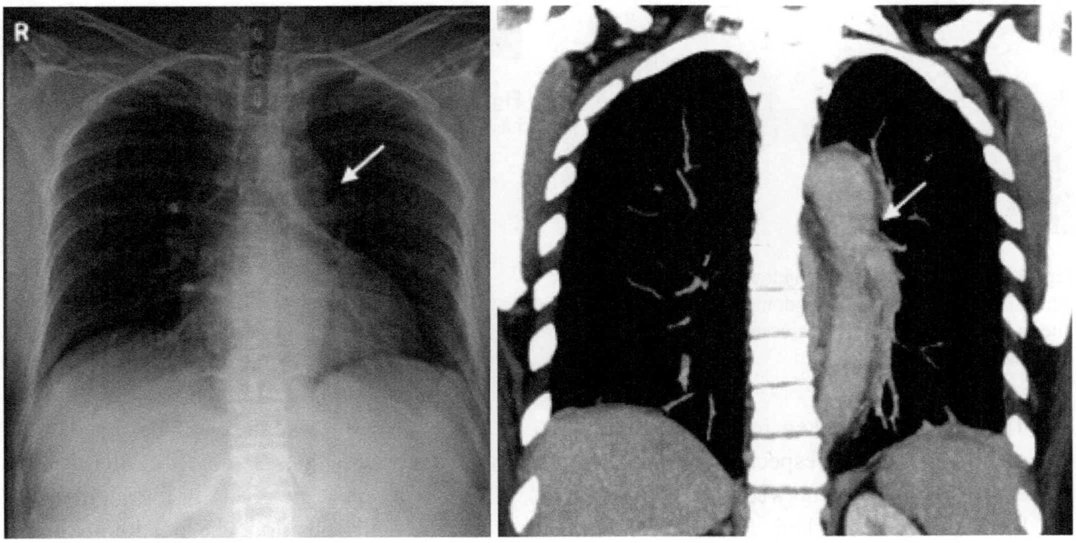

Fig. 3.16 The left hilar shadow is masked by the descending thoracic aorta (arrow) and the shadow of the left ventricle

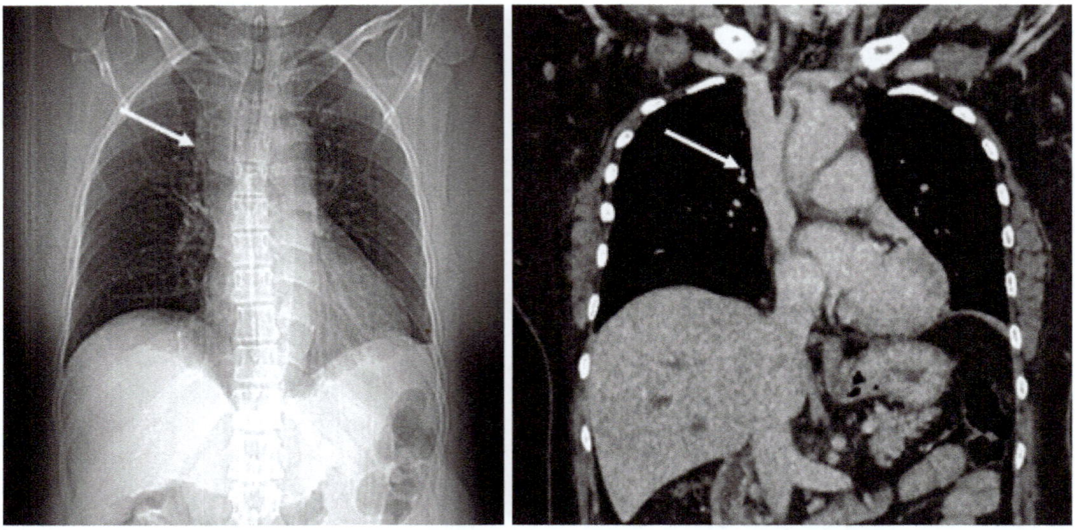

Fig. 3.17 The right hilar shadow is masked by the superior vena cava (arrow)

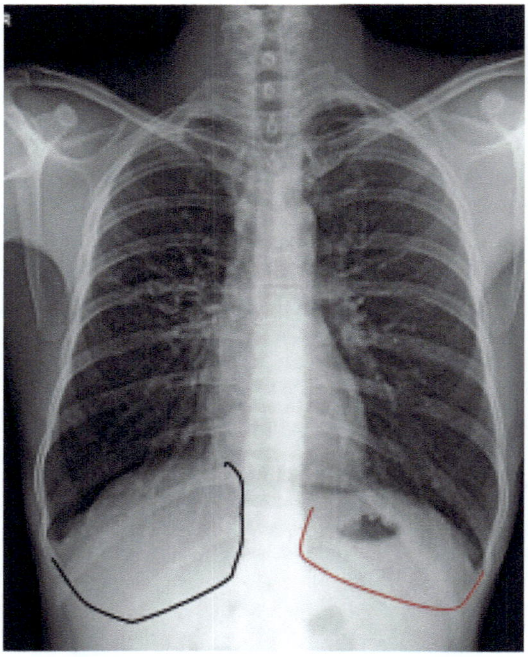

Fig. 3.18 Note the lucent shadows of the lower lobes which extend into the upper abdomen. These shadows are due to lower lobe parenchyma occupying the deep posterior costophrenic sulcus

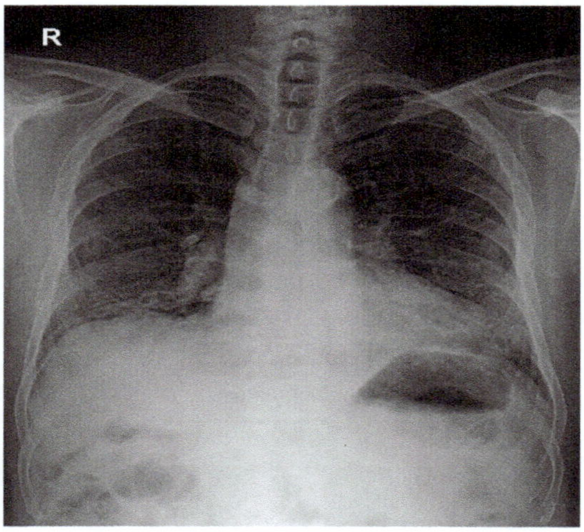

Fig. 3.19 Chest x-ray of an elderly patient showing fine basal fibrosis and elevated diaphragms

This may be mistaken for consolidation or pleural pathology, especially if the difference in densities between the upper and lower zones is marked. Breast shadows in lactating patients or in elderly males may be problematic and need to be remembered as a possible cause of increased density in the lower chest. In these cases, if the technician tries to overcome the problem by increasing the penetration, it results in the darkening of the upper zones. One needs to get used to such situations and remember that breast shadows will make the bases hazy and might also obscure the CP angles. Alternatively, one can repeat the X-ray in the supine position. In this position, the pendulous breast shadows normally fall to the side, thereby

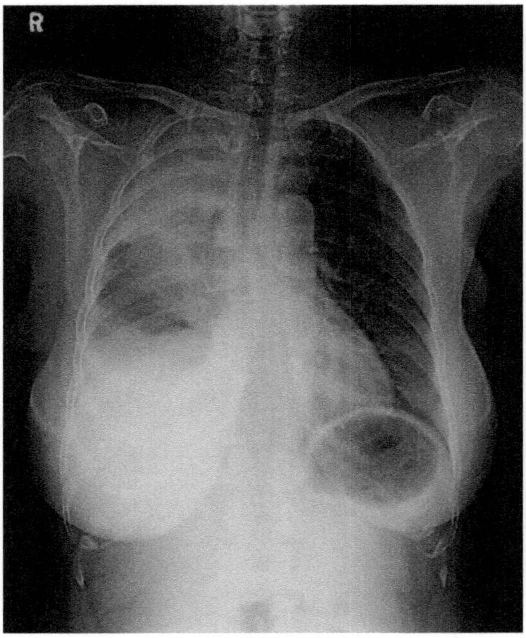

Fig. 3.20 Breast shadows obscuring the right base. The technician increased the exposure, yet the breast shadow on the right could not be sufficiently penetrated. This was because there was a mass in the right breast. On the other hand, the increased penetration blackened the left lung field

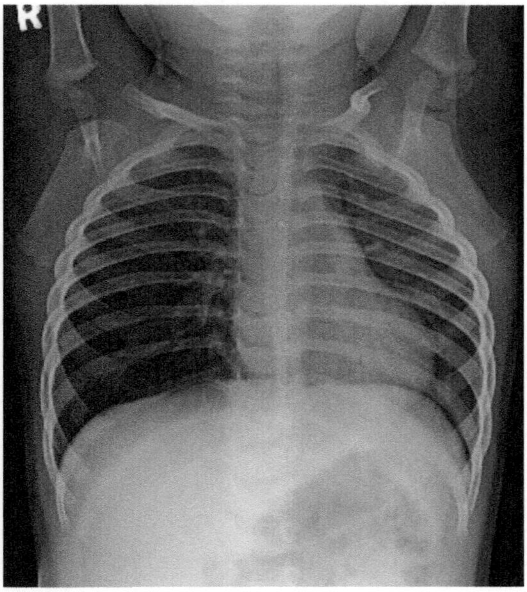

Fig. 3.21 In a small or restless child, an x-ray obtained in the supine position is often sufficient. Note the increased lucency and increased size of the right lung as compared to the left, in this case of foreign body lodged in the right main bronchus

improving the visibility of the lower lobes and pleura.

17. **X-Rays of Children:** The child's X-ray should be well-centred and obtained with deep inspiration. This can be achieved by holding the child firmly and pressing the exposure button when there is a momentary pause in between the act of crying (Fig. 3.21). Alternatively, in slightly older children, either by asking them to distend the abdomen and holding in this position for a moment or by using ultrashort exposure times, good X-rays can be obtained even without giving any breathing instruction. Nonetheless, obtaining a good X-ray of a child is easier said than done! The child may refuse to cooperate or stay still during the exposure. A film obtained in expiration appears hazy and simulates pathology. This is the reason why a film with deep inspiration is preferred. The right lower chest shows normal pulmonary vessels very well. These are often mistaken for chest infections. The heart size in children appears larger than in adults with an acceptable CT ratio of 60%.
18. **Other Structures Seen in a Chest X-Ray**

    A chest X-ray can show the thyroid gland indenting the trachea (Fig. 3.22), a dilated fluid-filled oesophagus as in achalasia cardia, an oesophagal diverticulum, a diaphragmatic hernia, mediastinal fat causing haziness in the lower chest and pathology of the bones and upper abdomen. Therefore, careful evaluation of all that is included in the chest X-ray is essential (Fig. 3.22).

    A systematic approach will enable proper evaluation of the chest X-ray PA view. However, other views, such as lateral and dedicated views, may be needed for further evaluation. If need be, obtain a CT scan of the chest for further evaluation.

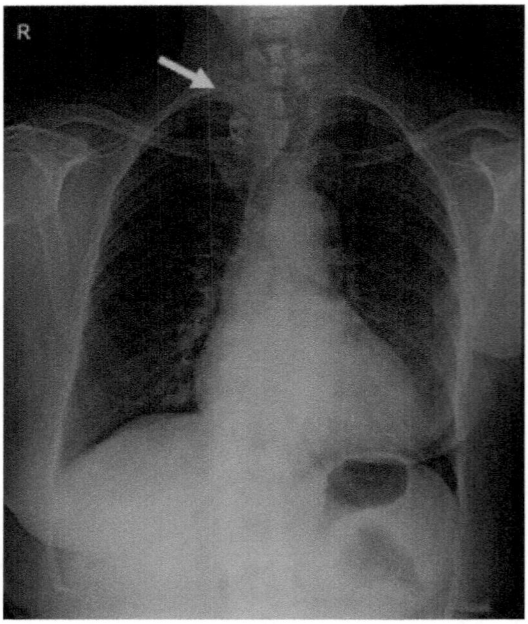

Fig. 3.22 Chest x-ray showing a partially calcified nodule in the right lobe of the thyroid gland indenting the trachea. Also, note the asymmetric position of the breast shadows, the left being at a higher level than the right. This observation needs clinical correlation

Reference

1. Furlow PW, Mathisen DJ. Surgical anatomy of the trachea. Ann Cardiothorac Surg. 2018;7(2):255–60. https://doi.org/10.21037/acs.2018.03.01. PMID: 29707503; PMCID: PMC5900092.

4 Systematic Interpretation of Chest X-Ray

Abstract

The interpretation of a chest X-ray not only requires a methodical approach but also basic clinical and radiological knowledge for the interpretation of different findings. One fundamental observation common to all diseases is that they can replace air within the air spaces, and thicken the supporting lung architecture, thereby distorting the normal arrangement of the lung tissues, and making the normally invisible matrix visible. They can affect blood vessels, pleura, diaphragm, mediastinal structures and bones in various ways. To these observations, which can be shared by all diseases, by adding clinical and laboratory data, one tries to tease out a diagnosis from the list of differential diagnoses.

Keywords

Chest X-ray · Interstitium · Radiological observations

Coming to interpretation, a method of systematically examining the X-rays must be developed. We can either start analyzing the X-ray from the periphery of the chest and proceed inwards towards the mediastinum or begin from the mediastinum gradually shifting our gaze outwards towards the periphery. We must also examine from the superior to the inferior edge of the X-ray film. A side-to-side comparison of the right and left hemithorax is also essential as any difference in lung density or architecture needs explanation.

The chest wall comprises bones such as ribs, scapula, clavicle, shoulders, spine and soft tissues, which include muscles, fat, skin, diaphragms and breast shadows.

A brief description is provided as to how one can approach the chest X-ray.

- Begin with the skin and subcutaneous tissues, then the bony structures, that is the ribs, the upper end of the humerus, shoulder joint, clavicle, scapula, cervical spine and the dorso-lumbar spine included in the X-ray. Look for fractures, both acute and unsuspected/old fractures (Fig. 4.1), and any evidence of bone destruction. Occasionally, a congenital anomaly such as an accessory cervical rib or a bifid rib may present as a mass lesion in the chest wall. A scoliotic spine may also result in an abnormal bulge of the chest wall (Fig. 4.2).
- Then check out the stomach bubble (Figs. 4.3 and 4.4), the subdiaphragmatic soft tissues and the soft tissues of the neck. The reason is that sometimes unexpected but important findings may be observed which may completely alter the diagnosis. One can occasionally detect a growth in the fundus air bubble of the stomach, an enlarged calcified thyroid

R. Gothi, *Radiographic and Imaging Techniques for Radiology Residents and Technologists*,
https://doi.org/10.1007/978-981-96-4816-0_4

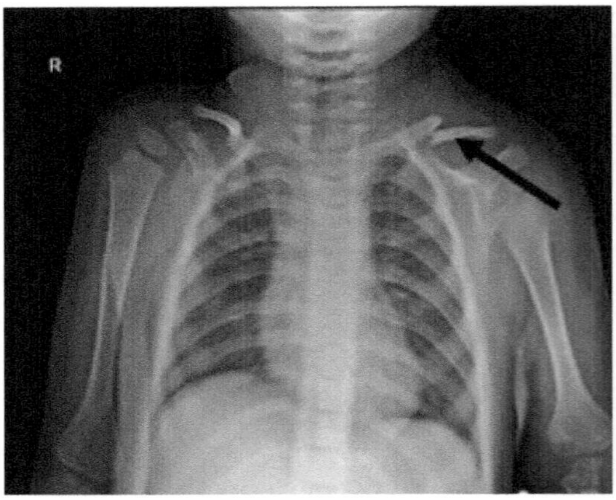

Fig. 4.1 A supine chest x-ray of a child showing a fractured left clavicle (arrow)

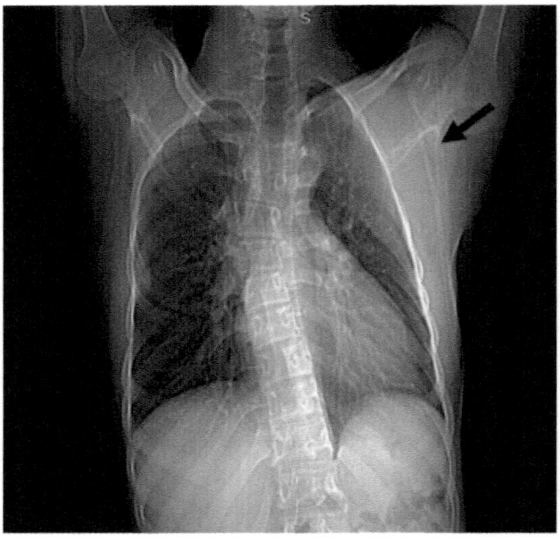

Fig. 4.2 Scanogram of the chest showing a scoliotic spine. Notice the soft tissue shadow over the left axilla widening the space between the ribs and the left scapula (arrow)

nodule and even air under the diaphragms. The absence of a fundus gas bubble is often noticed in cases of achalasia cardia. A grossly distended stomach bubble suggests gastric outlet obstruction.

- The superior surface of the liver may bulge upwards and can elevate the diaphragm smoothly (Fig. 4.5). A diffusely enlarged right lobe may also bulge upwards underneath a diaphragmatic hump (Fig. 4.6).

The position of the liver may be reversed along with the stomach bubble, suggesting

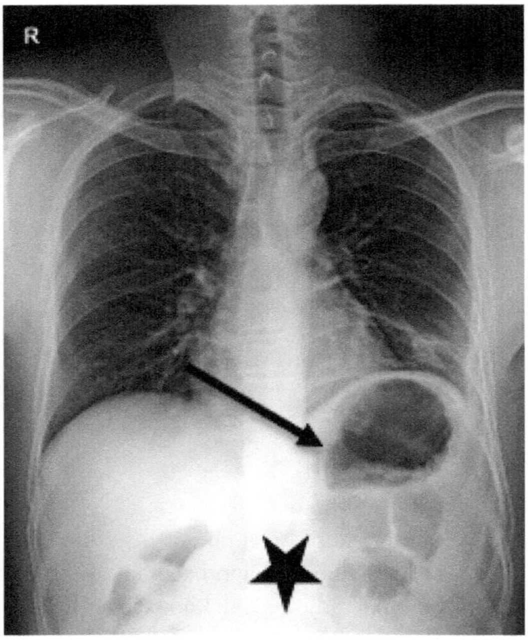

Fig. 4.3 X-ray chest showing air bubble in the gastric fundus and proximal body (arrow). Note that the stomach shadow has also been lifted up by a distended transverse colon (asterisk)

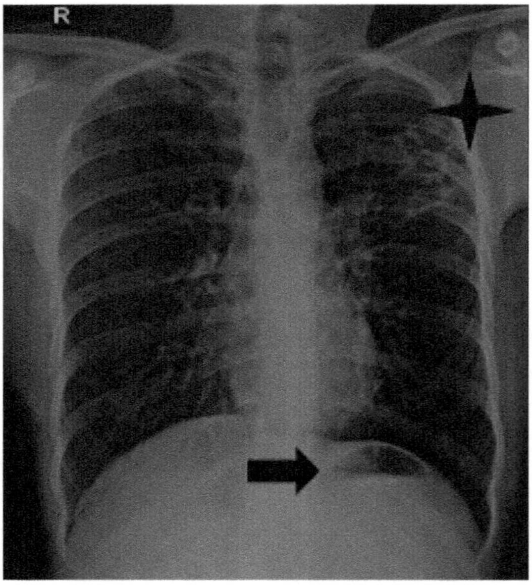

Fig. 4.4 The gastric fundus shows an air bubble with a fluid level (arrow) in this radiograph. Fluid level may be seen if the patient has had fluid recently or if there is gastric outlet obstruction. The space intervening between the fundus bubble and the left diaphragm is the combined shadow of the diaphragm and stomach wall. This space can increase if there is an interposition of the left lobe of the liver, a collection in this region or a fungal growth. Note the lesion in the left upper lobe of the lung (asterisk)

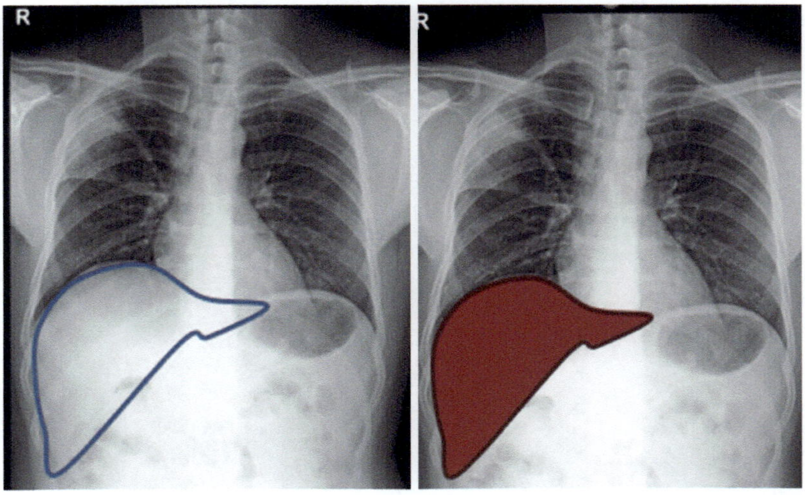

Fig. 4.5 Shadow of a normally positioned liver seen in a chest X-ray. Note it's sharp inferior edge outlined by bowel gas shadows

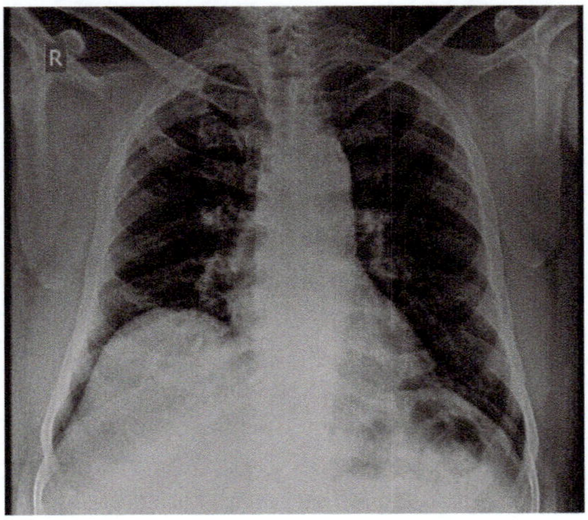

Fig. 4.6 Humped right dome of the diaphragm. The shape of the right lobe of the liver is altered in these cases and a part of the right lobe is accommodated within the diaphragmmatic hump

situs inversus. Focal or diffusely calcified lesions or cysts with calcification in their walls may also be seen in the upper lobe of the liver included in the chest X-ray. Right subphrenic gas-filled bowel loops can be seen interposed between the diaphragm and liver in a chest X-ray.

- Evaluate the breast shadows. If not seen or if they appear unusually asymmetric, on the chest X-ray, check with the patient for any previous surgery, any breast lesion or if the patient is lactating. Chest wall lesions, including solid masses, cold abscesses and callus formation around fractures may mimic focal breast lesions. The nipple may cast a shadow in the lower lung zone, resembling a pulmonary nodule. An absent breast shadow will result in increased lucency of the ipsilateral lung parenchyma (Fig. 4.7). Skin nodules can also mimic coin shadows or lung nodules. Hence, make it a practice to talk to or examine the patient, if anything is unusual is noticed, before suggesting any further investigations.
- Now examine the pleural spaces. The normal pleura, which surrounds the lung parenchyma, is not visible. The pleura becomes visible if it is calcified (Fig. 4.8) or when the lung is white, as in cases of pulmonary alveolar microlithiasis, which produces what is called "the black pleura sign".
- Examine the diaphragmatic outlines. The right diaphragm is normally one to one and a half intercostal space higher than the left. The outlines of the diaphragms should be well defined (Fig. 4.9). Occasionally, unusual elevations and localized bumps may be seen due to eventration, traction caused by fibrosis, phrenic nerve palsy or a subdiaphragmatic pathology.

After the diaphragms, it is the turn of the lung fields. **(Note process of examining a chest X-ray may vary from person to person, the goal being to examine every structure shown in the X-ray film/image.)**

- The lungs appear dark gray due to the presence of several structures which go to make

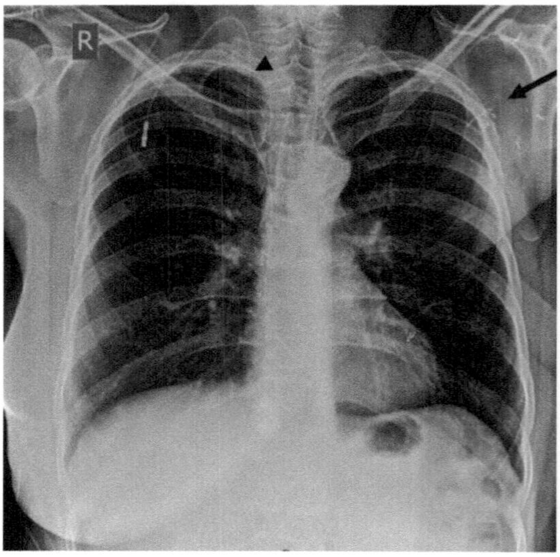

Fig. 4.7 Left breast shadow. Note the shadows of surgical clips in the left upper chest (arrow) and the presence of a chemoport over the right upper chest (arrowhead)

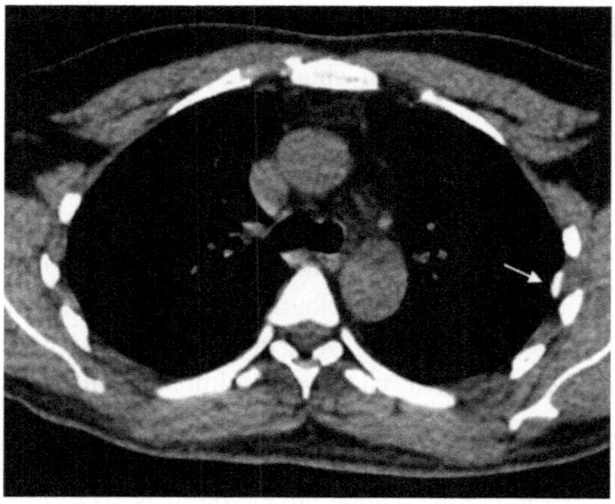

Fig. 4.8 CT scan of the chest showing a calcified pleural plaque (arrow). Such a small plaque may not be visible in a chest x-ray

them. These include the lung matrix or latticework (i.e., the interstitium), blood vessels, lymphatics, air spaces and bronchi. Therefore the normal lung should neither be too dark nor too light in density. They should be dark gray in density.

The normal white structures within the lung parenchyma include:

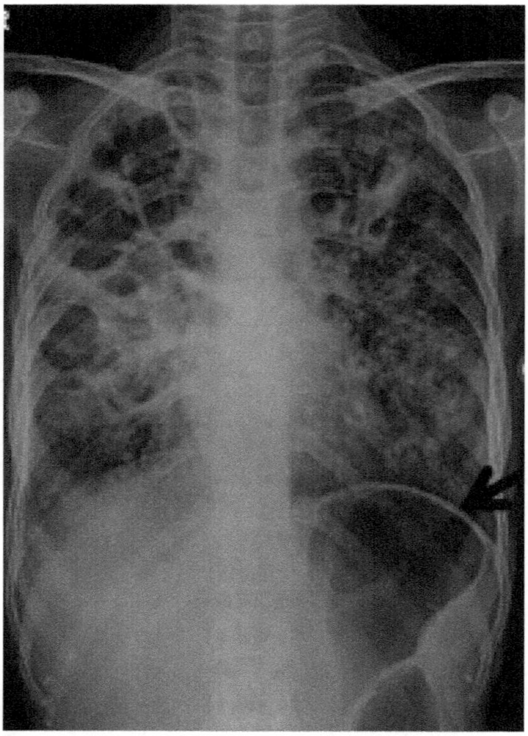

Fig. 4.9 The outline of the left diaphragm is seen between the left lung and gastric fundus gas bubble

1. Pulmonary arteries, which taper from the hilum towards the periphery.
2. Pulmonary veins which are directed towards the left atrium and are more apparent in the lower lobes as compared to the upper, especially in the erect films.
3. The outlines of bronchi, which are seen as parallel lines white, encasing an dark air column. They may also appear as ring-like shadows within the lung parenchyma.
4. Interlobar pleural fissures appear as thin white lines separating the different lobes of the lungs.
5. Small intrapulmonary nodes may often be seen, especially in cross-sectional imaging studies. They are usually located near the fissures and are round to geometrical in shape [1].
6. Any other white area seen within the lung field is most likely pathological and may

be the result of air space lesions such as consolidation, presence of a mass or collapse of a lung segment or lobe.

- **Consolidation:** This means solidification and happens because of the replacement of air in the air-spaces with fluid such as inflammatory fluid, blood or a mass lesion (Fig. 4.10). The consolidated segment appears as a whitish (opaque) area/patch, against the surrounding normal dark gray aerated lung parenchyma. It does not show loss of volume and may, in fact, enlarge the involved lobe or segment. It may show the presence of branching air-filled bronchi (air bronchogram) or air-filled alveolar spaces (air alveologram) within it. A CT scan may also detect fluid-filled dilated bronchi within an area of consolidation.
- **Collapse:** This means loss of volume with the inability of the lobe or segment to expand during breathing. It appears as a dense white area and may involve a subsegment, a segment, a lobe or the entire lung parenchyma. Loss of volume is recognized by the ipsilateral shift of adjoining pulmonary broncho vascular markings, mediastinum or pleural markings including fissures. Significant loss of volume due to fibrosis will lead to either tubular or tapering bronchial dilatation within the collapsed lung parenchyma. The tubular dilatation is called traction bronchiectasis and is usually seen when there is fibrosis. There might also be upward retraction of the hilum and diaphragm, crowding of the ribs and compensatory overexpansion of the adjoining lung segments. When there is a loss of volume of the upper lobes, the trachea may be pulled towards the atelectatic lobe, but unlike in a fibrosed shrunken lobe, it will not show kinking (Fig. 4.11).
- **Micronodules, Nodules and Masses** [2, 3]
A micronodule is less than 3 mm in size but can be up to 1.0 cm. A nodule is a round well or slightly ill-defined lesion measuring up to 3 cm. A mass is a well or ill-defined lesion measuring above 3 cm in maximum diameter.

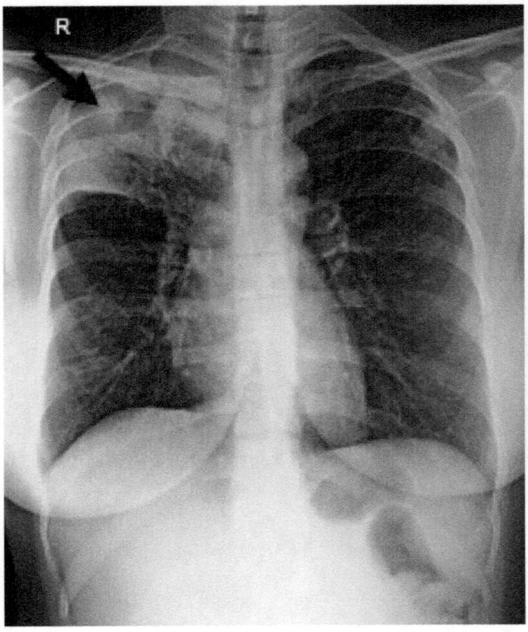

Fig. 4.10 Right upper lobe consolidation (arrow) outlined inferiorly by the horizontal fissure

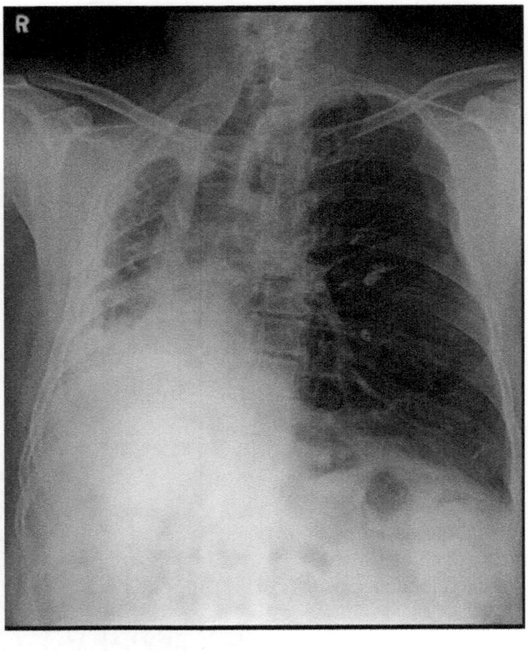

Fig. 4.11 Partial collapse of the right lung with ipsilateral (same side) shift of the trachea and mediastinum, including the cardiac shadow, thereby resulting in compensatory overexpansion of the left lung. Note the presence of calcified lesions in the left lung, indicating the possibility of an old granulomatous pathology, being the aetiology for the collapse. Note also the crowding of right-sided rib shadows

A mass of size above 5 cm, needs to be followed up, as the risk of malignancy increases with large-sized lesions. A nodule of 8 cm or more should always be followed by a CT scan of the chest and, if need be biopsied or reexamined by an early follow-up CT scan after 30 days to see what has become of it [4].

Pulmonary nodules can be distributed along lymphatics (perilymphatic nodules), in the air spaces (centrilobular nodules) or in the interstitium. They can be distributed across various spaces and tissues of the lung and are then called randomly distributed nodules. This distribution is appreciated in chest CTs and may not be distinguishable in an X-ray of the chest.

Micronodules such as those seen in miliary TB and several other diseases are usually randomly distributed. This means that they can be present anywhere or everywhere in the lung parenchyma. These nodules are very small in size, sometimes difficult to appreciate on an X-ray and may just cause haziness of the lung parenchyma.

Centrilobular nodules are ill-defined, soft tissue density nodules located in the centre of the secondary pulmonary lobule. They appear as faint soft tissue density opacities in a chest X-ray (Fig. 4.12).

Nodules 3 cm in size can have soft tissue density, can be calcified or show mixed densities (Fig. 4.13). They are usually round to ovoid but may have variable shapes. They can be seen in several infective and non-infective diseases. The management of these lesions will be determined by the clinical data.

Masses (Fig. 4.14) are more than 5 cm in size and are usually suspicious for malignancy. They need to be vigorously followed and may need a CT scan and if need be, biopsy to establish the diagnosis.

Careful interpretation of normal and abnormal features in a chest X-ray is a prerequisite for making a correct diagnosis. For this to happen, there has to be a systematic approach combined with clinical and laboratory inputs.

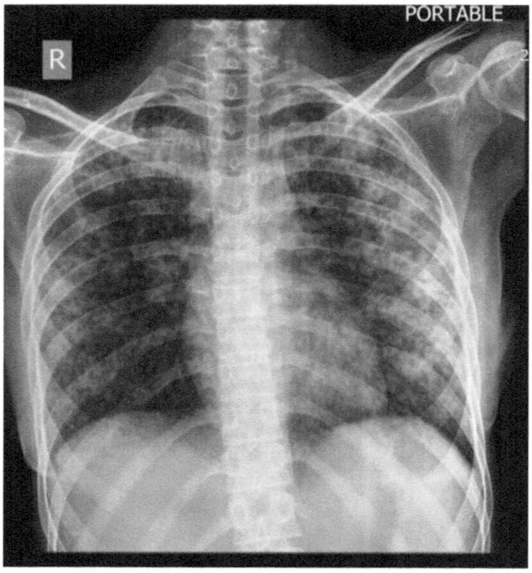

Fig. 4.12 Ill-defined centrilobular ground-glass density nodules distributed throughout the lung parenchyma

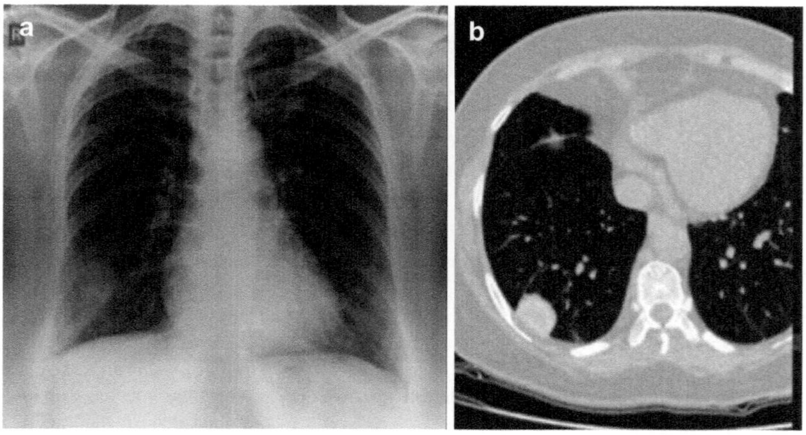

Fig. 4.13 (**a**, **b**) Chest x-ray (**a**) shows a soft tissue density nodule in the right lower lobe. Corresponding CT (**b**) is provided for comparison

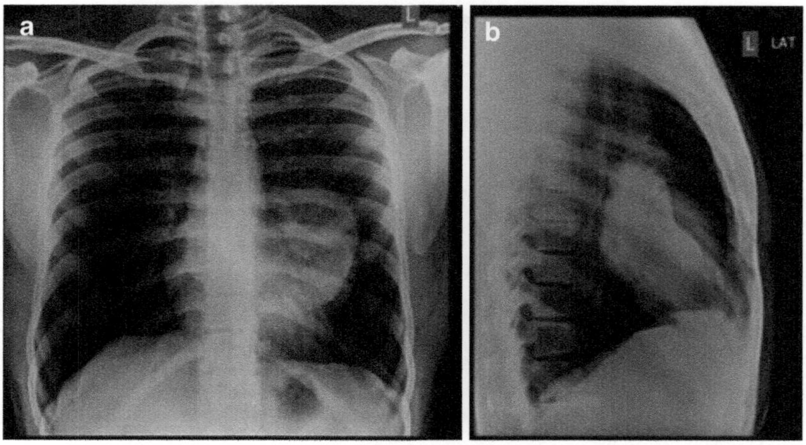

Fig. 4.14 (**a, b**) Chest x-ray PA and lateral view showing a mass in the left thorax

References

1. Schreuder A, Jacobs C, Scholten ET, van Ginneken B, Schaefer-Prokop CM, Prokop M. Typical CT features of intrapulmonary lymph nodes: a review. Radiol Cardiothorac Imaging. 2020;2(4):e190159.
2. Loverdos K, Fotiadis A, Kontogianni C, Iliopoulou M, Gaga M. Lung nodules: a comprehensive review on current approach and management. Ann Thorac Med. 2019;14:226–38.
3. Larici AR, Farchione A, Franchi P, Ciliberto M, Cicchetti G, Calandriello L, Del Ciello A, Bonomo L. Lung nodules: size still matters. Eur Respir Rev. 2017;26(146):170025. https://doi.org/10.1183/16000617.0025-2017.
4. Yankelevitz DF, Gupta R, Zhao B, et al. Small pulmonary nodules: evaluation with repeat CT—preliminary experience. Radiology. 1999;212:561–6.

5 Interpretation of Lung Lesions

Abstract

There are several diseases (Garg et al., Pol J Radiol 84:e205–e213, 2019) which cast abnormal shadows in the chest. They may resemble one another radiologically as well as in a CT scan. It is therefore very important to know the clinical background of the referred patient. The clinician should provide a reason for requesting a particular investigation. It is also the duty of everyone responsible for performing and reporting the investigation to find out the reason for requesting the investigation. This way, not only can the study be tailored to fulfil the requirement of the case but one can also suggest an alternative and a more appropriate step in arriving at the diagnosis.

Keywords

Pneumonia · Segmental · Lobar

Now let us discuss some of these diseases and their radiological [1] appearances.

- **Pneumonia:** Pneumonias can present themselves as lobar consolidation, bronchopneumonia and interstitial pneumonia based on the distribution in the lung field.

Segmental/Lobar Pneumonia: These appear as a white pulmonary segment or lobe. The air-filled gray lung parenchyma is replaced by consolidation, which could be made of inflammatory tissue, pus, accumulated blood or a mass. Cases of community-acquired pneumonia (CAP) are mostly lobar or segmental. They are caused by an infective organism, commonly Streptococcus pneumoniae. These are usually considered simple types of pneumonia and can affect children, healthy individuals, patients with low immunity, those with other comorbidities or frail elderly people, particularly during the winters. They can also be a consequence of other locally prevalent bacterial or viral infections seen during a change of season. Simple pneumonia can usually be diagnosed by history and physical examination. The lung involvement may not be visible in the X-ray chest taken on the first day of infection. The pneumonia may take a few days or up to a week or more to manifest in an X-ray. However, it may be visible earlier in a CT scan of the chest. Radiological clearance of pneumonia also takes time. Therefore, re-evaluation by an X-ray should be deferred for a later date once the treatment as well as clinical symptoms have subsided. This helps in convincingly demonstrating clearance or regression of the lung opacity. In

R. Gothi, *Radiographic and Imaging Techniques for Radiology Residents and Technologists*,
https://doi.org/10.1007/978-981-96-4816-0_5

those cases where the pneumonia is still visible despite completing the treatment, a repeat X-ray or even a CT scan may be performed after 3 months or even earlier. A CT scan may also be needed to rule out underlying causes of pneumonia, especially in smokers. The affected lung parenchyma in the case of simple pneumonia will not be accompanied by loss of volume or cavitation. It may show an air bronchogram if the airway within it is patent. The air bronchogram should be carefully examined. It should be smooth and uniformly tapering in a simple community-acquired pneumonia. If it is irregular in outline and tubular in shape, consider the possibility of surrounding fibrosis. Abrupt termination of an air bronchogram could be due to thick secretions, a foreign body or an endobronchial lesion.

Bacterial pneumonia can be unilateral or bilateral. The lower lobes are more often affected but any lobe can be involved (Fig. 5.1a, b).

In gram-negative infections, the volume of the consolidated lobe may increase. This can be made out by appreciating the bulging outlines of the adjoining pleural fissures. Pneumonias may be associated with parapneumonic effusion. In these cases, it may become difficult to distinguish simple pneumonia from other causes of consolidation. In such cases, ultrasonography or a CT scan of the chest and follow-up studies may be needed.

Hilar or mediastinal nodes may also be seen with simple pneumonias. They are often reactive and usually are not large, their size ranging between 1 and 2 cm. These reactive nodes are generally not visible in a chest radiograph till they enlarge or alter the density and outline of the hilum and mediastinum. The area of consolidation may show air-filled bronchi (air bronchogram sign) (Fig. 5.2).

Rarely, fluid may accumulate in the bronchi obscuring the air-bronchogram sign. When this happens, the bronchi are no longer visible in a chest X-ray. They may be seen in a CT scan as fluid-filled hypodense branching structures. Fluid within bronchi could be due to accumulated purulent secretions, mucus, blood or watery discharge (bronchorrhoea). Whenever fluid-filled bronchi are seen, one must look carefully for any proximal bronchial obstruction.

In the case of pneumonia, it is always prudent to repeat the X-ray after a course of appropriate treatment. If the pneumonic shadow does not resolve within 6–12 weeks at the maximum (Fig. 5.3), then other causes of non-resolving pneumonia such as congenital abnormalities (e.g., sequestrated lung seg-

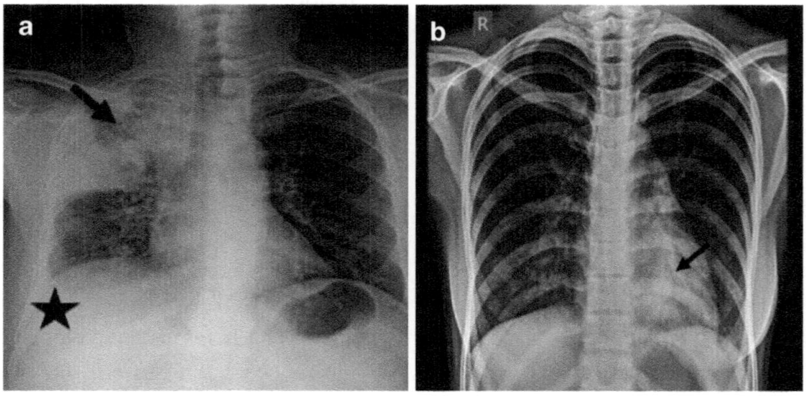

Fig. 5.1 (**a, b**) A case of right upper lobe consolidation (**a**) with some areas showing cavitation/breakdown. Note the air bronchogram (arrow) and blunting of the right CP angle (star) due to associated parapneumonic effusion. A 12-year-old girl with pain in her left lower chest (**b**), note a small retrocardiac density (arrow) which is suggestive of left lower lobe pneumonia

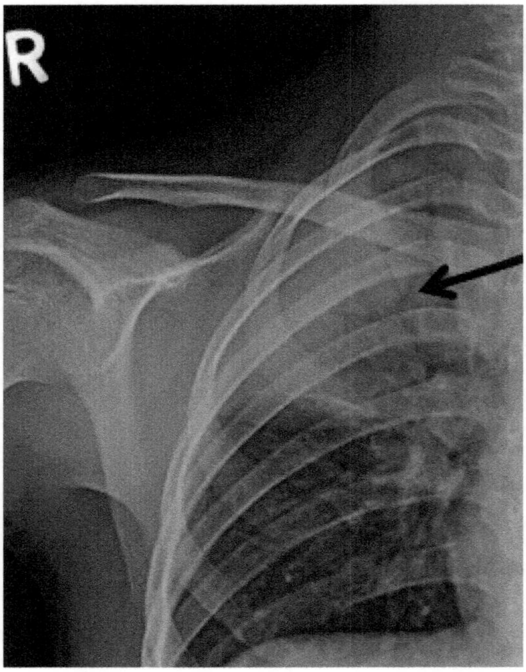

Fig. 5.2 Air bronchogram (arrow)is seen in this case of right upper lobe consolidation. The presence of air in the bronchi indicates patency of the airways

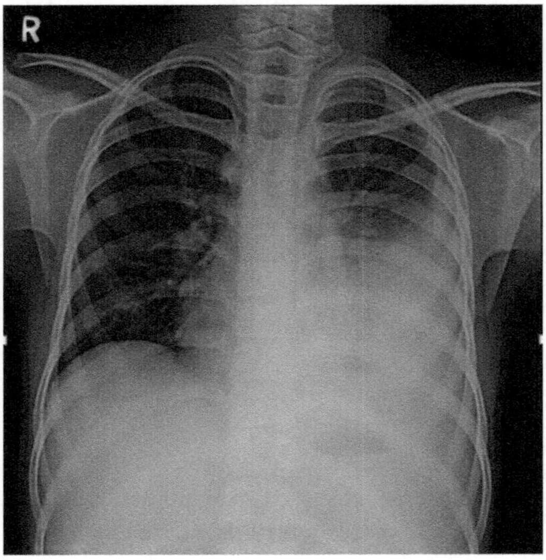

Fig. 5.3 A case of left lower lobe consolidation obscured by pleural effusion. Such cases must be followed up till complete clearance of the findings, otherwise an underlying/associated pathology may be missed. Alternatively, an ultrasound of the chest or a CT scan can also be carried out for further evaluation

ment), underlying parenchymal airways or airspace abnormality, foreign body causing occlusion and distal consolidation, atypical infections such as fungal, TB, or malignant lesions should be considered.

- **Bronchopneumonia:** These are opacities involving the bronchi and their surrounding parenchyma. The process is usually infective but can be inflammatory or due to a malignancy. The disease may involve any bronchopulmonary segment. It is more commonly seen in the periphery of the lung fields where the small calibre bronchi reside. These bronchi are unable to eject any fluid accumulated within them, hence they distend and become visible as nodular opacities in the lung periphery, which are called "tree-in-bud lesions". If the disease progresses, it can lead to the development of segmental or even lobar pneumonia. Any type of organism, from bacterial to viral or fungal can cause bronchopneumonia. The appearance of bronchopneumonia is nonspecific and needs to be correlated with other clinical and laboratory findings (Fig. 5.4).
- **Collapse (Atelectasis):** Collapse or loss of volume of a pulmonary segment or lobe, appears as a parenchymal opacity. There is crowding of bronchovascular markings in the collapsed segment or lobe. The adjoining pleural fissures come closer. Sometimes, the collapsed segment may blend with the mediastinal shadow or diaphragm and not be easily visible, unless carefully looked for. The bronchi within the collapsed segment may show air if they are unobstructed. However, they may be devoid of air in long-standing collapse and obstruction proximal to the collapsed region. Also, where there is proximal bronchial occlusion, the distal bronchi in the collapsed lobe may fill up with secretions. The lung parenchymal around the collapsed area may show consolidation or compensatory overexpansion with spread-out vascular markings, closer approximation of the pleural fissures and increased lucency. Collapse

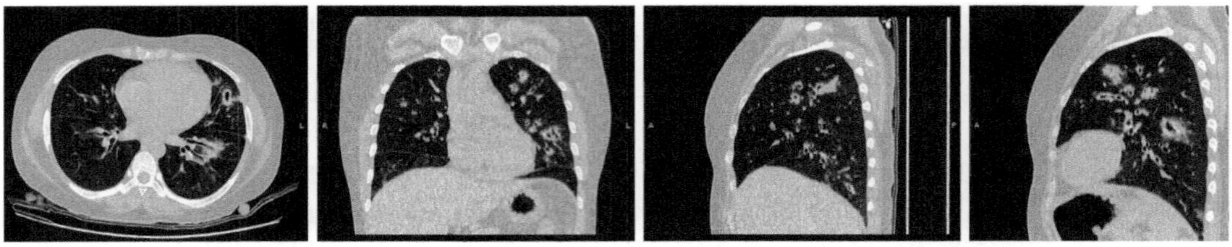

Fig. 5.4 CT scan images in multiple planes (axial, sagittal, and coronal planes) show thickening and inflammatory changes in the bronchial walls with extension of the inflammation into the adjoining pulmonary parenchyma

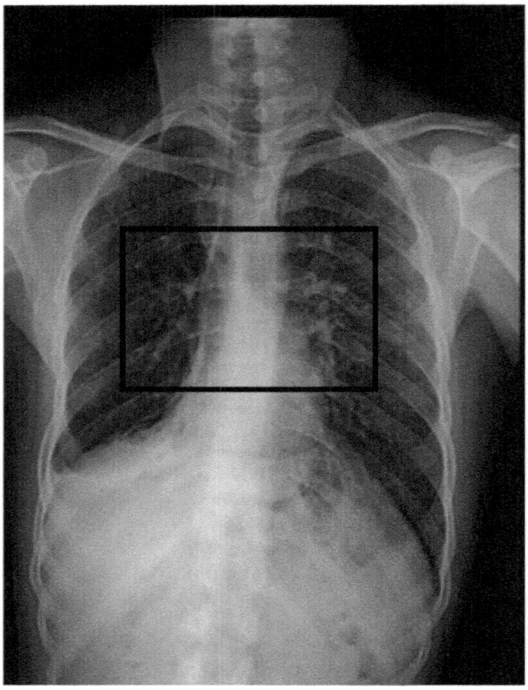

Fig. 5.5 A case of collapse right lower lobe with compensatory overexpansion of the right upper and middle lobes. Note the inward retraction of the right hilum (box), which is merging into the mediastinum, as compared to the left hilum which is visible. Also, note how the collapsed right lower lobe is merging into the mediastinum and diaphragm

can occur due to an intrapulmonary (endobronchial or parenchymal) pathology or an extraneous cause compressing the lung from outside. There are several intrapulmonary causes of collapse such as exo- or endobronchial lesions, foreign body ingestion, bronchostenosis and masses. Occasionally, thick viscid mucus plugs, especially in patients with bronchial asthma or mucoviscidosis, can result in collapse. Occasionally, in a segment which is collapsed due to fibrosis, the crowded mildly dilated bronchi show irregular outlines. This type of bronchial dilatation is called traction bronchiectasis. Recent collapse may be a reversible phenomenon if it is due to inspissated secretion, a foreign body ingestion a removable mass or if resulting from external compression caused by pleural effusion. A chronically collapsed segment may not regain its previous normal appearance. A lung lobe or segment which is chronically collapsed, especially due to long-standing pleural thickening, empyema or pneumothorax, may not re-expand despite a chest tube placement. This results in what is called "a trapped lung" (Fig. 5.5).

When both the middle and lower lobes are affected, the site of the occlusive bronchial lesion is usually the bronchus intermedius (Fig. 5.6).

Extrapulmonary causes of collapse are usually pleural-based pathologies, such as exudative pleural effusion, which cause compressive atelectasis of the underlying lung segment or lobe (Fig. 5.7).

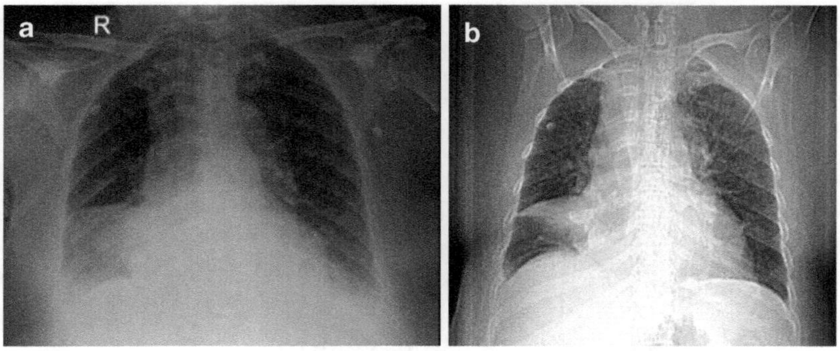

Fig. 5.6 (**a, b**) A case of middle lobe collapse. Figure (**a**) is a supine chest AP projection where the middle lobe is seen as soft tissue opacity outlined above by the horizontal fissure, obscuring the right heart border. Figure (**b**) is a CT scanogram film which resembles a lordotic view, and clearly shows middle lobe collapse

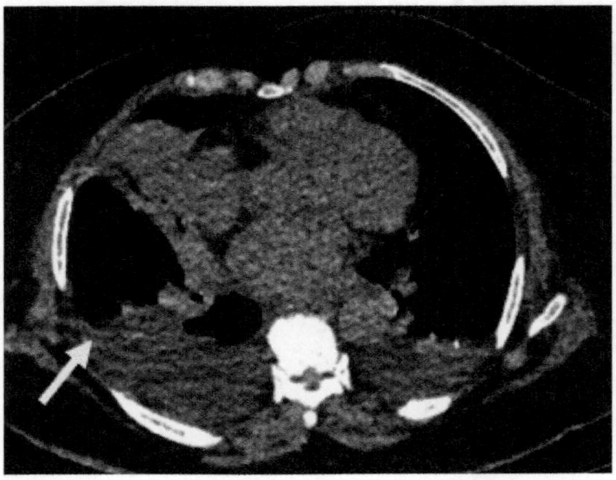

Fig. 5.7 CT scan of the chest showing right lower lobe compressive atelectasis (arrow) caused by pleural effusion. The left base is also compressed by the effusion

5.1 Granulomatous Lesions

5.1.1 Tuberculosis

Tuberculosis is a granulomatous disease caused by Mycobacterium tuberculosis (MTB). There are atypical varieties of tuberculosis also, which are caused by Mycobacterium avium complex (MAC), Mycobacterium abscessus and Mycobacterium kansasii. Diseases showing fibrosis, cavitation, calcification, multiple lobe involvement especially apical lung lesions, bronchiectasis and pleural effusion both unilateral and, occasionally bilateral, should be considered as possibly tubercular. Tuberculosis, causing shrinkage of the upper lobes secondary to fibrosis, can pull the trachea and the hilum upwards towards the fibrosed lung segment or lobe. The entire lung or at least a major part of it can be destroyed by TB. There may also be pleural calcification, lymph nodal calcification, destruction of ribs and spine, miliary shadows in the lungs and large pneumonic patches, due to MTB. Consider tuberculosis as one of the causes of chest infection and parenchymal lung lesions if the patient is a diabetic. Occasionally one may find complications of TB such as aspergillomas which appear as a mobile ball of soft tissues in a tubercular cavity. There may be focal bronchostenosis which may lead to the collapse of a segment or lobe. Rarely a malignancy may develop on a tubercular scar. This is called a scar carcinoma. Even lymphoma can develop in a patient having longstanding tubercular empyema [2]. However, not all upper lobe fibrosis is due to TB. Fibrosis may be seen in cases of Sarcoidosis, Silicosis, chronic obstructive airway disease, collagen disorders, fibrosing type of hypersensitivity pneumonia and after radiation for lung or breast cancers. Follow-up of confirmed cases of tuberculosis should be with x-rays every 3 to 6 months till completion of treatment (Figs. 5.8 and 5.9). Other important mimics of tuberculosis are histoplasmosis and fungal infections.

Some features of active tuberculosis may be suspected from a chest X-ray and CT scan. These

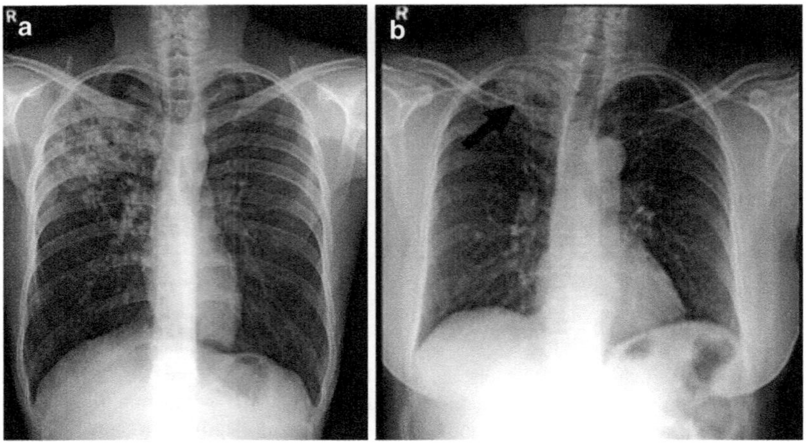

Fig. 5.8 (**a, b**) A case of infiltrative pulmonary Kochs, affecting the right upper lobe (**a**). Follow-up after 3 months shows (**b**) reduction in the extent of lung lesion (arrow)

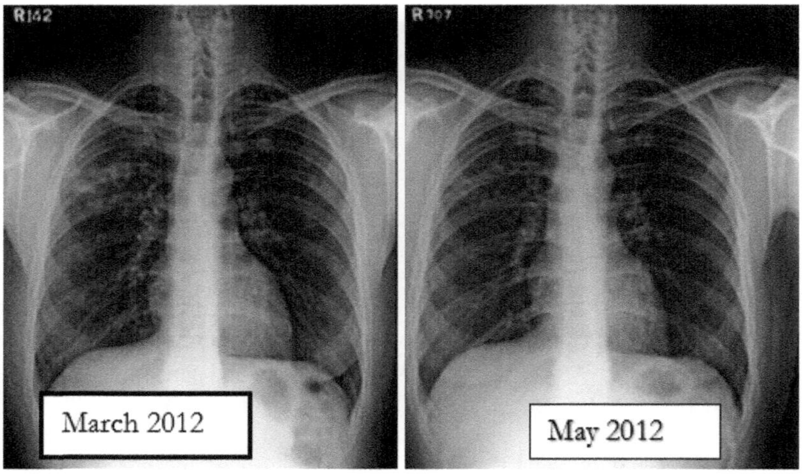

Fig. 5.9 Follow-up radiographs of another patient, obtained after adequate treatment with anti-tubercular drugs, show significant resolution of the lung lesion

include the presence of dense consolidation with cavitation, thick-walled cavities showing bronchial communication, ground-glass haze, bronchial involvement, miliary nodules and tree-in-bud lesions in the lung parenchyma (seen in CT chest). These lesions can be smear-positive. Enlarged necrotic hilar or mediastinal nodes and pleural effusion [3, 4] may also be associated with active TB.

Tuberculosis may involve a single pulmonary segment, a single lobe or multiple segments and lobes (Fig. 5.10). It has a predilection for involving the upper lobes and apical segment of the lower lobe. Old cases of TB leave behind fibrotic scars in the affected lung segments, bronchiectasis, pleural thickening and reactive nodes (Fig. 5.11).

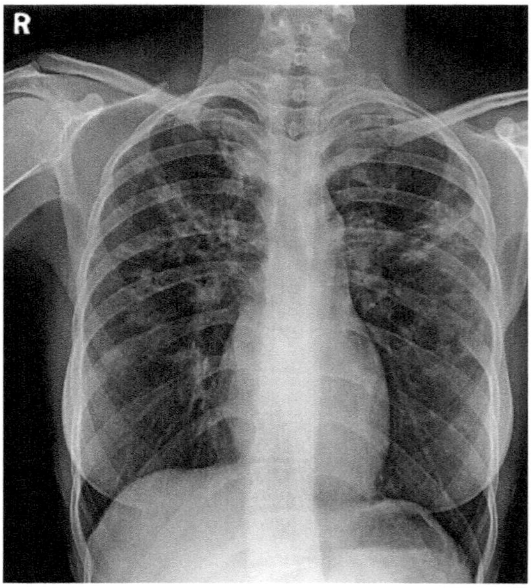

Fig. 5.10 A case of pulmonary Kochs involving both upper lobes. The DD would also include, histoplasmosis, fungal infection, sarcoidosis and COPD in this patient

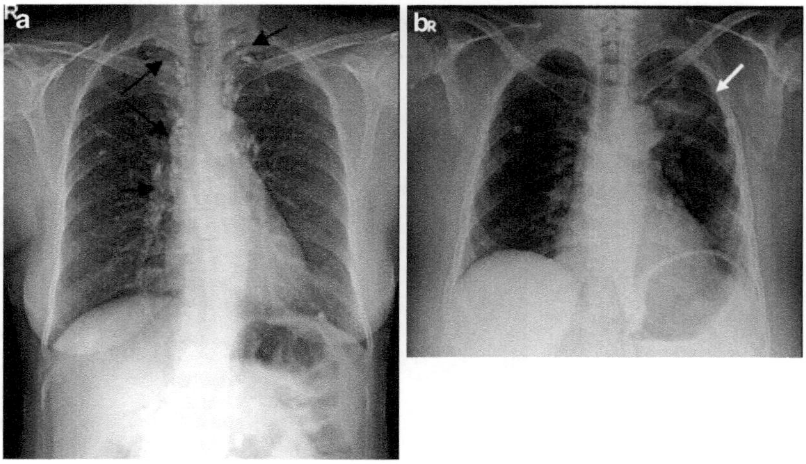

Fig. 5.11 (**a**) Old case of TB shows multiple calcified lymph nodes in (arrows) the mediastinum, neck and hilum. (**b**) Finger in glove appearance (arrow), indicative of allergic bronchopulmonary aspergillosis

5.1.2 Sarcoidosis

This is a non-tubercular granulomatous lung disease causing pulmonary fibrosis with predominantly upper lobe predilection. The fibrosis is peribronchovascular and subpleural with associated nodules distributed predominantly in the same regions. There may also be the presence of mediastinal and bilateral hilar nodes. Rarely focal peripheral consolidation, pleural effusion or ground-glass haze may be seen in a high-resolution CT. Histopathology of these lesions shows fibrosis and several compact non-caseating granulomas. These findings are contrary to the diagnosis of TB, where, one sees caseating granulomas, as well as contrary to the diagnosis of hypersensitivity pneumonia, which shows ill-formed granulomas. Sometimes, sarcoidosis may present in an atypical manner, such as large areas of consolidation.

5.2 Fungal Lesions

The appearance of fungal lesions may be variable and mimic several diseases. The lesions typically involve the upper lobes but can involve all lobes. There may be peribronchial consolidation, bronchiectasis, nodules, masses, cavitation and fibrosis. There may be areas of ground-glass opacities, especially around the lesions, which are often seen with invasive aspergillosis, mucormycosis and cryptococcosis. Other signs associated with fungal infections include finger in glove appearance (seen in allergic bronchopulmonary aspergillosis), bird nest sign (seen in mucormycosis), air crescent sign (seen in aspergillomas in cavities) and reverse halo sign (earliest reported with cryptococcosis). Wedge-shaped infarcts and pleural effusions can also be seen in patients with haematological disorders [5]. In these patients, MRI or CT pulmonary angiogram may demonstrate the “vessel occlusion sign”. Fungal infections may involve several organs [6], hence correlation with other clinical findings is essential. Amongst the various fungal infections, Histoplasmosis may mimic TB and needs to be kept in the differential diagnosis, especially if patients are coming from endemic areas [7].

5.3 Lung Abscesses

These are thick-walled cavities containing air/fluid/or both within them. Abscesses, which are thick-walled (Fig. 5.12), are usually of recent origin and are formed by liquefaction within an area of consolidation. They can be single or multiple. The inner wall of the abscess should be carefully evaluated. If smooth, it is probably benign but if it appears irregular or nodular, consider the possibility of malignancy. The presence of air within an abscess cavity usually suggests bronchial communication. Air can also enter by drifting from the adjoining air spaces. Thin-walled abscess cavities are called pneumatoceles and are

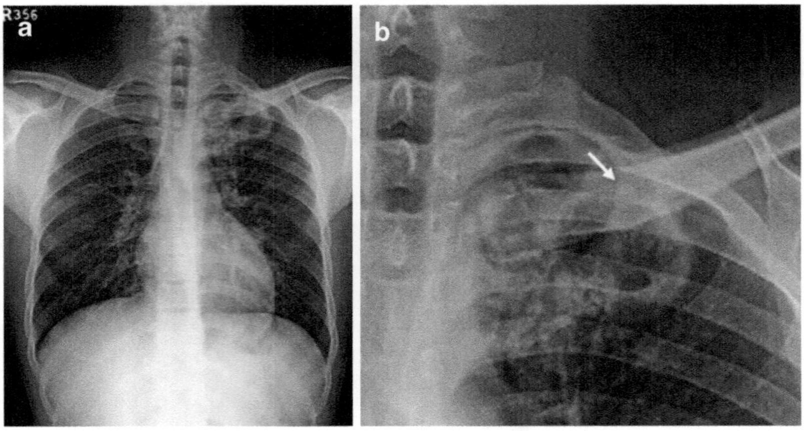

Fig. 5.12 (**a**, **b**) A thick-walled abscess is seen in the left upper lobe (**a**). Magnified view of the abscess (**b**)

usually the remains of a previous abscess. They can mimic cysts. Hence a detailed history as well as a correlation with previous records is essential.

There are various causes of lung abscesses. These include:

- Staphylococcal Infection: The abscesses form in an area of lobar consolidation by liquefaction necrosis of the infected lobe. They are thick-walled in the acute phase, becoming thinner in due course. They may develop in any lobe and may be accompanied by empyema. Sometimes it is difficult to differentiate a large peripherally located lung abscess from an empyema. In such cases, a CT scan is helpful. A lung abscess is typically spherical [8] in all views, as compared to an empyema which appears differently shaped in different views. It may look round in the PA view and ovoid in the lateral view. The abscess, being intraparenchymal, usually displaces the surrounding vessels, which, the empyema, being extra parenchymal, compresses the underlying lung parenchyma thereby causing crowding and convergence of vessels towards the empyema (the comet tail sign). The wall of the abscess is thick [9, 10] and uneven while in an empyema, the walls are usually thin and smooth as they are located between the visceral and parietal pleura.
- Malignancy: Squamous cell carcinoma of the lung may resemble a thick-walled abscess. It usually has a nodular inner wall formed by the liquefaction necrosis of the central part of the tumour. Absence of symptoms of infection, age and history of smoking help in furthering the diagnosis. Other malignancies which can look like abscesses include, primary pulmonary lymphoma, Hodgkin's lymphoma and metastatic squamous cell carcinoma.
- Klebsiella Abscess: This develops during a chest infection. It is usually single but can be multiple and is seen in an area of consolidation. It may mimic an acute staphylococcal abscess. Many other gram-negative infections can also result in the development of lung abscesses (Fig. 5.13).
- Tubercular Abscess: The abscess is a focal bronchiectatic cavity, usually small but can be large, thick-walled and may show bronchial communication. Bronchial communication is best seen in a CT scan. The diagnosis can be considered if there are associated features of TB, such as scarring, calcification and infiltration (Fig. 5.14).
- Fungal Abscess: Histoplasmosis, nocardiosis, aspergillosis, mucormycosis and actinomycosis may also produce abscesses or necrotic lesions. They can be of any size and may develop anywhere. They are often seen in an immunocompromised or diabetic patient (Figs. 5.15 and 5.16).
- Infected Hydatid Cyst: A hydatid cyst may appear as a round soft tissue density shadow. Once infection supervenes, then the lesion shows surrounding consolidation or air within it. Helpful features of a ruptured hydatid cyst are

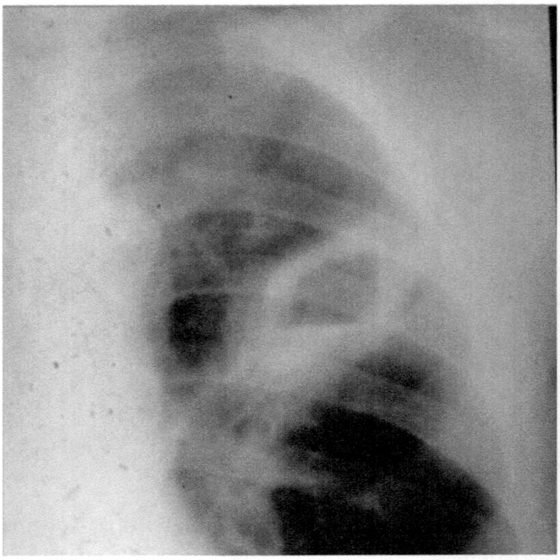

Fig. 5.13 A case of lung abscess. Pseudomonas was cultured from the sputum

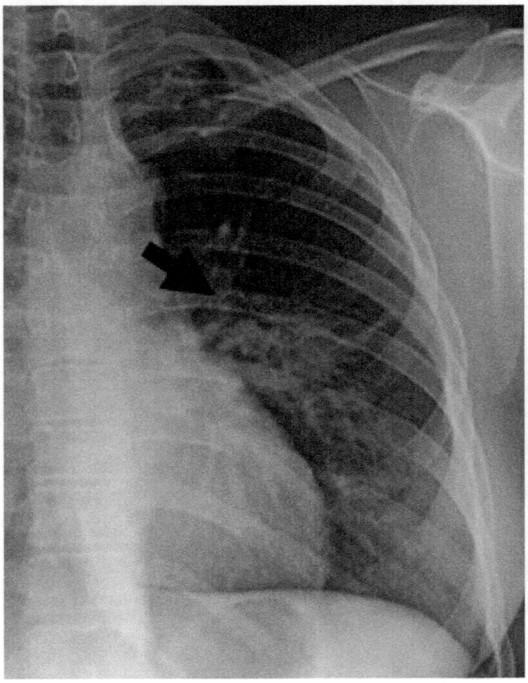

Fig. 5.14 A case of juvenile diabetes mellitus with a thick-walled abscess in the apical segment of the left lower lobe (arrow). Sputum examination showed acid-fast bacilli

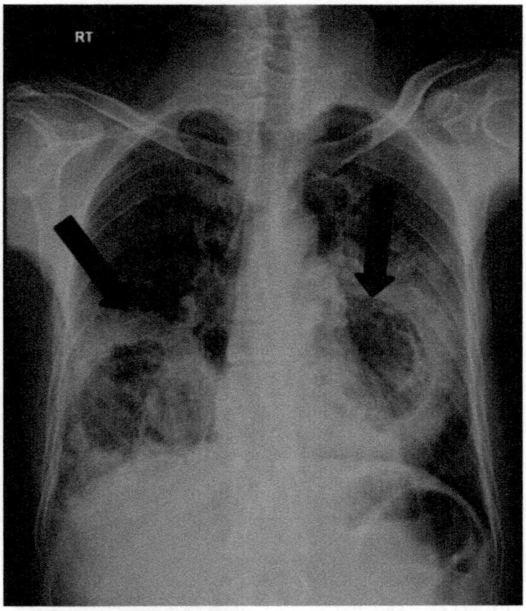

Fig. 5.15 A case of uncontrolled diabetes mellitus showing fungal abscesses due to mucormycosis (arrow) producing a "bird nest" sign

a history of the sputum expectorated being fluidic (bronchorrhoea) in consistency or coughing out membranes in the sputum. Previous films, if available, are very helpful in these cases.

The contents of an abscess may be pus, necrotic tissue, blood clot or a fungal ball. The latter is generally mobile. Rarely a malignancy may develop in an abscess. An abscess is a source of chronic ill health and may be associated with haemoptysis (Fig. 5.17).

- **Bronchiectasis:** Bronchiectasis is a disorder of the intrapulmonary bronchi. The bronchi are dilated with deformed walls. They may appear tubular, fusiform or saccular in appearance (Figs. 5.18, 5.19 and 5.20). The dilated bronchi lose their mucociliary function and may retain secretions which can get infected, resulting in the development of cavities with air-fluid levels. Bronchiectatic cav-

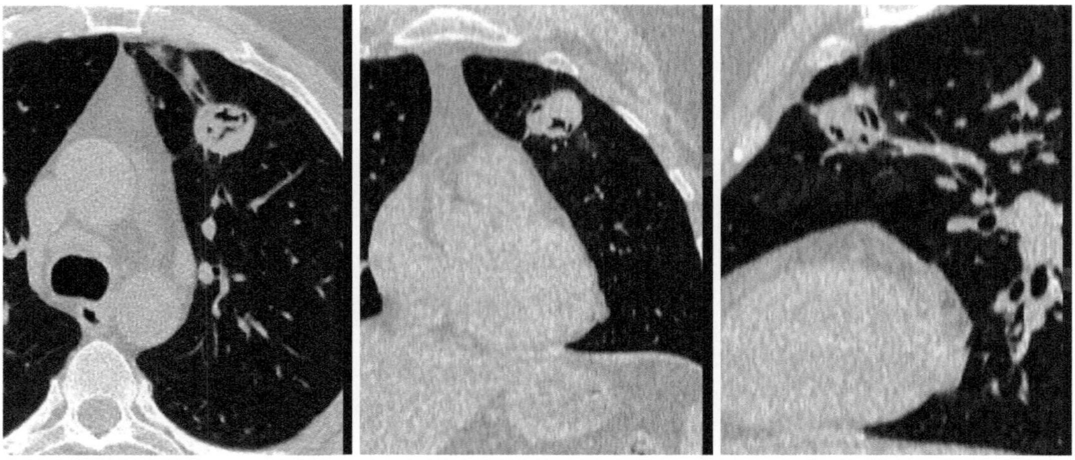

Fig. 5.16 CT scan of a small tubercular abscess in the left upper lobe, showing surrounding consolidation. Note the unchanged shape of the abscess in all (axial, coronal and sagittal) views

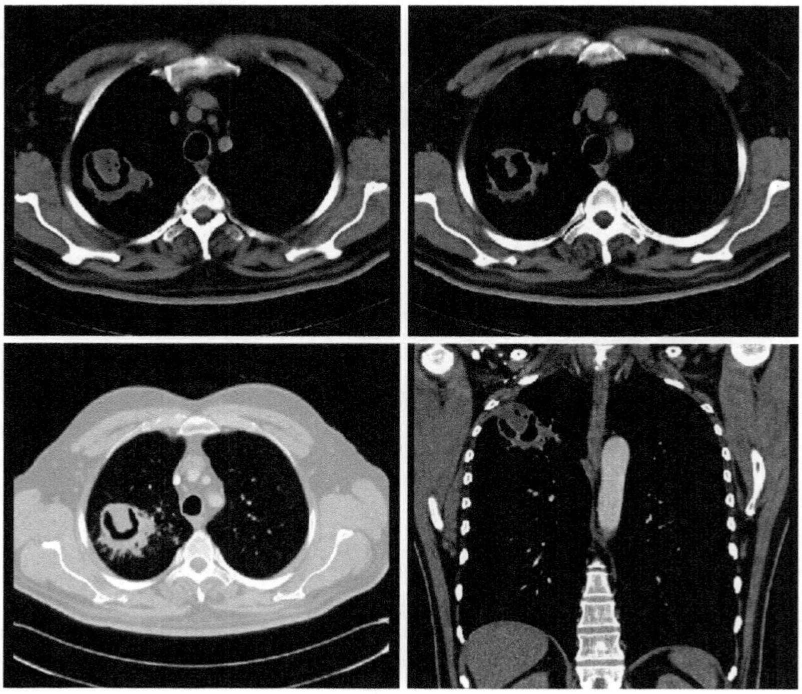

Fig. 5.17 Axial and coronal CT scan images in lung and mediastinal windows of a case of necrotizing pneumonia showing a thick-walled abscess in the RUL with a mass suspended within it. Because this mass within the cavity is adherent to the non-dependent wall, the possibility of an aspergilloma is unlikely which is usually mobile and changes position on turning the patient supine

ities may also contain fungal balls. The adjoining air spaces may show opacities caused by organization and fibrosis, resulting in loss of volume of the lobe/segment. If a patient has repeated chest infection in the same region, has attacks of haemoptysis, clubbing of fingers or brings out foul sputum, then think of underlying bronchiectasis. Look for the involvement of multiple segments and lobes, in which case the bronchiectasis could be due to fungal infection, tuberculosis or even mucoviscidosis and surgical treatment may not be an option. If it is localized to a segment which also shows volume loss, think of endobronchial lesions like foreign bodies, an extrinsic node compress-

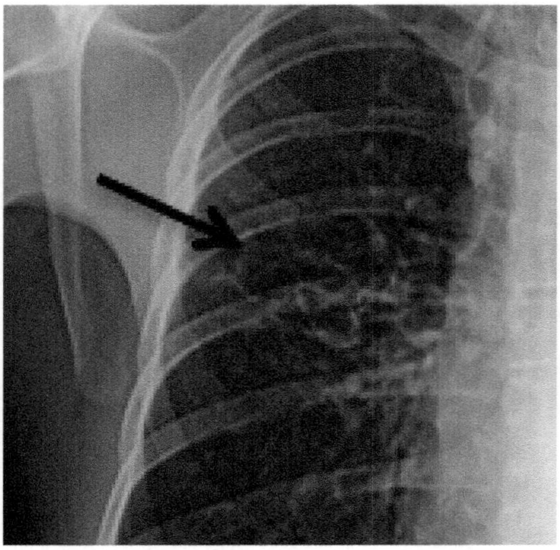

Fig. 5.18 Right upper lobe cystic bronchiectasis (arrow)

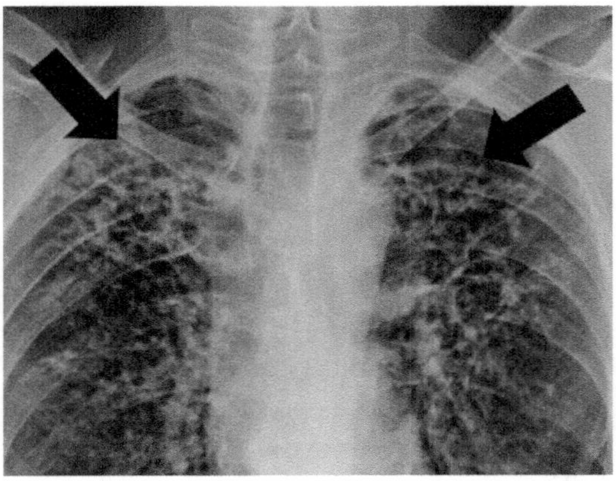

Fig. 5.19 Post-tubercular fibrosis (arrows) causing traction bronchiectasis in both upper lobes. The traction bronchiectasis could be tubular or varicoid in shape and is non-tapering

ing on the bronchus, a broncholith or an endobronchial mass lesion. Look at the adjoining areas carefully for other abnormalities such as fibrosis, mass lesion, calcification and pleural pathology. The dilated bronchus may appear opaque due to the accumulation of inspissated secretions which might appear hyperdense in a CT scan. A finger-in-glove opacity in the upper lobes can also be due to an underlying fungal infection causing bronchiectasis. Allergic bronchopulmonary aspergillosis results in opaque tubu-

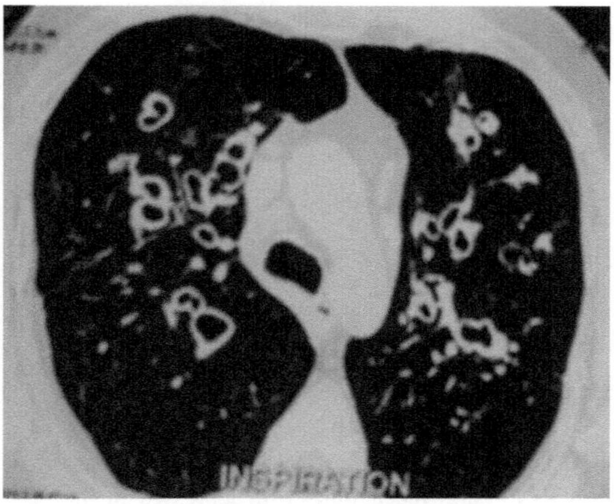

Fig. 5.20 CT scan of the chest showing thick-walled bronchiectatic cavities having saccular and tubular shapes

lar shadows, predominantly in the upper lobes and central lung fields, migrating from one segment to the other at various times.

- **Emphysema:** This is diffuse air space disease. There is destruction of the parenchyma, compensatory overexpansion of remaining air spaces and thickening and luminal narrowing of the small airways. It is an obstructive pulmonary disease with a loss of elasticity. Air can enter but may not easily find an exit. The loss of airspaces affects the exchange of gases. The patient therefore is likely to be out of breath in the advanced stage of the disease. The trapped air causes expansion and increase in the lung volume as well as tubular narrowing of the mediastinum, flattening and depression of the diaphragms and, in advanced cases, pulmonary artery hypertension.

Think of emphysema when the lungs are large and lucent, with sparse, stretched out thin peripheral vascular markings, with flattened or depressed diaphragms, narrow mediastinum and a bulging sternum (which is seen in the lateral chest X-ray) (Figs. 5.21 and 5.22).

Findings of emphysema are usually extensive in chronic smokers and even in patients with subacute hypersensitivity pneumonia. Large air spaces are called "bulla (which are air spaces without visible walls) or emphysematous cavities (air spaces with a thin visi-

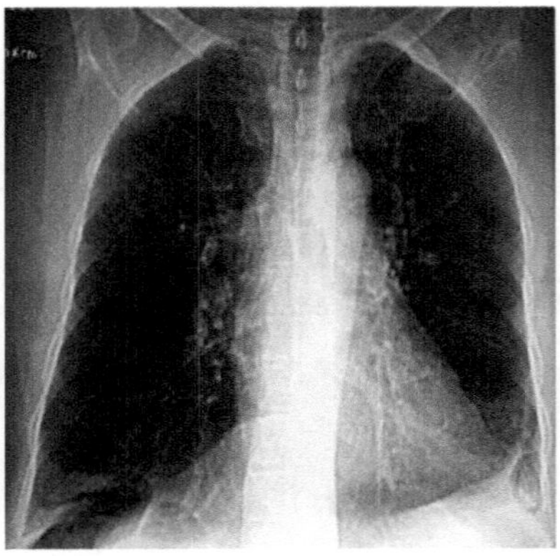

Fig. 5.21 Large lucent lungs with depressed diaphragms, consistent with overinflation secondary to emphysema

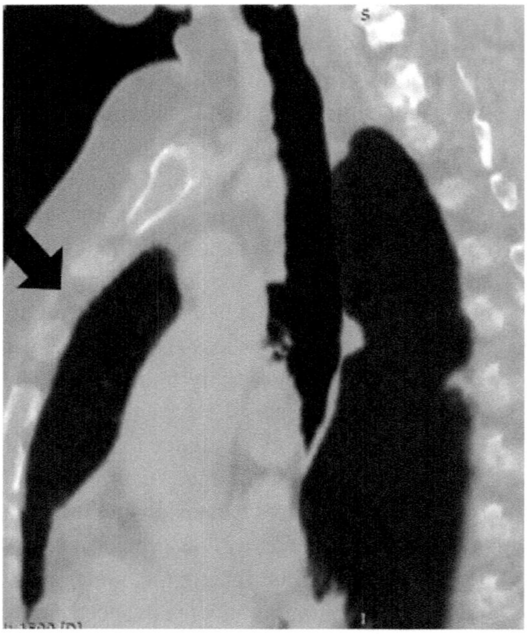

Fig. 5.22 Sagittal section of a CT scan showing a bulging sternum with increased retrosternal translucency (arrow) caused by retrosternal herniation of overinflated lung lobe

ble wall having variable appearance). These may be along the pleura or occupy the entire lobe. They may cause a pressure effect on the adjoining blood vessels and interstitium, displacing and compressing them. They can get infected and may show fluid levels within them. There may also be smaller air-containing lucent spaces with poorly defined or non-visualized walls with vascular shadows in their centre. These are called centrilobular emphysematous bulla. Emphysema can be associated with fibrosis and when that happens, it is called "combined pulmonary fibrosis with emphysema (CPFE)". Localized emphysema restricted to a lobe or segment, can be a sequela of a focal lesion obstructing the bronchus. In these cases, an expiratory film is helpful. The obstructed lung/lobe/segment will stand out as a lucent (dark) area, unchanged in size and outline due to trapped air within it., while the non-obstructed may show a ground-glass haze (Fig. 5.23).

- **Lung Masses** Any lesion above 3 cm in diameter is a mass. Lung masses, both benign and malignant, can present in various ways.
- Most benign masses are single, maybe completely solid, mixed or cystic and may contain fat and/or calcification. They may be avascular, hypovascular or highly vascular. They may not always be round. Vascular lesions may have a lobular or round appearance and may show an enhancement pattern with a density similar to the contrast-opacified blood vessels in different phases of a multiphase CT. Malignant lesions may be primary lung tumours or metastatic deposits. Primary tumours presenting as focal ground-glass opacities or a part solid nodule may not be visible in a chest X-ray. They may be seen in lung window setting in a low-dose CT scan using high-resolution sharp algorithm. They may also appear as soft tissue density nodules with smooth, spiculated or

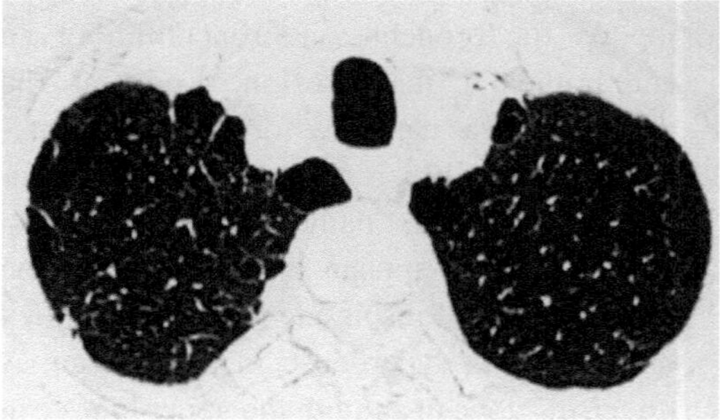

Fig. 5.23 Emphysematous bulla at the periphery of both lung fields

lobulated borders. Larger masses may have a necrotic centre thereby resembling an abscess. They can present as non-resolving consolidation, which is why a pneumonia-like shadow should be kept under observation and followed till it resolves completely. A primary lung neoplasm may exert a mass effect and cause bulging of the pleural fissures. They may involve the chest wall and diaphragm resulting in fixity to the chest wall as well as diaphragm findings, best appreciated on fluoroscopic screening. The diaphragmatic excursion may also be lost if the phrenic nerve is involved in the neck, upper chest (right phrenic nerve) or mediastinum (left phrenic nerve). The hemithorax may be completely opaque, either due to the presence of a large mass or secondary to accompanying pleural effusion opacifying the hemithorax and causing contralateral mediastinal shift. The lesion may also cause rib (Fig. 5.24) or vertebral destruction with intraspinal extension. So, scrutinize the bones thoroughly.

Primary lung cancers can sometimes be multiple—either synchronous or metachronous, that is by the timing of their appearance. They can be smooth in outline and appear as coin shadows. They are usually spiculated in outline and show strands called pleural tags which reach out to the pleural surface. If the lesion has one of these attributes, it could either be a fibrotic lesion or a lung cancer. Ask for a history of smoking, weight loss, loss of appetite, blood in sputum, chronic cough, change in voice or pain in the chest. Occasionally, the lesion may be small and hidden within the shadow of the adjoining or overlying bones. The lesion may be hilar in location and may be missed unless large. A hilar lesion may be suspected when there is distal volume loss. A careful look at all hidden and visible areas is needed to unmask the lesion. An associated large pleural effusion may obscure an underlying parenchymal tumour. Hence a PET scan is needed to detect a small mass which may be seen only due to their FDG uptake.

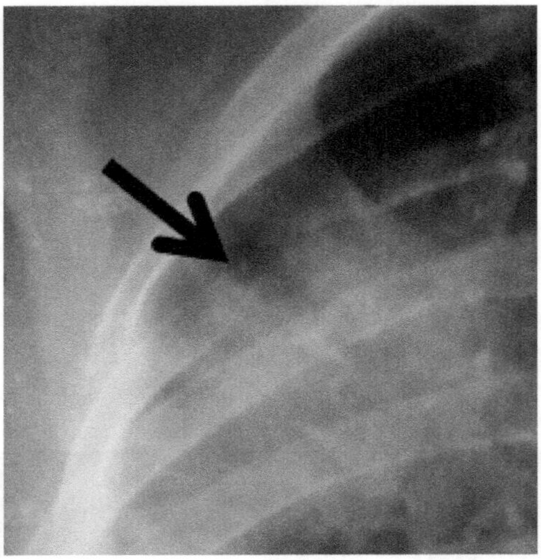

Fig. 5.24 Lung cancer presenting as a mass in the right upper lobe. Note the bone destruction (arrow). Patient gave a history of smoking for several years, recent onset of pain right upper chest, cough and occasional haemoptysis. There was no history of fever. History, therefore, is very important. Other causes of bone destruction associated with lung lesions could be actinomycosis, a fungal infection, TB or metastasis

A patient with primary lung cancer will often be a chronic smoker, although even non-smoker men and women can develop primary lung cancer. Think of lung cancer if there is a change in the appearance and size of a lesion which was also present in a previous film (hence the importance of comparing and obtaining old films!). Lung cancers are usually primary bronchogenic carcinomas, if single or metastatic deposits, if multiple. Other tumours of the lung could be primary lymphomas or undifferentiated lung tumours.

Metastatic deposits are usually well circumscribed, located peripherally and can be of varying sizes ranging from miliary shadows to cannon ball-sized lesions.

- **Pulmonary Nodules:** A pulmonary nodule is an opacity having either soft tissue or calcific density and measuring less than 3 cm in maximum diameter. Smaller nodules, 1–3 mm in size are called miliary nodules. Nodules larger than 3 cm are called masses. Miliary nodules are very fine and sometimes hard to see if not carefully looked for. They fill the lucent air-space between the rib shadows. The lung parenchyma looks hazy when filled with miliary nodules with indistinct vascular markings. Miliary nodules are randomly distributed in the lung field. They may be associated with mediastinal or hilar lymph nodes and pleural effusion. They may also be associated with hypodense nodules in the liver and spleen. The aetiology of miliary nodules is non-specific but is most often due to pulmonary tuberculosis. Slightly larger and denser nodules can be seen in conditions such as pneumoconiosis, sarcoidosis, silicosis, fungal infection and metastatic deposits. Larger nodules, especially if located in the periphery of the lungs suggestive of deposits, collagen vascular diseases and septic emboli. Solitary nodules could be both benign, (such as hamartomas, granulomas, fungal lesions (Fig. 5.25), nocardiosis) or malignant—both primary (Fig. 5.26) and secondary deposits. Nodules with cavitation could be fungal, tubercular, malignancies, granulomatosis with polyangiitis and atypical infective lesions.

- **Interstitial Lung Disease (ILD):** The pulmonary interstitium is the framework of fibro collagenous tissue (Fig. 5.27). It is the latticework which encloses and supports air spaces, vessels and central bronchi (Fig. 5.28). This network is composed of connective tissue, lymphatics and bronchovascular structures. The interstitium also exists in the membranes outlining the alveolar spaces and adjoining pulmonary capillary endothelium. The histological components of this interstitium are collagen, elastin and mucopolysaccharides which form a gelatinous strand. The interstitium can be divided into three zones, axial (peribronchovascular), parenchymal and peripheral (subpleural). Normally, it is very fine and unless thickened, may be difficult to appreciate in a chest X-ray. It may be visible in the lung apices or bases in a high-resolution CT scan of the chest, particularly in older patients or whenever there is interstitial lung involvement due to any cause. Interstitial lung diseases are predominantly in the periphery of the lung fields, called the lung cortex, but are also commonly seen affecting the bases, as in cases of idiopathic pulmonary fibrosis. The disease can also be predominantly central, as there is plenty of interstitial tissue along the bronchovascular structures. There are several

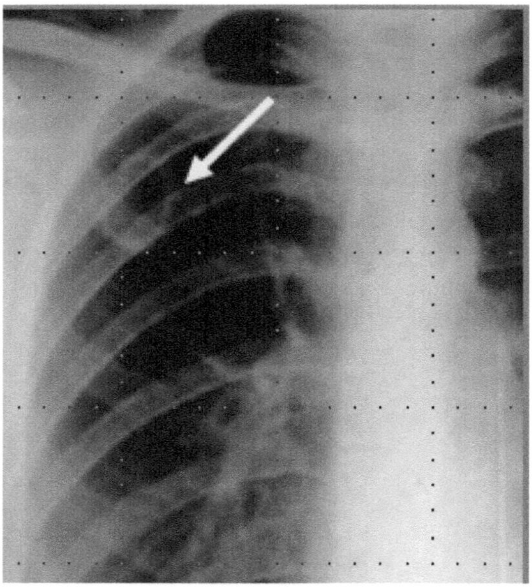

Fig. 5.25 A case of chronic coccidioidomycosis presenting as a thin-walled cavitating nodule

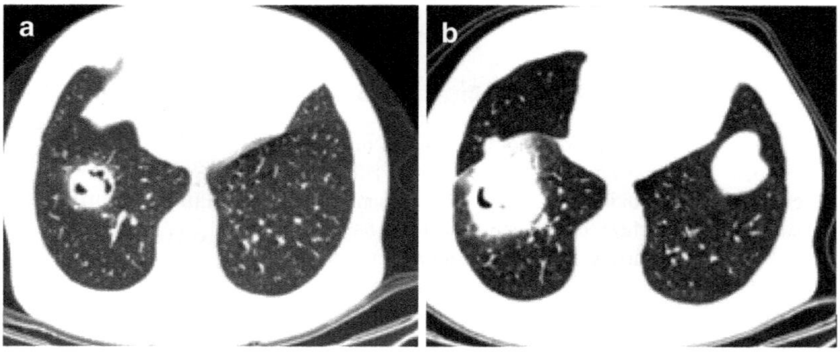

Fig. 5.26 (**a, b**) Scans of a 59-year male smoker taken 3 months apart. Figure (**a**) shows a cavitating lesion in the right lower lobe (**a**). (**b**) Shows an increase in the size of the lesion within 4 months

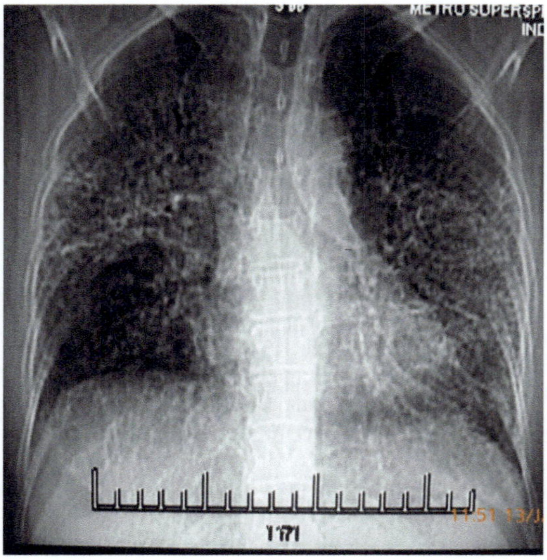

Fig. 5.27 Chest X-ray shows diffuse interstitial thickening

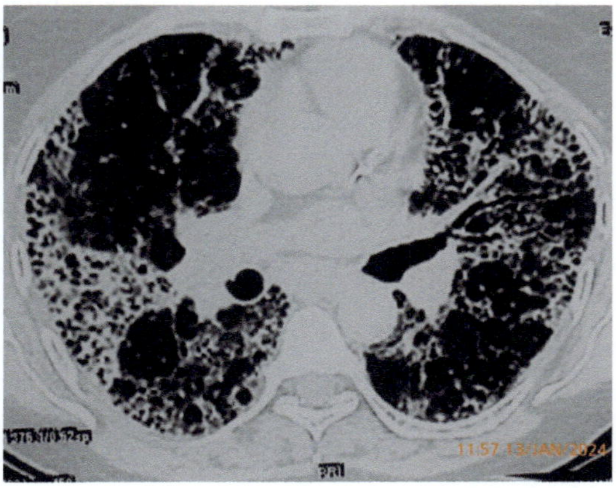

Fig. 5.28 HRCT chest of a case of diffuse interstitial lung disease

central diseases which affect the bronchovascular interstitium. These include sarcoidosis, chronic hypersensitivity pneumonia, lymphangitis carcinomatosa and connective tissue disorders. In many fibrotic interstitial lung diseases, the subpleural or peribronchovascular interstitium is involved. The peripheral pleura and fissures appear thick, distorted and sometimes nodular. The bronchovascular outline appears thick and spiculated. Diffuse interstitial thickening also reduces lung volume and blurs the outlines of the diaphragmatic and mediastinal pleura. When these findings are seen, think of interstitial lung disease. Also, whenever there is interstitial involvement, search for other abnormalities, such as dilated main pulmonary artery (suggestive of pulmonary artery hypertension), lymphadenopathy (could be a case of sarcoidosis), pleuro-pericardial involvement (connective tissue disorder, oesophageal dilatation (progressive systemic sclerosis), bony abnormality or any other systemic disorder. Hilar and mediastinal nodes can also be seen in lymphangitis carcinomatosis, silicosis and sometimes as a reactive phenomenon due to the associated lung disease. While most interstitial lung diseases lead to loss of volume, a few of them are associated with an increase in lung volume. These include Langerhans cell histiocytosis, lymphangioleiomyomatosis and combined fibrosis with pulmonary emphysema.

- **Langerhans Histiocytosis** predominantly involves upper zones and the patients are young smokers. Small nodules turning later on into bizarre-shaped cysts are noted in this condition. They are scattered all over the lung, but less common in the bases and costophrenic angle area.
- **Tuberous Sclerosis:** These are thin-walled uniform-sized cysts. Other clinical features including kidney lesions such as angiomyolipoma, skin, bone and brain involvement may be seen.
- **Lymphangioleiomyomatosis:** It almost exclusively affects females of childbearing age and results in the development of cysts which are few to numerous. The intervening parenchyma is normal. All regions of the lung, except the peripheral lung parenchyma near the CP angle and mediastinum [11] may be involved in the disease process.
- **Neurofibromatosis:** Typically involves lower zones.

Quite clearly, there are many ways in which diseases of the chest can manifest themselves. The observations often overlap and the final diagnosis may not be easy or possible to arrive at, simply by looking at the images. The chest X-ray may give clues but many times, it is the CT scan which is more helpful in not only detecting abnormalities but also in suggesting a differential diagnosis. Taking a step further, a CT scan also helps in safely performing interventional procedures such as biopsies and chest tube placement.

References

1. Garg M, Prabhakar N, Gulati A, Agarwal R, Dhooria S. Spectrum of imaging findings in pulmonary infections. Part 1: bacterial and viral. Pol J Radiol. 2019;84:e205–13. https://doi.org/10.5114/pjr.2019.85812.
2. Ueda T, Andreas C, Itami J, Miyakawa K, Fujimoto H, Ito H, Justus E. Roos pyothorax-associated lymphoma: imaging findings. Am J Roentgenol. 2010;194(1):76–84.
3. Wetscherek MTA, Sadler TJ, Lee JYJ, et al. Active pulmonary tuberculosis: something old, something new, something borrowed, something blue. Insights Imaging. 2022;13:3. https://doi.org/10.1186/s13244-021-01138-8.
4. Bhalla AS, Goyal A, Guleria R, Gupta AK. Chest tuberculosis: radiological review and imaging recommendations. Indian J Radiol Imaging. 2015;25(3):213–25. https://doi.org/10.4103/0971-3026.161431.
5. Lewis RE, Stanzani M, Morana G, Sassi C. Radiology-based diagnosis of fungal pulmonary infections in high-risk hematology patients: are we making progress? Curr Opin Infect Dis. 2023;36(4):250–6. https://doi.org/10.1097/QCO.0000000000000937.
6. Orlowski HLP, McWilliams S, Mellnick VM, Bhalla S, Lubner MG, Pickhardt PJ, Christine O. Menias imaging spectrum of invasive fungal and fungal-like infections. RadioGraphics. 2017;37(4):1119–34.
7. Semin Chong A, Lee KS, Yi CA, Chung MJ, Kima TS, Han J. Review pulmonary fungal infection: imaging findings in immunocompetent and immunocompromised patients. Eur J Radiol. 2006;59:371–83.
8. Hassan M, Asciak R, Rizk R, et al. Lung abscess or empyema? Taking a closer look. Thorax. 2018;73:887–9.
9. Stark DD, et al. Differentiation lung abscesss from empyema. https://ajronline.org/doi/pdf/10.2214/ajr.141.1.163?download=true.
10. Williford ME, Godwin JD. Computed tomography of lung abscess and empyema. Radiol Clin North Am. 1983;21(3):575–83. https://doi.org/10.1016/S0033-8389(22)01106-X.
11. Weerakkody Y, Kogan J, Silverstone L, et al. Lymphangioleiomyomatosis. Radiopaedia.org. https://doi.org/10.53347/rID-7334.

Pleural Pathology

6

Abstract

The lung parenchyma is encased by visceral and parietal pleura, which are normally not visible unless diseased. The pleura often gets involved in various diseases which usually take the form of fluid, air in the pleural cavity, mass lesions or calcification. Pleural pathology can cause respiratory distress, pain, fever and symptoms, depending upon the nature of the pathology. In this chapter, we will look at various manifestations of pleural diseases.

Keywords

Pleura · Effusion · Pneumothorax · Masses · Pleural calcification

The pleura is often an overlooked aspect of the chest unless affected by disease.

In this chapter, we will go through some common radiological findings found in various pleural diseases.

- **Pleural Thickening and Calcification:** The normal parietal and visceral pleura, surrounding the lung parenchyma, is not visible by any imaging modality, be it an X-ray, a CT scan of the chest or an MRI. This is because it is very thin, measuring between 0.2 and 0.4 mm [1] and perpendicular to the X-ray beam. It can, however, be seen between the lung lobes as a fissural line. Once the pleura thickens (Fig. 6.1) or calcifies, it becomes visible. It also manifests itself as an opacity in the event of fluid/mass/air being present between its layers.

  The extrapleural space is a potential space where fat, fluid or a mass arising from outside the pleura can accumulate. This may produce a "pseudo-pleural pathology" appearance.

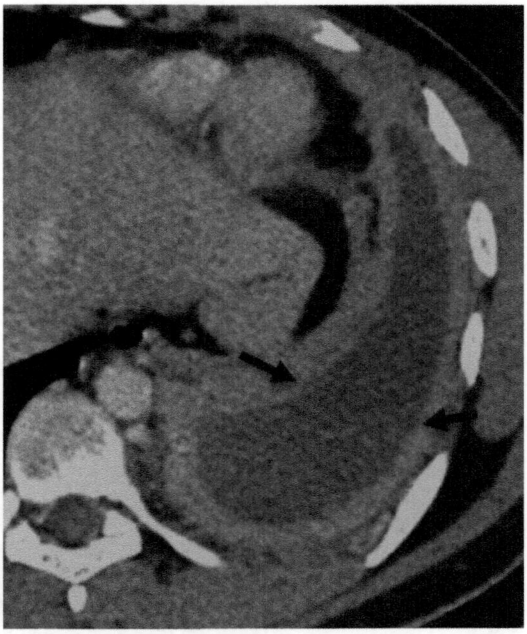

Fig. 6.1 CT scan of a case of exudative pleural effusion showing pleural thickening. The thickened visceral and parietal pleura (arrows) are separated by the pleural fluid, producing the "split pleura sign"

R. Gothi, *Radiographic and Imaging Techniques for Radiology Residents and Technologists*,
https://doi.org/10.1007/978-981-96-4816-0_6

Pleural thickening may be focal or diffuse. It can be seen along the lateral chest wall, over the lung apices, along the diaphragm, mediastinum or in the fissures. The entire hemithorax may be affected by pleural pathology. The hemithorax may show a reduction in volume as compared to the opposite side because of fibrosis or collapse of the enclosed lung. The diaphragm may be pulled upwards and appear tented. The ribs may come together and look crowded. Apical pleural thickening, if asymmetric with a difference of more than 5 mm, is suspicious for a mass and needs CT evaluation. A thickened pleura may occasionally calcify. This can happen in chronic infections such as tuberculosis or asbestosis. An increase in pleural thickening over time is a finding which needs further evaluation. A tumour of the pleura such as a mesothelioma, a lymphoma or a metastatic deposit may have developed, resulting in the gradually increasing pleural thickening. The pleural outline, in these cases, may be lobulated. Multiple lobulated shadows along the pleural surface could either be due to multiple pleural fluid loculations, multiple extrapleural fluid collections or nodules as in neurofibromatosis, or due to metastatic deposits. Solitary lobular mass can be due to a benign pleural pathology called a "solitary fibrous tumour of the pleura". Interstitial lung diseases can cause asymmetric pleural retraction with fatty infiltration from the chest wall into the extrapleural space.

- **Pleural Fluid Collection:** Pleural fluid collection can be visualized in a chest X-ray, USG chest, CT and MRI (Fig. 6.2).

Normally there is approximately 10–20 pleural fluid [2]. Pleural effusion is a pathological condition, resulting in the accumulation of more than normal amounts of fluid between the visceral and parietal pleura.

The quantity of fluid accumulated in the pleural space can be estimated in a chest X-ray, in a CT scan as well as in an ultrasound image of the chest. In a chest X-ray PA view, if the pleural fluid is about 200 cc, the costophrenic angle is obscured and if the volume increases to 500 ml or more, the diaphragm is obscured [3]. Similarly, there are several ways of ascertaining pleural effusion by USG [4] and CT scans [5].

In the early stages, when pleural fluid begins forming, it may go unnoticed in a chest X-ray PA view. If a lateral view is obtained, even effusions as small as 50 ml can be detected [3]. The fluid could be a transudate (low in protein), exudate (high in protein with echoes or septa seen in ultrasound) (Fig. 6.3), haemorrhagic, chylous (that is, containing chylomicrons) or frankly purulent (empyema). All pleural fluid collections look alike in a chest X-ray. Ultrasound of the chest can show internal septa, masses and small nodules

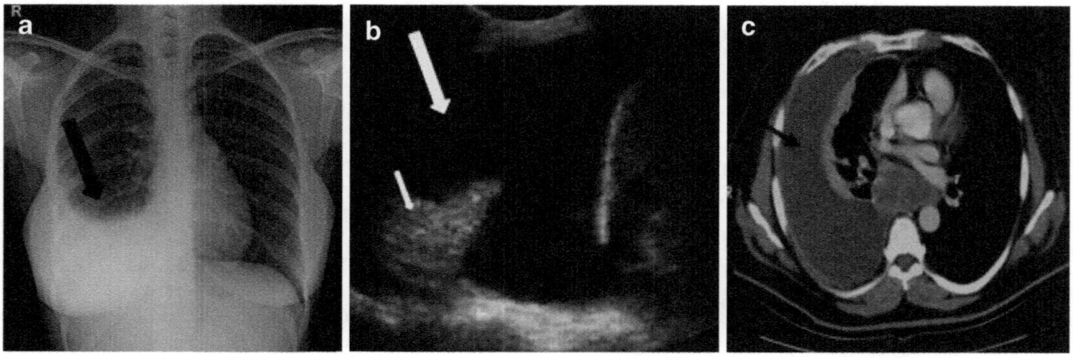

Fig. 6.2 Chest X-ray erect PA view showing a right pleural effusion, obscuring the diaphragm and producing a meniscus sign (**a**). USG chest showing pleural effusion, note the collapsed lung (small arrow). (**b**) CT scan of the chest (**c**) showing right pleural effusion (arrow)

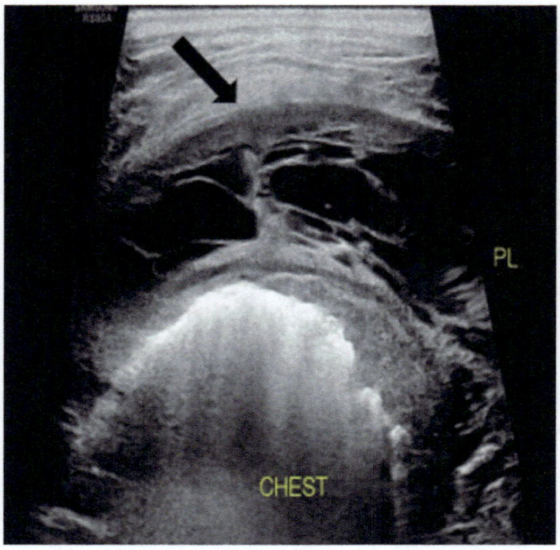

Fig. 6.3 USG chest showing exudative pleural effusion with thick septa. Note also the thickened visceral pleura (arrow)

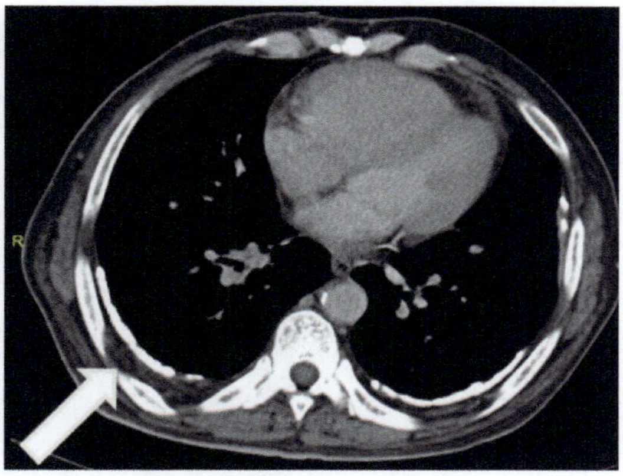

Fig. 6.4 CT scan of the chest showing pleural calcification on both sides. Note the extrapleural soft tissue (arrow). A history of exposure to asbestosis or old granulomatous pathology must be sought if pleural calcification is present

adherent to the pleural surface. An MRI of the pleura is also useful in detecting septa, nodules and masses. A non-contrast CT scan can help identify blood clots as they are denser than normal fluid, whereas a contrast-enhanced PET-CT scan may show pleural nodules and masses, not visible in a conventional CT study.

Calcification in a pleura can be identified in an X-ray chest as well as in a CT scan (Fig. 6.4).

The pleural space can be expanded either by fluid collection or a mass between the visceral and parietal pleural layers. Pleural fluid accumulates first in the deepest portion of the pleural cavity which is the posterior costophrenic sulcus (Fig. 6.5). This is the place, seen best in a lateral chest X-ray, where even a small quantity of pleural fluid, if present, will blunt the posterior costophrenic angle. The posteriorly located free fluid also obscures the posterior segment of the lower lobe which occupies this region., making it appear hazy.

The normal gray zone of the posterior segment of the lower lobe is seen below the diaphragms, extending behind the shadow of the liver, on the right side. It is better appreciated on the right side as compared to the left, as it contrasts well with the soft tissue shadow of the anteriorly located liver. When the quantity of fluid increases to 50 ml or more, the lateral costophrenic angle becomes blunted. Further increase of fluid will produce a soft tissue density shadow with a superomedial concavity (the meniscus sign). The increasing volume of fluid will increase the pressure effect on the underlying lung and compress it. If the disease becomes long-standing, the compressed lung may undergo fibrosis and scarring. It may then not be able to re-expand. When the pleural effusion is large, not only can the underlying lung collapse, but the mediastinum can also shift towards the opposite side. The diaphragmatic cupola may gradually flatten and finally invert, resulting in pushing the liver and spleen downwards and making them clinically palpable. In these situations, the best way to demonstrate diaphragmatic inversion is with a chest CT or ultrasound scan. Pleural fluid may be loculated along the chest wall and in the fissures, appearing as spindle or oval-shaped soft tissue density shadows. The outline of these loculations is sharp and taper towards their ends. Loculated effusions may get sealed off between the thickened pleural layers and persist for a long time. Recent loculations can disappear once the causative factor, especially cardiac failure, is quickly taken care of. In such cases, they are known as "vanishing tumours" of the lung.

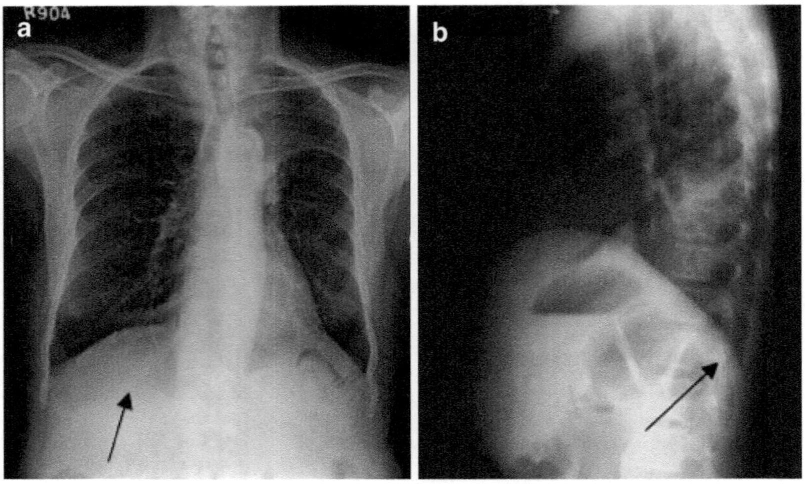

Fig. 6.5 PA view of the chest showing the posterior segment of the lower lobe, occupying the deepest part of the chest (arrow in **a**) and extending behind the soft tissue density shadow of the liver which is anterior to it. Lateral chest X-ray demonstrating the deepest part of the chest (arrow in **b**)

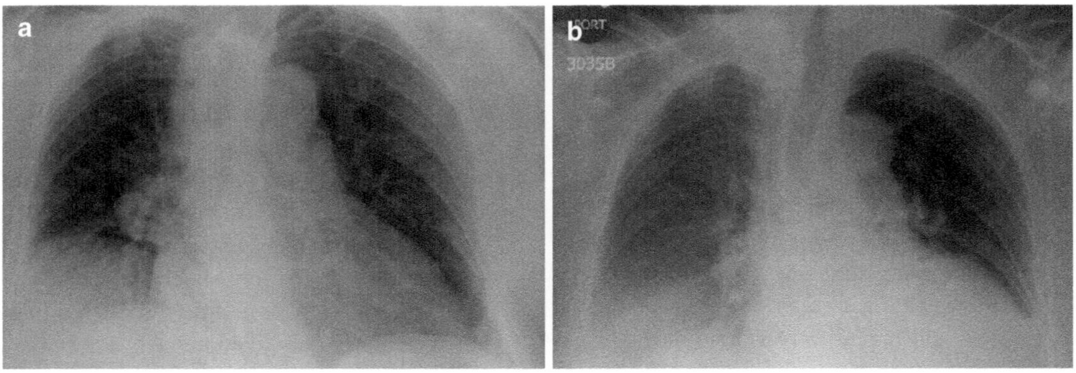

Fig. 6.6 X-ray chest in sitting (**a**) and in the supine position (**b**). Note the haziness of the right lung field in the supine X-ray. This is due to the pleural fluid forming a layer beneath the dependent posterior aspect of the lung, thereby making it appear hazy in an X-ray chest AP view

Pleural fluid collection can also be recognized in a supine AP X-ray. Free fluid spreads out into the hemithorax, surrounds the lung bases, thereby making the lung appear hazy (Fig. 6.6).

- **Pneumothorax:** The presence of air within the pleural space is called pneumothorax. It appears as a black stripe along the lateral chest wall, separating the parietal from the visceral pleura with concavity towards the lung surface. Since the normal pleura is not visible in a chest X-ray, separation of the chest wall from the lung field, by a lucent shadow having no bronchovascular markings, is suggestive of the presence of air in the pleural space. The inner margin of the pneumothorax is sharp being outlined by the visceral pleura. The outer margin is not visible as the parietal pleura merges with the soft tissues of the extrapleural space. This is known as an absent "double wall sign", which helps distinguish an encysted pneumothorax from a peripheral bulla, in which the double wall sign will be present [6]. A bulla can also be distinguished from an encysted pneumothorax by the fact that it is usually confined to a lung lobe, will have an identical shape in all views and will be convex towards the lung. An encysted pneumothorax will extend beyond the borders of the lobe which is not likely to happen with a bulla. Although there may be no vascular markings in the pneumothorax, occasionally there may be a few or many thin or thick septa which might be seen within the pneumothorax. These septa are usually found if there has been an underlying complication such as bleeding or infection. A longstanding pneumothorax can get loculated, especially if the underlying lung is pathological [7] and does not re-expand despite the presence of a chest tube for 5 days or more. Pneumothorax, when free, extends from the apex of the chest to the diaphragm. Air can also accumulate along the mediastinal pleura separating the lung from the cardiac silhouette. When it accumulates there, it may sharply delineate the superior vena cava (SVC) and azygos vein on the right and the superior intercostal vein and subclavian artery on the left. Pneumothorax can extend beneath the sternum in the supine film and when it accumulates in the anterolateral costophrenic sulcus and extends downwards towards the hypochondrium, it can produce a "deep sulcus sign" [8]. Pneumothorax can develop following a rib fracture, a ruptured emphysematous bulla, a subpleural cyst or following an interventional procedure. Rarely a pneumoperitoneum may ascend through congenital defects in the diaphragm into the pleural cavity and produce pneumothorax [9]. A pneumothorax may occasionally show a fluid level, due to accumulated serous fluid, pus or blood. A large pneumothorax can result in depression of the dome of the diaphragm and contralateral mediastinal shift. Such a pneumothorax is called "tension pneumothorax" (Fig. 6.7).

- **Hydropneumothorax:** As the name suggests, hydropneumothorax is the accumulation of air and fluid in the pleural space (Fig. 6.8). This can happen due to reasons, such as after pleural tapping, following chest wall trauma, or secondary to a bronchopleural fistula.
- **Pleural Thickening:** The pleura can be thickened due to chronic granulomatous and non-granulomatous infections, asbestos exposure and both benign as well as malignant tumours. Pleural thickening can be appreciated in a chest X-ray especially if accompanied by a blunted costophrenic angle. It appears as a soft tissue space between the ribs and lung parenchyma (Fig. 6.9).

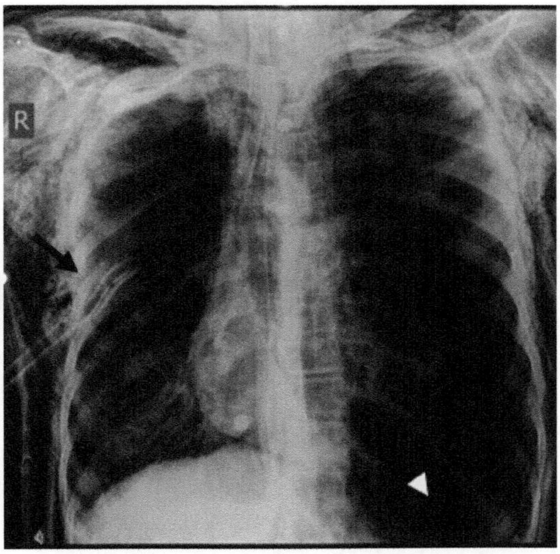

Fig. 6.7 Left-sided tension pneumothorax (arrowhead), obscuring the lung markings, shifting the mediastinum to the right and inverting the left diaphragm. Note the chest tube on the right side (arrow), inserted for evacuating the right pneumothorax, along with the presence of subcutaneous emphysema

Besides USG, both CT scan (Fig. 6.10) and MRI can show pleural thickening and pleural-based masses. Administered intravenous contrast may show enhancement in both acute inflammation of the pleura and pleural-based masses in a CT scan. These acute or subacute pathologies may also show avid FDG uptake in a PET scan.

Chest ultrasound (Fig. 6.11) can show a thickened pleura as well as the contents, such as nodules, masses and septa encased by the thickened pleura.

While a chest X-ray may show effusion or extrapulmonary mass, because of the similar density of thickened pleura, pleural effusion and pleural-based or extrapleural mass in a chest X-ray, an ultrasound should be carried out as the first investigation to see the nature of the pleural-based lesion. Ultrasound beam can easily travel through fluid and hence is suited to display the composition of the pleural shadow (Fig. 6.12).

- **Pleural Masses:** These appear as soft tissue density opacities in the chest radiograph and may be mistaken for a loculated pleural effu-

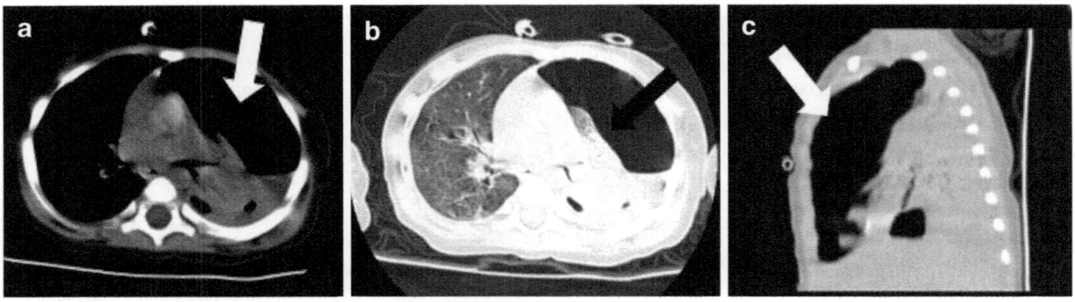

Fig. 6.8 A case of left-sided hydropneumothorax. (**a**) mediastinal window, (**b**) lung window and (**c**) parasagittal view showing pneumothorax (arrow) located beneath the anterior chest wall with collapse of the left lower lobe

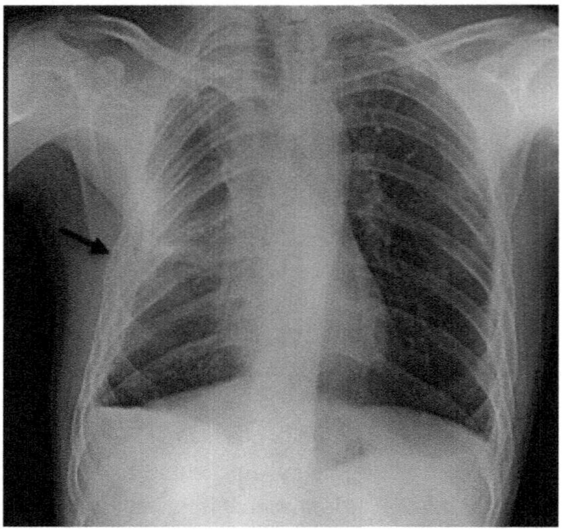

Fig. 6.9 Chest X-ray showing right-sided pleural thickening with blunted right CP angle. Note the widening of the space between the chest wall and lung caused by the thickened pleura (arrow)

sion. A tangential beam X-ray may enable localizing them to the extrapulmonary space. Extrapulmonary masses, both pleura-based and extrapleural, have an indistinct border on the side away from the lung tissue. This is because, unlike the inner border which is silhouetted by the air-containing lung parenchyma, the outer border merges with the surrounding soft tissue density. This is called the "incomplete border sign" [10]. The easiest way to quickly detect pleural masses is to do a chest USG. If the rib overlying the lesion is destroyed or the intercostal space is widened, think of the extrapulmonary extension of pleural lesion or empyema necessitans.

- **Role of PET-CT and MRI in Pleural Diseases** [11]

  Metabolically active disease involving the pleura will show increased uptake, in an FDG PET scan. Both malignant tumours and inflammatory pathologies may be PET avid. A malignant lesion may show a higher SUV (systemic uptake value) as compared to a benign pathology. Nevertheless, a PET scan is non-specific as far as determining the aetiology of a PET avid lesion goes. An important advantage of a PET scan is that it helps in guiding biopsy towards the most accessible metabolically active lesion.

  MRI (Fig. 6.13) allows excellent evaluation of the pleural space and its contents. There are various sequences as well as contrast studies which enable excellent evaluation of not only the pleura but also the adjoining bones, soft tissues and lung parenchyma. However, the images may be degraded in a breathless or unstable patient. Hence respiratory or cardiac gating may be needed to get better images. The main drawback is the cost and time factor of doing an MRI scan.

  In conclusion, the pleural space can be a source of many diseases and can be evaluated by all modalities. It is important to distinguish a pleural from a pulmonary and extrapleural lesion. The availability of ultrasound has made examination and management of most pleural lesions, especially fluid collection or pneumothorax more easy. In complex cases, a CECT, MRI and even a PET scan may be needed.

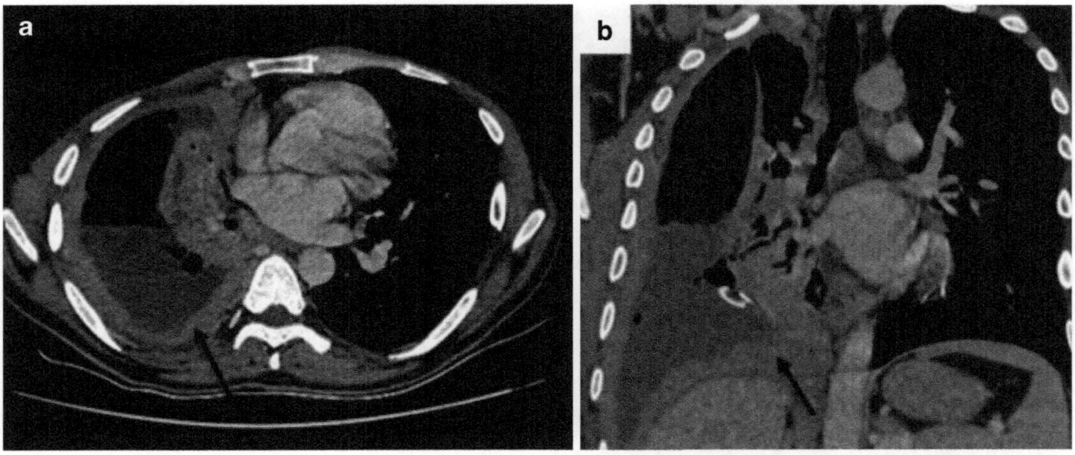

Fig. 6.10 Axial (**a**) and coronal sections (**b**) of a case demonstrating right-sided pleural thickening with hydropneumothorax. It was caused by the diffuse spread of pleural-based metastasis

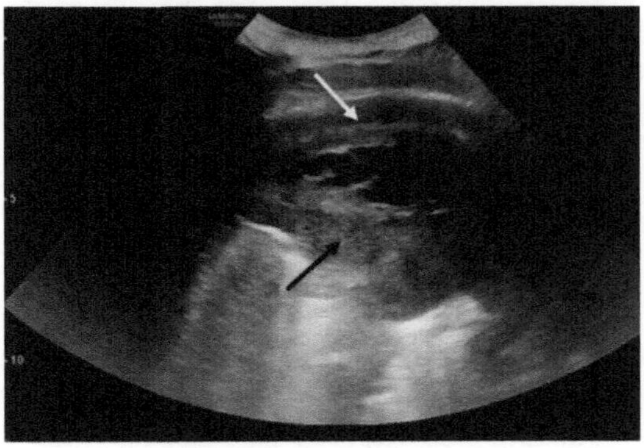

Fig. 6.11 USG of the chest. Note pleural thickening (arrows) with effusion with septa in the pleural fluid

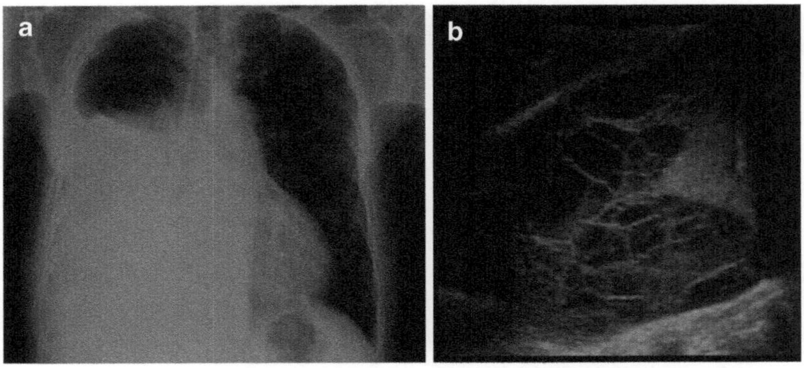

Fig. 6.12 A case of right-sided pleural effusion. Note that the X-ray chest (**a**) does not reveal anything other than opaque right lower thorax. It is the meniscus along the chest wall, which tells us that it is fluid. However, nothing else can be made out of this opacity. Ultrasound of the same case (**b**) shows septated contents within the pleural cavity

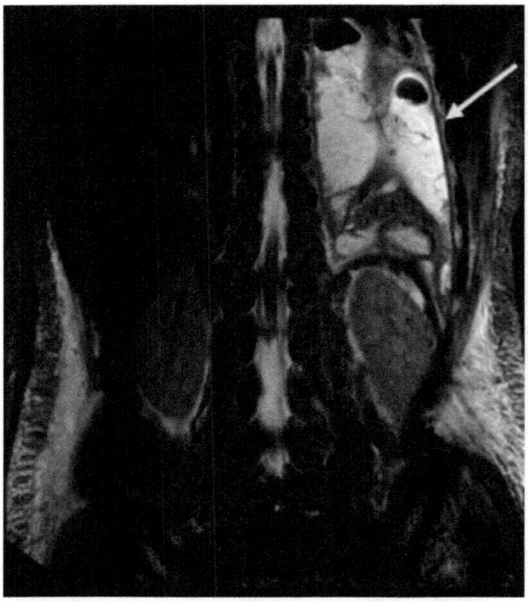

Fig. 6.13 MRI chest showing left pleural effusion with air bubbles and septa within the pleural fluid collection (arrow)

References

1. Sureka B, Thukral BB, Mittal MK, Mittal A, Sinha M. Radiological review of pleural tumors. Indian J Radiol Imaging. 2013;23:313–20.
2. D'Agostino HP, Edens MA. Physiology, pleural fluid. [Updated 2023 Aug 28]. In: StatPearls. Treasure Island, FL: StatPearls Publishing; 2024. https://www.ncbi.nlm.nih.gov/books/NBK513353.
3. Blackmore CC, Black WC, Dallas RV, Crow HC. Pleural fluid volume estimation: a chest radiograph prediction rule. Acad Radiol. 1996 Feb;3(2):103–9. https://doi.org/10.1016/s1076-6332(05)80373-3.
4. Ibitoye BO, Idowu BM, Ogunrombi AB, Afolabi BI. Ultrasonographic quantification of pleural effusion: comparison of four formulae. Ultrasonography. 2018;37(3):254–60.
5. Hazlinger M, Ctvrtlik F, Langova K, Herman M. Quantification of pleural effusion on CT by simple measurement. Biomed Pap Med Fac Univ Palacky Olomouc Czech Repub. 2014;158(1):107–11. https://doi.org/10.5507/bp.2012.042.
6. Nair A, Bhat R, Aggarwal P. Multi-loculated pneumothorax post COVID-19 pneumonia. Vis J Emerg Med. 2022;26:101260. https://doi.org/10.1016/j.visj.2021.101260.
7. Tufman A, Winter H, Kahnert K, Reu S, Müller-Lisse U, Hube RM. A persistent pneumothorax? 5-year follow-up after diagnosis of Swyer–James–MacLeod syndrome. Breathe. 2016;12(2):e55–E58. https://doi.org/10.1183/20734735.000316.
8. Kong A. The deep sulcus sign. Radiology. 2003;228(2):415–6.
9. Chae MS, Kwak J, Roh K, et al. Pneumoperitoneum-induced pneumothorax during laparoscopic living donor hepatectomy: a case report. BMC Surg. 2020;20:206. https://doi.org/10.1186/s12893-020-00868-8.
10. Hsu CC-T, Henry TS, Chung JH, Little BP. The incomplete border sign. J Thoracic Imaging. 2014;29(4):W48. https://doi.org/10.1097/RTI.0000000000000088.
11. Hallifax RJ, Talwar A, Wrightson JM, Edey A, Gleeson FV. State-of-the-art: radiological investigation of pleural disease. Respir Med. 2017;124:88–99. https://doi.org/10.1016/j.rmed.2017.02.013.

7 Evaluation of the Heart

Abstract

The cardiac shadow is the centrepiece of a chest X-ray. While the prime position in cardiac evaluation has gone to echocardiography and angiography, the plain X-ray chest is still a very valuable tool in the evaluation of cardiac-related diseases. In this section, the cardiac shadow, both normal and abnormal, as seen in the chest X-ray, will be discussed.

Keywords

Cardiac shadow · Echocardiography

The cardiac shadow is located in the middle of the chest and lies predominantly in the middle mediastinum. Almost two-thirds of the cardiac silhouette is towards the left side of the midline while the remaining one-third extends into the right chest.

The cardiac shadow normally appears larger in a child as well as in an anteroposterior (AP) view of the chest. The shape and size of the shadow alters if there is any pathology. A heart size over 16 cm and an aorta over 3.5 cm are large. The normal cardiothoracic ratio in an X-ray chest posteroanterior (PA) view is less the 0.55 in an adult (Fig. 7.1).

It is important to ensure that the CT ratio is properly calculated to clearly define cardiomegaly. The CT ratio must be obtained during maximum inspiration, as it increases in the expiratory phase due to the elevation of the diaphragms. If a person is unable to hold breath in deep inspiration, then the CT ratio is likely to be fallacious.

The CT ratio may also be fallacious if the patient is rotated especially to the left. In an obese patient, there may be abundant epicardial fat deposited around a normal-sized heart, which can result in pseudo-enlargement of the cardiac silhouette. Therefore, it is best to say that the cardiac silhouette appears prominent, instead of reporting it as cardiomegaly, which is a disease. The finding of prominent cardiac shadow must be correlated with clinical and other relevant data. Also never forget to compare with previous X-rays, if available.

Once it is agreed that there is cardiomegaly and most likely due to a pathology, one can go further with the interpretation of various features of cardiac and extracardiac abnormalities. Pathological enlargement of the heart could be due to pericardial or cardiac pathology. We will go through some of these conditions in the subsequent sections.

Pericardium and Pericardial Diseases The normal pericardium is approximately 2 mm thick [2] and may be visible in a lateral chest X-ray as a thin line separated by fat on its either side. It can also be seen in a PA view of the chest when it is calcified or whenever there is a pneumopericardium.

R. Gothi, *Radiographic and Imaging Techniques for Radiology Residents and Technologists*,
https://doi.org/10.1007/978-981-96-4816-0_7

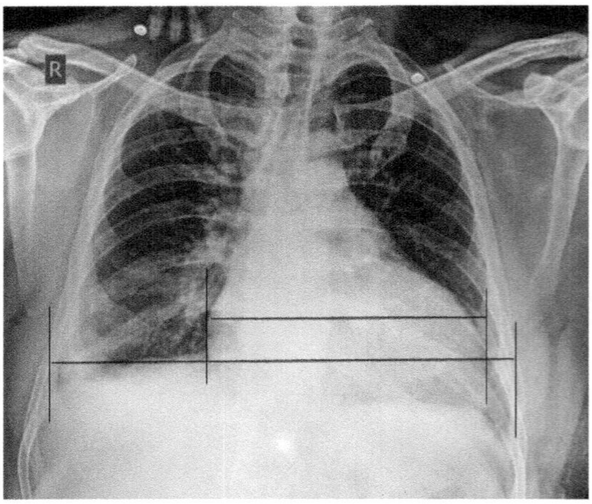

Fig. 7.1 Cardiothoracic ratio. The ratio of the distance between the right and left heart borders and the maximum width of the thoracic cage, obtained in maximum inspiration in an erect PA chest, is calculated as shown in the image above, and the CT ratio is obtained. The CT ratio does not vary significantly between different phases of the cardiac cycle [1].

Pericardial diseases include constrictive pericarditis, pericardial effusion, pericardial involvement by a systemic disease or a pericardial mass.

- **Pericardial effusion**: Normally, there is 15–50 ccs of pericardial fluid. This fluid is seen either at the base of the heart overlying the diaphragm or in pericardial recesses, which are located in the superior mediastinum where the pericardium wraps around the aorta and pulmonary artery (Fig. 7.2).

  Fluid accumulation beyond this range is suggestive of pericardial effusion. However, to be visible in a chest X-ray, it should be at least 250 ml.

  When there is pericardial effusion, the cardiac shadow enlarges and often the borders appear smooth. This is because the cardiac pulsations are unable to reach the pericardium and affects its outlines. The shape of the fluid-filled pericardium could be globular, like a hot water bottle. It may produce an "oreo-cookie sign", which is seen in the lateral chest X-ray [3] as a vertical pericardial fluid collection encased between substernal paracardial and epicardial fat. The enlarged pericardium can widen the carinal angle. Pericardial effusion may obstruct the superior vena cava (SVC) and inferior vena cava (IVC) due to increased pericardial pressure, and thereby causing dilatation of the SVC and IVC. Fluid in the pericardial cavity can be a transudate as in uremic pericarditis, and secondary to acute myocardial effusion (MI) (which is also called "Dressler syndrome"). Pericardial fluid could be a transudate as seen in cardiac failure, uremia , or hypoalbuminemic states. It could be an exudate as seen in TB of the pericardium, and haemorrhagic (hemopericardium), which is seen in malignancies or following rupture of an aortic or a coronary artery aneurysm within the pericardial cavity. The contours of the heart in pericardial effusion are smooth. The cardiac pulsations are obscured during fluoroscopic examination, as they are masked by the pericardial fluid.
- **Pericardial thickening: The** pericardium may be thickened (Fig. 7.3) in cases of constrictive pericarditis.

  The heart size may be normal or enlarged. The contour may appear normal or globular, especially in cases of associated pericardial effusion. Pericardial thickening may compress the right heart and cause a tamponade. The SVC and IVC may distend and become visible along the right heart border because of raised pericardial pressure as well as increased right heart pressure. In a chest X-ray, SVC distension will cause mediastinal widening. Obstruction of the IVC will lead to distension of the hepatic veins and hepatic venous congestion, thereby causing diffuse hepatic parenchymal enlargement. Ascites could develop in cases of chronic constrictive pericarditis. When the thickened pericardium calcifies, it becomes visible either as a localized dense shadow in the atrioventricular (AV) groove or as diffuse calcific density enveloping the heart shadow. Calcific pericarditis may be seen in cases of tubercular pericarditis. However, the calcification could also be idiopathic and sequelae to viral pericarditis [4].
- **Pericardial masses:** Pericardial masses are usually solid. They could be cystic if there is a lesion such as a hydatid cyst or a loculated exudative collection entrapped within the pericardial layers. These lesions can cause

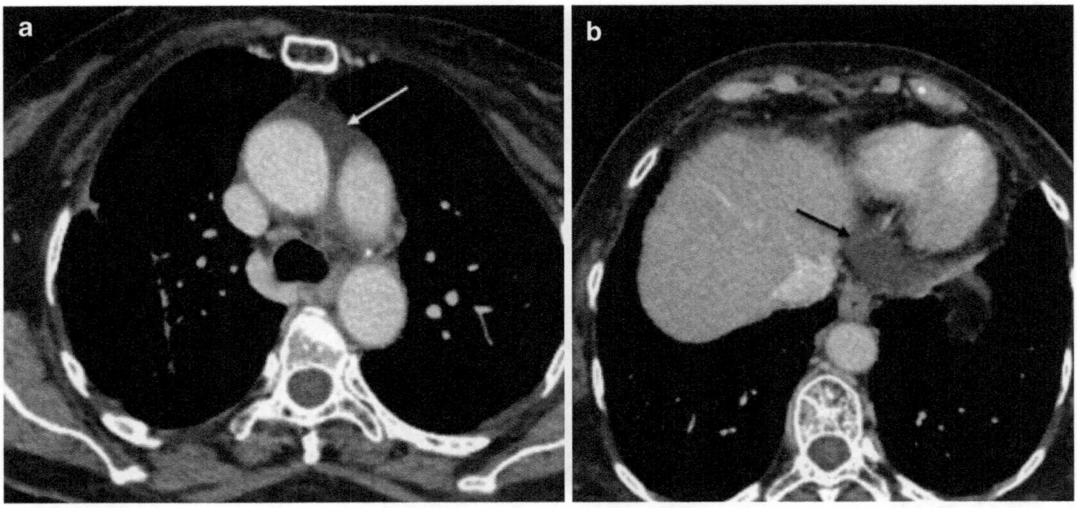

Fig. 7.2 Fluid-filled superior pericardial recess (**a**) wrapping around the aorta and main pulmonary artery (arrow). This is a normal finding. Fluid at the base (**b**) of the heart (arrow) is also a normal finding

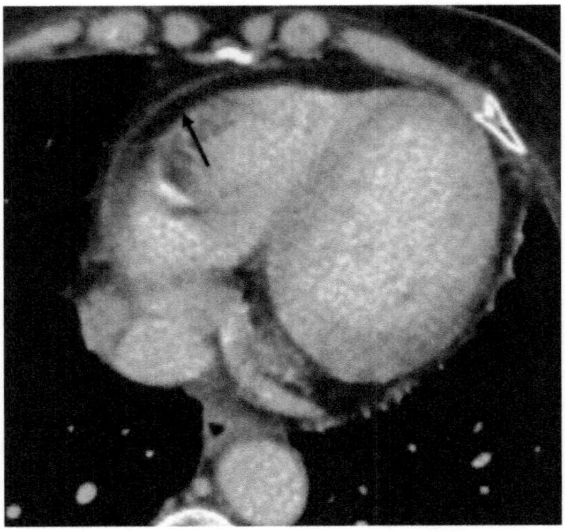

Fig. 7.3 CT scan showing thickened pericardium (arrow)

flattening or focal depressions on the cardiac contour, resulting in tamponade. Most pericardial masses resemble pericardial effusion. They may have been discovered incidentally or due to their compressive effect on the underlying cardiac chamber. Echocardiography followed by cross-sectional imaging will be needed to investigate such an abnormal bulge [5]. Masses of the pericardium could be primary pericardial tumours such as mesothelioma, haematogenous metastatic deposits from a distal primary or due to local spread of primary lung or oesophageal lesion. Both CT and MRI can be performed for further delineation of the size and composition of these masses. If the pericardium appears thick and irregular, the possibilities include a tumour, adhesions, chronic inflammation or a multisystem disease such as Erdheim–Chester disease.

- **Other pericardial disorders:** These could be congenital or post-operative pericardial defects, pericardial diverticulum, post-op pericardial fat flaps, pneumopericardium following trauma or pericardiocentesis and secondary to fistulous communication with the stomach. Focal pericardial fat necrosis and also be detected on CT scans [6].
- **Myocardial pathology:** Enlargement of the heart could be due to hypertrophy of the cardiac muscles or dilatation of the cardiac chambers. Hypertrophic cardiomyopathy or hypertrophy of the cardiac muscles is a diagnosis which cannot be made from a plain chest X-ray. On the other hand, dilatation of the cardiac chambers can be assessed from X-rays. The right atrium (RA), left atrium (LA), right ventricle (RV) and left ventricle (LV) can be figured out on a PA and a lateral view of the chest.
- **The right atrium (RA):** The RA is located behind and slightly to the right of the right ventricle (Fig. 7.4). RA enlargement may be

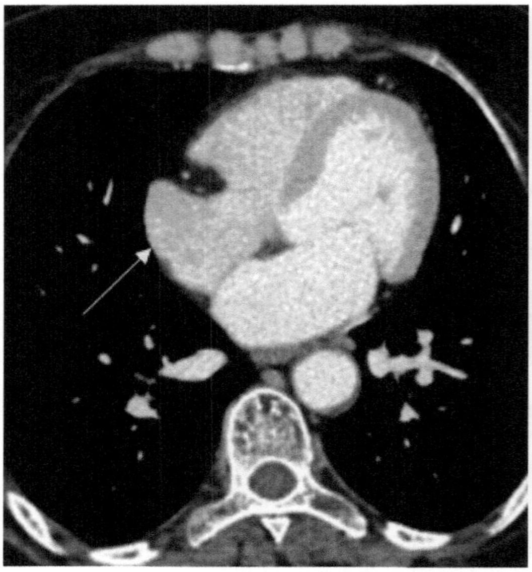

Fig. 7.4 Note the position of the right atrium (arrow) in this CT scan. It is located behind the right ventricle, and protrudes slightly more to the right

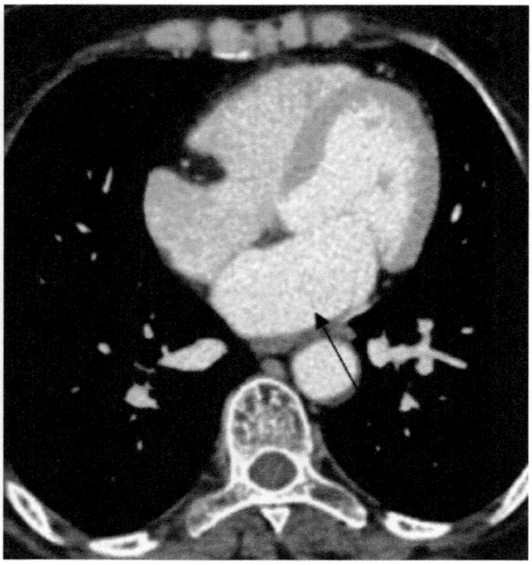

Fig. 7.5 The left atrium (arrow) is seen behind the LV, separated from the right atrium by the interatrial septum and from the left ventricle by the mitral valve

difficult to diagnose from a chest X-ray. It can be suspected if the right heart border bulges more than 5.5 cm away from the midline. The other way to suspect it is by looking at the length of the right heart border. If it is more than 50% of the length of the right cardiovascular border, it can be considered enlarged [7]. **The left atrium (LA):** The LA is located behind the left ventricle (Fig. 7.5), below the carina and in front of the oesophagus (Fig. 7.6).

LA enlargement causes a double density below the carina, the shadow of the right atrium being superimposed on it. The left atrial bulge extends more into the right chest. There is an elevation of the left main bronchus because it is much closer to LA as compared to the right main bronchus, leading to the widening of the carinal angle. Enlargement of the LA may also be associated with a protrusion of the left atrial appendage. The left atrial appendage shows a convexity along the left heart border, just below the main pulmonary artery (Fig. 7.7).

- **The right ventricle**: The RV is located anteriorly behind the sternum (Fig. 7.8). RV enlargement pushes the cardiac apex upwards in the PA view of the chest. In the lateral view, the RV touches the sternum over a length of more than 7 cm, as measured from the diaphragm.
- **The left ventricle**: The LV is located behind and towards the left of the RV. LV enlargement pushes the apex, which is formed by the LV, downwards. In the lateral view, the LV, because of its posterior location, results in the cardiac shadow overlying the spine. Enlargement of all chambers suggests either advanced cardiac failure or dilated cardiomyopathy, while enlargement of one chamber suggests either a distal obstruction or fluid overload due to regurgitation from an incompetent atrioventricular (AV) valve. Enlargement of a combination of cardiac chambers and the respective outgoing blood vessels should raise a suspicion of valvular disease, congenital heart disease, or lung-related diseases. In case of an abnormal cardiac shadow is evident, obtain an echocardiogram for a definite diagnosis.

Do not forget that the heart can also enlarge due to fluid overload. Increased blood volume due to any cause may lead to cardiomegaly. Cardiac enlargement may also be seen in anaemia and hypothyroidism.

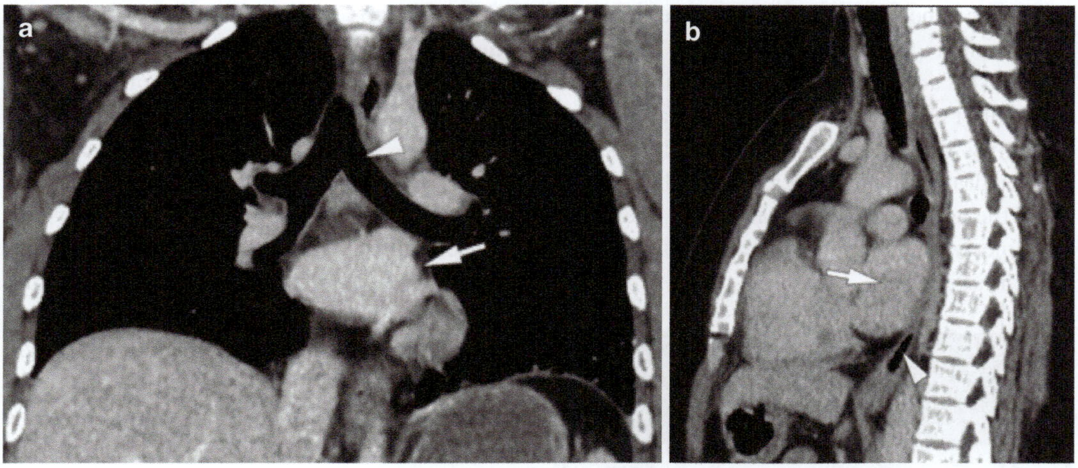

Fig. 7.6 (**a**) The LA (arrow) is seen below the carina (arrowhead). (**b**) The LA (arrow) is seen indenting the oesophagus (arrowhead)

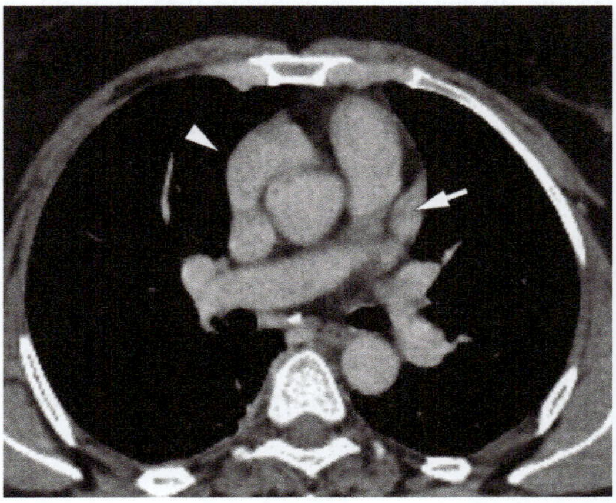

Fig. 7.7 Right atrial appendage (arrow) and left atrial appendage (arrowhead)

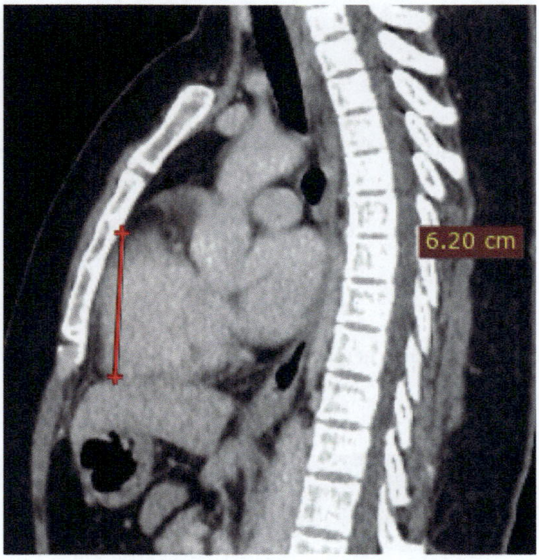

Fig. 7.8 Note the distance of the normal RV from the diaphragm to sternum. It is less than 7 cm

While looking at the heart, do not forget to look at the retrocardiac space (Fig. 7.9), the aorta, pulmonary artery and intrapulmonary vessels. Make sure the aortic knuckle is left and not right-sided. The main pulmonary artery (MPA) may enlarge in cases of pulmonary artery hypertension.

Always look out for any device related to the cardiac shadow, such as a pacemaker lead, implantable cardioverter defibrillator (ICD), any stent, a replaced mitral or aortic valve or a closure device for Atrial Septal Defect (ASD). Lookout for any complication [8] such as a broken pacemaker lead (Fig. 7.10a, b).

With many more devices coming up, such as intraaaortic balloon pumps, Extracorporeal Membrane Oxygenation (ECMO) and ventricular assist devices [8], it is important to discuss the images with the cardiologist.

Identification of Valves from a Chest X-Ray Sometimes multiple valves such as aortic and mitral valves are replaced and it becomes essential to differentiate the replaced mitral from aortic valves in a chest CT. In a PA view of the chest, draw a line from the right cardiophrenic angle to the inferior edge of the left hilum. The aortic and pulmonary valves lie to the right of this line, while the mitral and tricuspid valves lie to its left. In the lateral view, if a line is drawn from the carina to the cardiac apex, the aortic and pulmonary valves lie above this line while the tricuspid and mitral valves lie behind it [9].

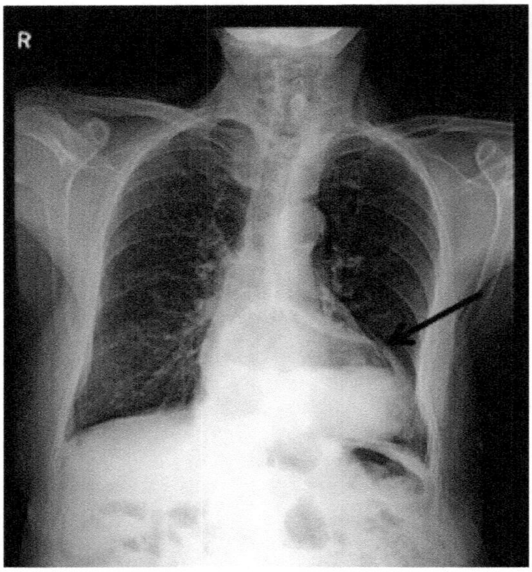

Fig. 7.9 Hiatus hernia (arrow) producing a retrocardiac density

Estimation of Cardiac Chamber Size from a Chest CT Scan When does one say that the cardiac size is enlarged? [10]. One of the easiest ways is to use the cardiothoracic ratio even in a chest CT. A single cardiac chamber enlargement can also be made by eyeballing. However, when it comes to defining the enlargement of individual cardiac chambers, there have to be some objective criteria also. A 4-chamber view of the cardiac shadow in a gated and even in a non-gated study can be used to determine the enlargement of individual cardiac chambers. In clinical practice, the difference in measurement between a gated and non-gated CT examination does not significantly change the measurements of chamber enlargement. However, in a gates study, the diameter of the cardiac chamber should be measured at end systole, to get a more accurate measurement of the diameter of a cardiac chamber.

All cardiac chambers are evaluated in the axial CT sections. Except for the LA diameter, which is anteroposterior diameter, the maximum transverse diameter is used to measure the rest of the chambers. The cardiac chambers are slightly smaller approximately 0.5 cm) in females as compared to males. An RA diameter greater than 6 cm, an RV diameter greater than 7 cm, an LA diameter greater

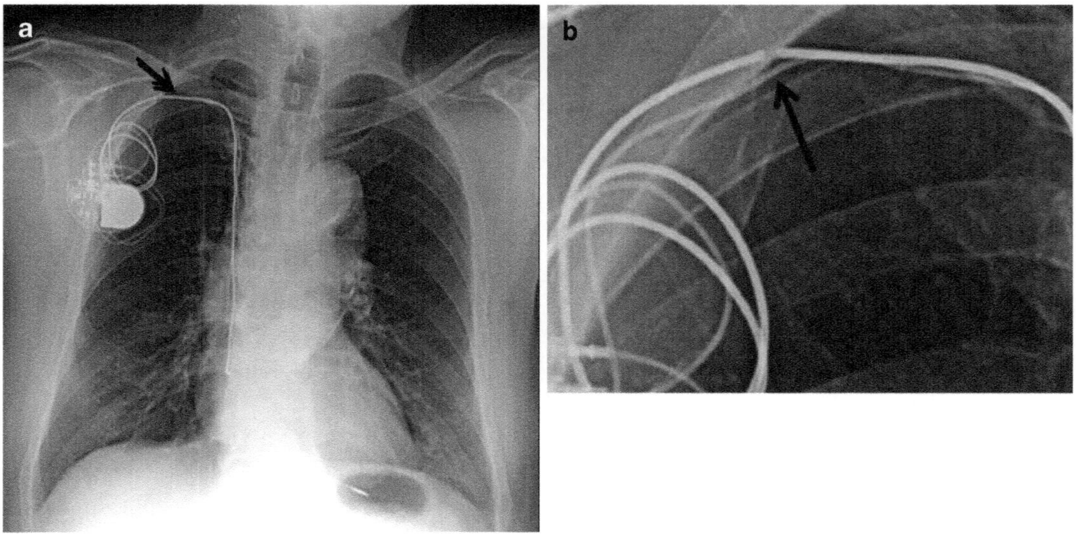

Fig. 7.10 Broken pacemaker lead suspected (**a**) (arrow). The magnified image shows the broken lead (**b**) (arrow)

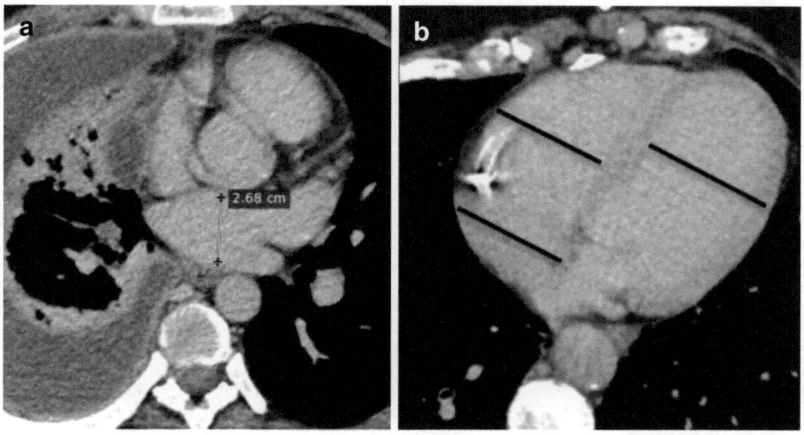

Fig. 7.11 Measurement of cardiac chambers in axial CT. (**a**) Shows the measurement of LA diameter in the AP axis and (**b**) shows the measurement of the rest of the chambers in the transverse axis

than 5 cm and an LV diameter greater than 6 cm are suggestive of enlargement in males (Fig. 7.11).

Summing up, a plain X-ray chest can provide plenty of useful information about the cardiac status. Both PA and lateral views are important, Often there can be difficulty identifying and distinguishing pericardial from cardiac diseases. In such situations, echocardiography may be used to distinguish the two. The role of CT and MRI in the evaluation of cardiac diseases is ever-increasing and, in this aspect, surpasses the value of plain films of the chest in the evaluation of cardiac diseases.

References

1. Baron MG. Radiology of the hear. Goldmans Cecil Med. 2012;1:264–71. https://doi.org/10.1016/B978-1-4377-1604-7.00053-1.
2. Munden RF, Carter BW, Chiles C, MacMahon H, Black WC, Ko JP, McAdams HP, Rossi SE, Leung AN, Boiselle PM, Kent MS, Brown K, Dyer DS, Hartman TE, Goodman EM, Naidich DP, Kazerooni EA, Berland LL, Pandharipande PV. Managing incidental findings on thoracic CT: mediastinal and cardiovascular findings. A white paper of the ACR incidental findings committee. J Am College Radiol. 2018; https://doi.org/10.1016/j.jacr.2018.04.029.
3. Li I, Greenstein J, Hahn B. Pericardial effusion with Oreo cookie sign. J Emerg Med. 2017;52(5):756–7. https://doi.org/10.1016/j.jemermed.2017.01.015.
4. Nguyen T, Phillips C, Movahed A. Incidental findings of pericardial calcification. World J Clin Cases. 2014;2(9):455–8. https://doi.org/10.12998/wjcc.v2.i9.455. PMID: 25232549; PMCID: PMC4163768.
5. Tower-Rader A, Kwon D. Pericardial masses, cysts and diverticula: a comprehensive review using multimodality imaging. Prog Cardiovasc Dis. 2017;59(4):389–97. https://doi.org/10.1016/j.pcad.2016.12.011. PMID: 28062266.
6. Ünal E, Karcaaltincaba M, Akpinar E, et al. The imaging appearances of various pericardial disorders. Insights Imaging. 2019;10:42. https://doi.org/10.1186/s13244-019-0728-4.
7. Tatco V. Right atrial enlargement on chest radiography (illustration): case study. Radiopaedia.org. https://doi.org/10.53347/rID-46377.
8. Mathew RP, Alexander T, Patel V, Low G. Chest radiographs of cardiac devices (part 1): cardiovascular implantable electronic devices, cardiac valve prostheses and Amplatzer occluder devices. SA J Radiol. 2019;23(1):1730. https://doi.org/10.4102/sajr.v23i1.1730.
9. Saxena P, Bhan A, Sharma RK, Mehta Y. Which valve is which? Ann Card Anaesth. 2015;18(4):587–8. https://doi.org/10.4103/0971-9784.166477.
10. Hota P, Simpson S. Going beyond cardiomegaly: evaluation of cardiac chamber enlargement at non–electrocardiographically gated multidetector CT: current techniques, limitations, and clinical implications. Radiol Cardiothorac Imaging. 2019;1(1):e180024.

The Intrathoracic Vasculature 8

Abstract

The major vessels in the chest are located in the mediastinum from where their branches traverse into the right and left hemithorax, upper limbs, neck and head. These vessels include the thoracic aorta and its branches, the main pulmonary artery, its right and left subdivisions, the azygos and hemiazygos veins, and the superior and inferior vena cava. The thoracic duct is small and difficult to see in a chest X-ray It can be seen in a CT scan of the chest (Liu et al., AJR Am J Roentgenol 187(6):1615–20, 2006). It lies close to the oesophagus in the thorax and behind the left common carotid artery at the level of the thoracic inlet.

Keywords

Aorta · Main pulmonary artery · Azygos vein · Thoracic duct

The major vessels arising from and related to the cardiac silhouette include the aorta and pulmonary artery. Smaller structures, such as the thoracic duct, are not seen in the chest X-ray [1].

In this chapter, we will look at the various structures present in the mediastinum.

8.1 The Thoracic Aorta

This is one of the most important mediastinal structures (Fig. 8.1). It belongs to the visceral compartment as per the International Thymic Management Interest Group (ITMIG) classification [2] and comprises the aortic root, the ascending aorta, the arch and the descending aorta.

The aortic root (Fig. 8.1) consists of (a) the aortic annulus (which is the ring-like ventricular-aortic junction), (b) the aortic valves, which have three leaflets or cusps, (c) the valve attachments, (d) the interleaflet triangles, (e) the right and left coronary ostia, (f) sinus of Valsalva and (g) the Sinotubular junction [3].

The aortic annulus or ring is ovoid-shaped and forms the site of insertion of the aortic valves.

Being normally a tricuspid valve, the valves or cusps are called the right, left and non-coronary cusps. The cusps form the floor of the sinus of Valsalva. The coronary arteries arise from the respective sinus of Valsalva, the right ostio being anteriorly positioned and the left posterior and towards the left. The purpose of the sinus of Valsalva is to prevent the coronary artery ostia from being closed during the systolic contraction of the left ventricle (Fig. 8.2).

The aortic root fuses with the tubular segment of the ascending aorta at the sinotubular junction

R. Gothi, *Radiographic and Imaging Techniques for Radiology Residents and Technologists*,
https://doi.org/10.1007/978-981-96-4816-0_8

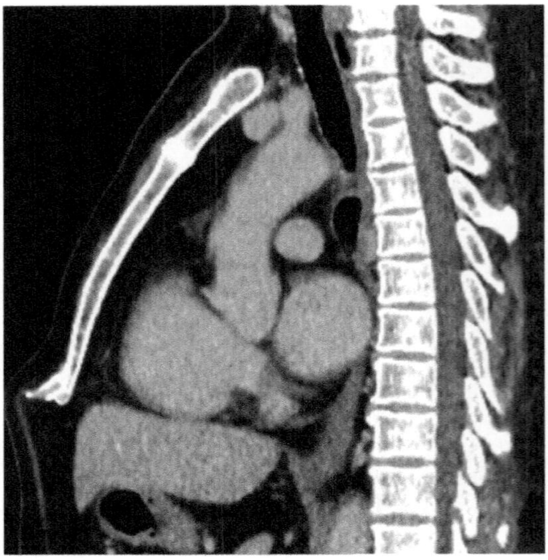

Fig. 8.1 Position of the aorta in the visceral space of the mediastinum

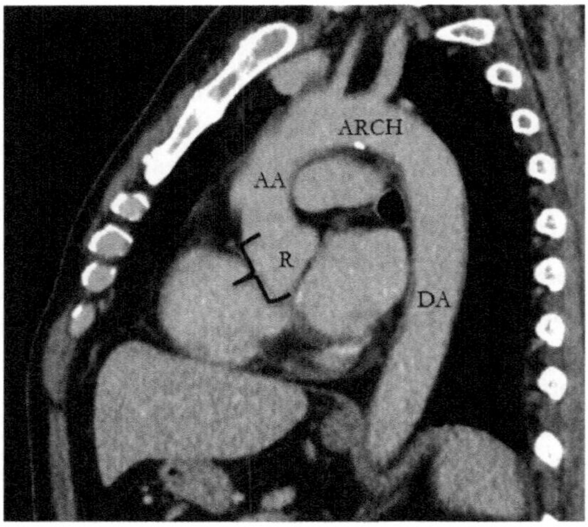

Fig. 8.2 The aortic root (R), ascending (AA), arch (ARCH) and descending aorta (DA) are seen in this contrast enhanced CT image

(Fig. 8.3). From here, it ascends anteriorly and to the right of the cardiac chambers, then turns posterior and towards the left, forming the aorta arch. The arch gives out the major vessels, the right brachiocephalic, the left common carotid and the left subclavian arteries and then continues posteriorly and leftwards to form the aortic knuckle. The aortic knuckle is that segment of the aortic arch, which is directed towards the left paraspinal region. It is seen as a round structure normally

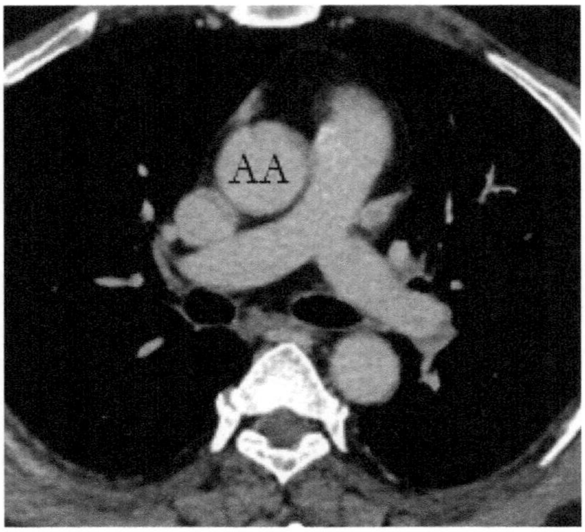

Fig. 8.3 The ascending aorta is located between the SVC and the main pulmonary artery. The descending aorta is located to the left of the vertebral bodies, and as mentioned above, behind the cardiac silhouette, in the posterior mediastinum

located to the left of the tracheal column, though sometimes, as a variation, it may be seen on the right side of the trachea. The normal aortic knuckle is under 3.5 cm in maximum diameter. The aortic knuckle continues as the descending thoracic aorta, which is located behind the cardiac shadow in the posterior mediastinum (Fig. 8.3). The descending aorta gives out intercostal arteries, which travel along the inferior margins of the ribs to supply the ribs and chest wall. It also gives rise to bronchial arteries. These commonly arise below the aortic knuckle but can arise ectopically from the ascending aorta, arch and branches of the aorta. The normally arising bronchial arteries enter the lung parenchyma through the hila. Their normal calibre is under 2 mm [4]. On enlarging, they are responsible for the rib notching as seen in cases of coarctation of the aorta. Enlarged bronchial arteries are often a cause of haemoptysis.

Aortic anomalies which can be appreciated on plain X-rays include (a) enlargement of the aortic dimension due to atherosclerosis, aortic aneurysms and aortic regurgitation, (b) aortic wall calcification, (c) abnormal position of the aortic arch, and (d) focal reduction in aortic diameter due to coarctation. A CT scan of the thorax with intravenous (IV) contrast can also show diffuse wall thickening due to inflammatory diseases of the aorta.

8.2 The Pulmonary Artery

The main pulmonary artery (MPA) (Fig. 8.4) is located along the left heart border below the aortic knuckle. It appears as a slight bulge, which may not be evident in every case.

However, in patients with pulmonary hypertension or chronic fibrotic lung diseases, the calibre may increase beyond the threshold of 3.0 cms.

The MPA gives out the right and left pulmonary arteries. These arteries are large and form the bulk of the pulmonary hilum. The pulmonary arteries normally do not show any calcification in their walls. This could be due to the high-pressure jets of blood flowing through them. When calcification is seen in the pulmonary arteries, think of a chronic thrombus or aneurysm. The right and left pulmonary arteries are normally smaller in calibre as compared to the main pulmonary artery. They may enlarge in cases of pulmonary artery hypertension, especially primary pulmonary hypertension, in right heart diseases, tumours of the pulmonary artery and acute pulmonary artery thrombosis. They branch into upper and lower lobe subdivisions and gradually taper towards the periphery. They can be traced up to within 5 mm of the lung periphery. The arterial branches are more prominent in the lower lobes as compared to the upper. Non-visualization of the peripheral pulmonary artery branches could be due to oligemia as in cyanotic congenital heart diseases (right to left shunt), lung pathology (small airway disease, emphysema), cysts or tumours. An embolus can also result in a distal vessel cut-off. In cases of pulmonary thromboembolism, occlusion of the central pulmonary artery may make the periphery of the lung appear lucent, due to diminished distal blood flow. The periphery may also show triangular area of opacities due to infarction. Enlargement of the proximal arteries indicates increased flow, increased peripheral resistance or thrombosis. Increased flow will enable visualization of arterial branches, as nodular shadows There will also be increased visibility of the vessels to the lung periphery. These features are usually seen in conditions causing hyperdynamic flow such as in cases of left to right shunts and are called as pulmonary plethora.

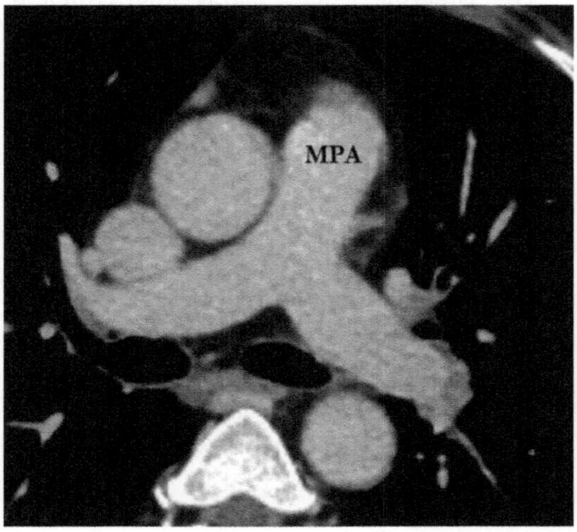

Fig. 8.4 The main pulmonary artery (MPA) lies to the left of the ascending aorta and is slightly smaller in width as compared to it

8.3 The Pulmonary Veins

The pulmonary veins have a variable anatomy [5]. They are normally visible in the lung bases and hilar regions in the standing position. The upper lobes veins can be seen if the X-ray has been taken in supine position. These veins drain into the left atrium (Fig. 8.5). Draining anywhere else is abnormal. The upper lobe pulmonary veins are smaller in calibre as compared to the lower lobe veins. When the upper and lower lobe veins are similar in size or the upper lobe veins look large, especially in a sitting or stand-

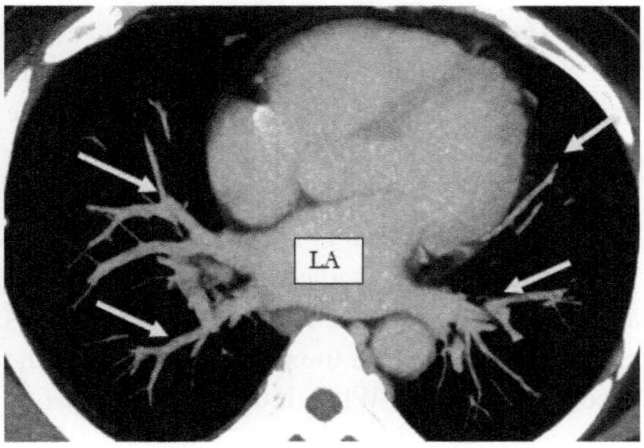

Fig. 8.5 The right and left pulmonary veins (arrow) are seen draining into the left atrium (LA)

ing X-ray chest, then think of a pathology which is directly or indirectly obstructing the pulmonary venous outflow. These conditions could be mitral valvular disease, left heart failure, a hilar mass or a stenotic lesion obstructing the venous outflow.

8.4 The Intercostal Arteries

These are not seen in a chest X-ray but can be seen in a CT aortic angiogram, especially when enlarged. The enlarged intercostal arteries can cause rib notching by their pulsatile action. Rib notching is commonly seen in coarctation of the aorta or severe aortic stenosis caused by a bicuspid aortic valve (remember, we discussed that the normal aortic valve is tricuspid!).

- Bronchial arteries are also not seen in a chest X-ray. They are seen in a CT aortogram, as small tortuous vessels arising normally from the descending aorta and traversing through the hila to reach the lungs. In cases of chronic pulmonary artery thrombosis/absence of pulmonary artery/hypoplasia or aplasia, the bronchial arteries form alternate pathways to supply blood to the lung parenchyma, beyond the occluded artery. Bronchial arteries can also dilate in diseases such as bronchiectasis and cause haemoptysis.

8.5 The Azygos and Hemiazygos Veins

The azygos and hemiazygos veins are located in the posterior mediastinum on either side of the descending thoracic aorta. The hemiazygos vein is located to the left of the aorta and crosses over the dorsal spine to drain into the azygos vein [6]. The azygos vein is cradled between the trachea and the right main bronchus. From here, it arches anteriorly to open into the posterior aspect of the superior vena cava. When it engorges, either due to superior or inferior vena cava obstruction, or cardiac decompensation, it manifests as a rounded shadow above the right main pulmonary artery (Fig. 8.6). It can also be seen in the upper zone of the right chest if there is an azygos lobe fissure. In these cases, it is seen as a comma-shaped structure in the fissure above the right hilum.

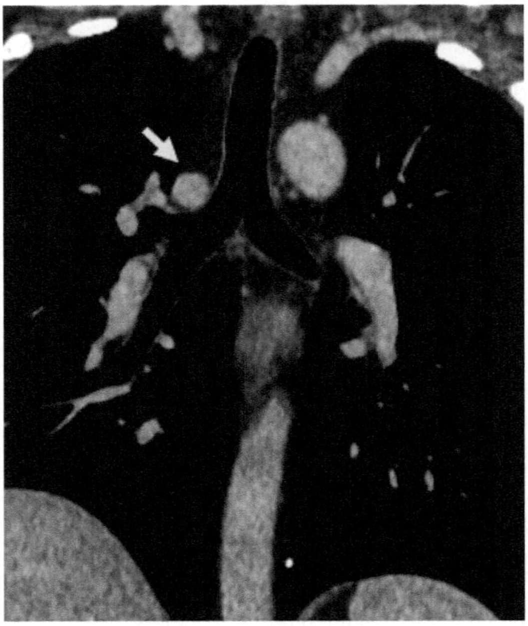

Fig. 8.6 Azygos vein (arrow) located between the right main bronchus and trachea

The superior vena cava is approximately 7 cm long and 2.1 cm wide [7]. It can be seen in the middle mediastinum (visceral space), located to the right of the aorta (Fig. 8.7) and extending from the thoracic inlet to the posterior aspect of the right atrium. It is often difficult to visualize in the chest X-ray as it may merge with the soft tissue density of the rest of the mediastinal structures. However, when it is distended or pushed outwards by the ascending aorta, it's outer wall can be seen as a linear shadow bordering the mediastinum to the right. The inferior vena cava is also difficult to see in the X-ray because it of its short intrathoracic course (Fig. 8.8).

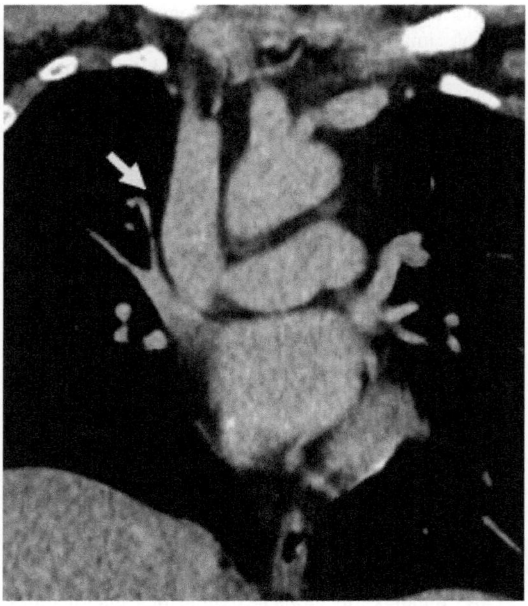

Fig. 8.7 SVC (arrow) located to the right of the aorta

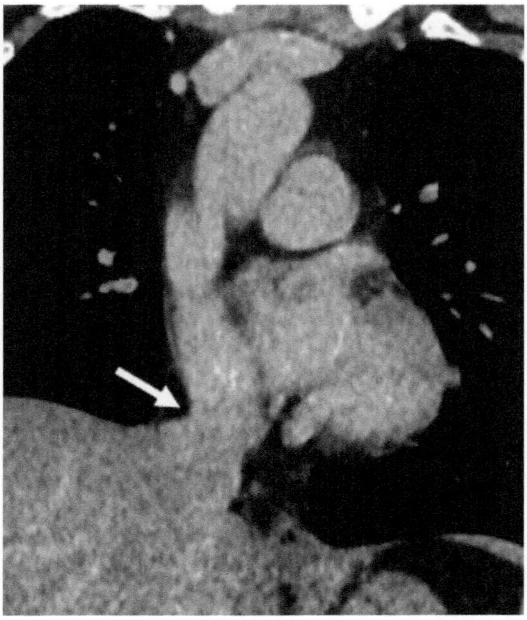

Fig. 8.8 The IVC (arrow) opening into the right atrium

8.6 Intrapulmonary Lymphatics

Normal intraparenchymal lymph nodes are usually not seen in the chest X-ray. They can sometimes be seen as sub centimetre round to ovoid structures in the lung fields in a chest X-ray . They can be seen a small nodules in the mediastinum in a CT scan. They can enlarge due to several reasons. These include infections, tumours, reaction to a chest infection and fluid overload caused by obstructing cardiac diseases such as mitral stenosis. They can be seen in diseases such as sarcoidosis, tuberculosis, histoplasmosis and malignancies, which affect lymph nodes. When the nodes are diseased, especially in malignancies, they are unable to drain the lymphatic fluid. The lymph therefore accumulates downstream within the lymphatics which distends either smoothly or if infiltrated by the disease process,irregularly. In all these cases, lymphatics can be seen within the perihilar peribronchialor in the parenchymal interstitium. Dilated lymphatics can also be seen in the lung periphery, perpendicular to the pleura, as septal thickening (Kerley B lines).

- **The thoracic duct**: The thoracic duct can be seen in 70% of patients in a CT scan of the chest. However, it may not be seen in its entirety [8]. The cisterna chyli can be seen as a tubular fluid-filled structure, located in the retrocrural space, at the T12 level, adjoining the aorta. The thoracic duct can also be imaged by a technique called "bipedal lymphangiography" in which an oil-based contrast is injected into the webs of the toes, using a thin needle and pressure injector. This is followed by early and delayed X-rays to delineate lymphatics in the early phase and nodal phase in the delayed study. This technique is now obsolete. Presently non-contrast MR using heavy T2 W sequences, CT/MR lymphangiography with contrast injection into the inguinal nodes are the methods that are considered acceptable procedures for lymphangiography.

In conclusion, a knowledge of the intrathoracic vascular system is essential for correct interpretation of findings, which might be related to them.

References

1. Liu M, Iv BFB, Whetstone J, Escott EJ. Normal CT appearance of the distal thoracic duct. AJR Am J Roentgenol. 2006;187(6):1615–20. https://doi.org/10.2214/AJR.05.1173.
2. Carter BW, Benveniste MF, Madan R, Godoy MC, de Groot PM, Truong MT, Rosado-de-Christenson ML, Marom EM. ITMIG classification of mediastinal compartments and multidisciplinary approach to mediastinal masses. Radiographics. 2017;37(2):413–36. https://doi.org/10.1148/rg.2017160095.
3. Charitos EI, Sievers H. Anatomy of the aortic root: implications for valve-sparing surgery. Ann Cardiothorac Surg. 2013;2(14):53–6. https://doi.org/10.3978/j.issn.2225-319X.2012.11.18.
4. Almeida J, Leal C, Figueiredo L. Evaluation of the bronchial arteries: normal findings, hypertrophy and embolization in patients with hemoptysis. Insights Imaging. 2020;11:70. https://doi.org/10.1186/s13244-020-00877-4.
5. Hassani C, Saremi F. Comprehensive cross-sectional imaging of the pulmonary veins. RadioGraphics. 2017;37(7):1928–54.
6. Piciucchi S, Barone D, Sanna S, Dubini A, Goodman LR, Oboldi D, Bertocco M, Ciccotosto C, Gavelli G, Carloni A, Poletti V. The azygos vein pathway: an overview from anatomical variations to pathological changes. Insights Imaging. 2014;5(5):619–28. https://doi.org/10.1007/s13244-014-0351-3.
7. Milner DM, Satinder P, Kamel A, Aal A. Comprehensive imaging review of the superior vena cava. Radiographics. 2015;35(7):1873–92.
8. Sun JD, Shum T, Behzadi F, Mark M. Hammer imaging findings of thoracic lymphatic abnormalities. Radiographics. 2022;42(5):1265–82.

9 The Mediastinum and Its Normal Structures

Abstract

The mediastinum has been divided into compartments based on organs which reside there. This division is still useful but was more prevalent when only X-rays were available. The advent of CT scans has not only reinforced the well-known anatomical divisions but upgraded the description based on the information gleaned from the CT images. In this chapter, we will look into the mediastinum and combine information acquired both from X-rays and CT scans.

Keywords

Mediastinum · Classification of mediastinum · X-rays of mediastinum · CT of mediastinal structures

The most well-known and widely recognized classification of the mediastinum was described by Benjamin Felson [1]. In this classification, using the lateral view of the chest, two lines are drawn, one along the posterior cardiac border and the other, 1 cm behind the anterior border of the dorsal vertebral bodies (Figs. 9.1 and 9.2). The soft tissues anterior to the line passing behind the cardia shadow and great vessels fall in the anterior mediastinum. The space between this line behind the heart and the line, 1 cm behind the anterior margins of the vertebral bodies, is the middle mediastinum. The soft tissues behind the vertebral line are inside the posterior mediastinum.

Recently, the International Thymic Malignancy Interest Group (ITMIG) [2] has introduced another way of dividing the mediastinum (Fig. 9.3a–c). By this method, the mediastinum is divided into a prevascular compartment, which contains the thymus, nodes, brachiocephalic vein and soft tissue in front of the great vessels and cardiac shadow. The middle compartment, also called the visceral compartment, contains the cardiac shadow, great vessels, trachea, oesophagus and nodes. The posterior boundary of the visceral compartment is a vertical line drawn 1 cm behind the anterior vertebral border. Behind this line, is the paravertebral space. Its posterior limit is formed by a line drawn along the anterior surface of the transverse processes of the dorsal vertebral bodies.

Let us now look at the various structures residing in the mediastinum.

R. Gothi, *Radiographic and Imaging Techniques for Radiology Residents and Technologists*,
https://doi.org/10.1007/978-981-96-4816-0_9

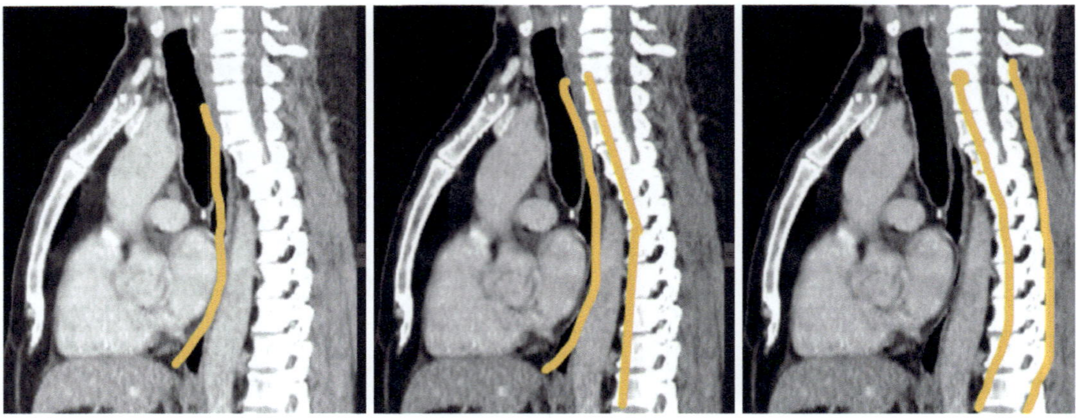

Fig. 9.1 Sagittal CT scan of the chest showing mediastinal division using Felson's method

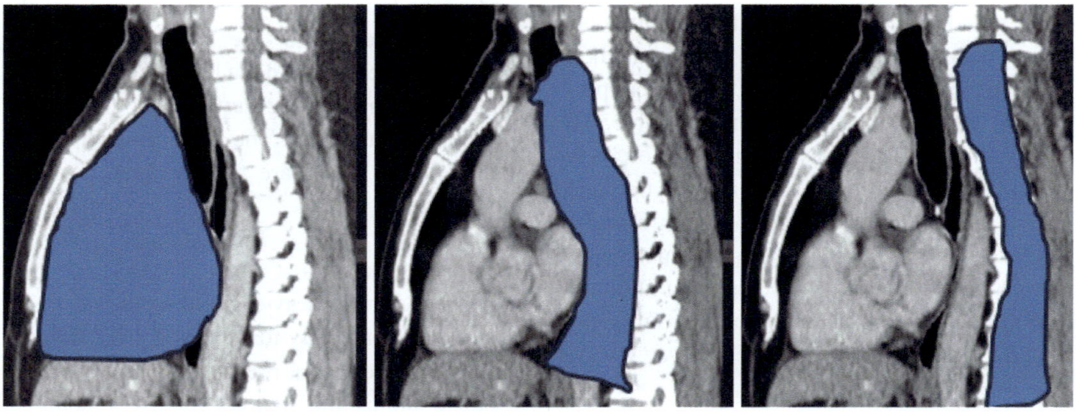

Fig. 9.2 Felson's classification of mediastinum using two lines, one behind the posterior heart border and the other approximately 1 cm behind the anterior vertebral margin

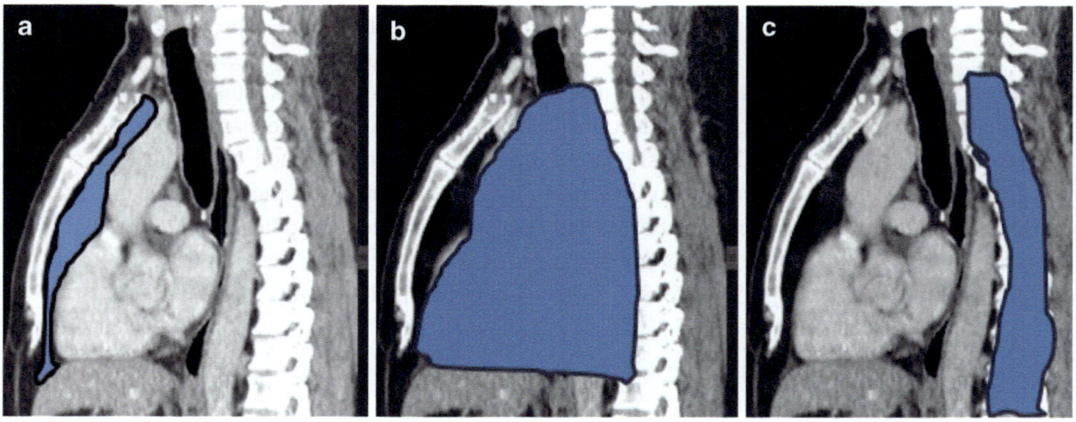

Fig. 9.3 (**a–c**) ITMIG model of mediastinal classification: prevascular space (**a**), visceral space (**b**), and paravertebral compartment (**c**)

9.1 Trachea and Bronchus

The trachea and both main bronchi reside in the visceral space of the mediastinum (Fig. 9.4). By using a high kV technique and increasing penetration [3], the trachea and bronchi are much better visualized as compared to the X-ray obtained using normal technical factors. This technique, used particularly for adults, also reduces the radiation exposure [4]. The kV is kept around 120–140 as compared to the normally used 60–70 kV. With the recent wide availability of selenium-based flat panel detectors in digital radiography, nearly the same results as with the high kV technique can be obtained along with reduction in radiation dose by adjusting the exposure factors [5].

The trachea begins in the neck at the level of the inferior surface of the cricoid cartilage and terminates in the thorax at the level of the carina (located at the T4 level). It may normally show a slight deviation to the right. It is uniform in calibre, with up to 3 mm thin wall [6]. It has 18–22 cartilaginous rings [6] surrounding the anterolateral walls (Fig. 9.5). The posterior tracheal wall does not have cartilage and is made of an inner layer comprising of tracheal membrane [6] and an outer layer formed by the trachealis muscle. The cartilaginous rings prevent the trachea from collapsing completely during expiration. The posterior membrane by ballooning outwards during inspiration, provides room for the distension of the tracheal lumen. During expiration, it is sucked inwards towards the tracheal lumen.

The trachea is indented on its left side by the aortic knuckle. If this indentation is missing, consider the possibility of a right sided aorta. The right main bronchus is relatively longer and enters the thorax below and behind the right main pulmonary artery. The left pulmonary artery is located above the left main bronchus. Hence the shadow of the left hilum, which is formed by the pulmonary artery is at a higher level as compared to the right hilar shadow. The right upper lobe bronchus is above and anterior to the right main

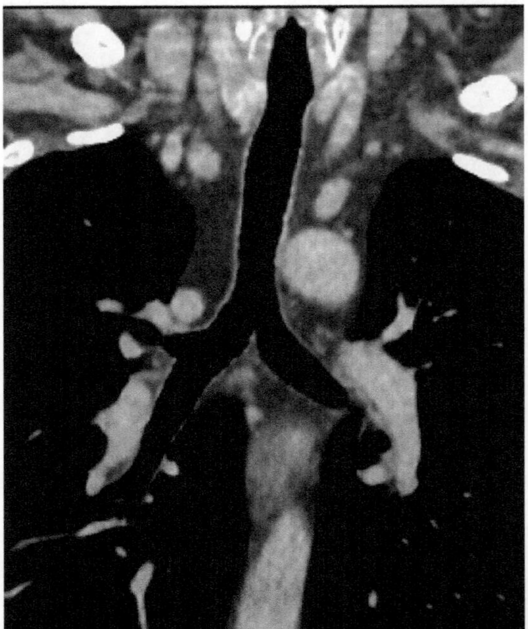

Fig. 9.4 CT scan showing trachea and both main bronchi. Note the thin walls of the trachea and the position of the two pulmonary arteries. The right pulmonary artery is located below the right main bronchus. The left pulmonary artery is above the left main bronchus

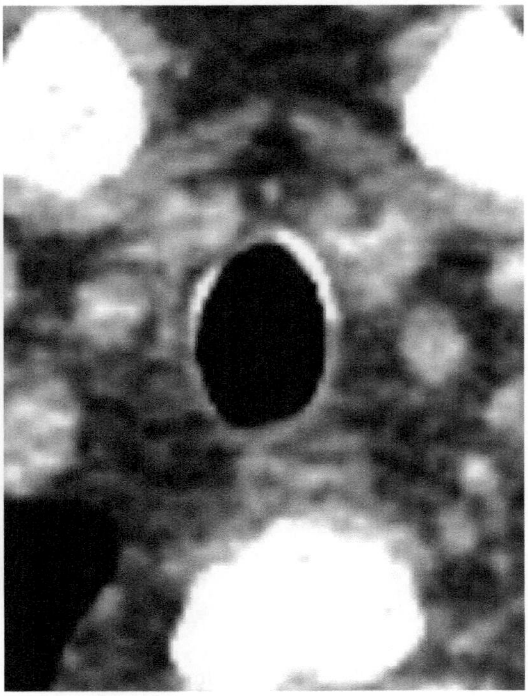

Fig. 9.5 Note the presence of partially calcified anterior and lateral walls of the trachea

pulmonary artery and is called the eparterial bronchus, while the left upper lobe bronchus is located below the left pulmonary artery and is called the hyparterial bronchus. The angle formed by the right and left main bronchus is called the carinal angle, which is normally less than 70°.

Both tracheal and bronchial walls are evident in X-rays and CT scans. Normally the bronchi and pulmonary arteries are nearly the same in size. Whenever there is a significant discrepancy in the sizes of the bronchus and pulmonary arteries, think of a pathology affecting either of the structures.

Look carefully into the air-filled tracheobronchial column for any filling defect or narrowing. Look for bronchial occlusion whenever the lung, a lobe, or a segment appears hyperinflated, shrunken, hyperlucent or opaque. In smokers, the trachea may appear narrow and slit-like. This appearance is called "sabre-shaped" trachea (Fig. 9.6) and is suggestive of softening of the tracheal rings secondary to chronic obstructive airways disease.

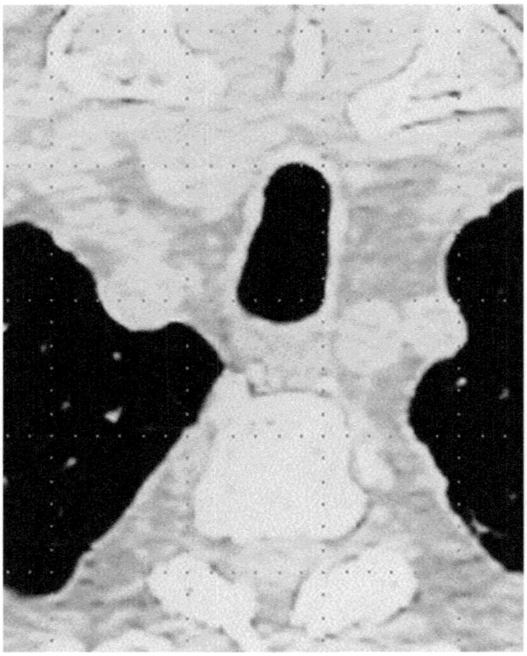

Fig. 9.6 The trachea is flattened from side to side. This appearance is suggestive of sabre-sheath trachea, and is often seen in patients of chronic obstructive pulmonary disease (COPD)

In tracheobronchomalacia (Fig. 9.7), tracheal lumen is reduced below 50% of normal appears slit like.

Widening of the trachea may be seen in patients on prolonged mechanical ventilation (Fig. 9.8) or in patients having bronchial asthma or diffuse fibrosing lung disease (Fig. 9.9).

Widening of both trachea and bronchi is called tracheo-bronchomegaly and may be seen in Mounier Kuhn syndrome.

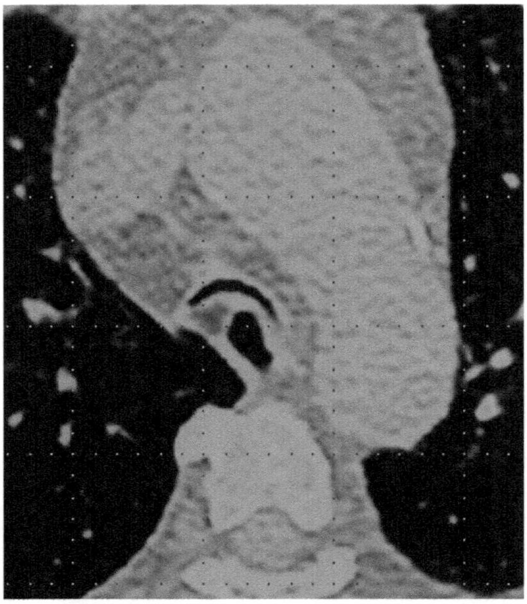

Fig. 9.7 CT scan showing a crescentic slit like trachea with a narrow lumen, suggestive of tracheomalacia

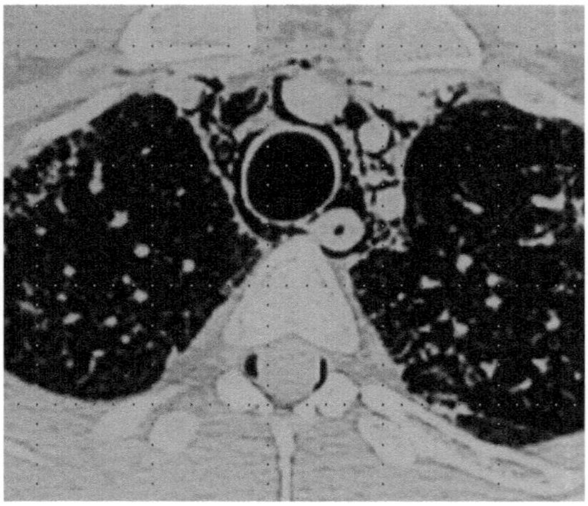

Fig. 9.8 A distended, round trachea with thick walls

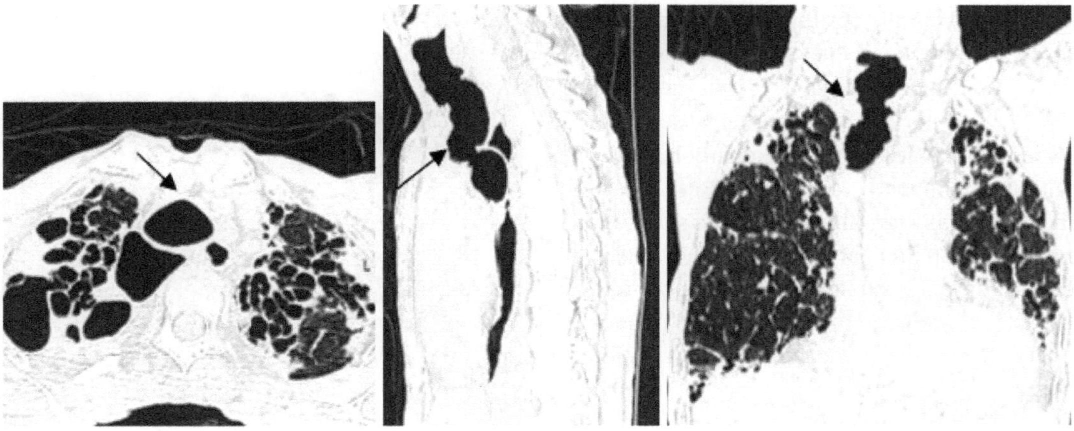

Fig. 9.9 Axial, sagittal and coronal scan showing a distorted and dilated trachea (arrow) in a case of diffuse fibrosing lung disease

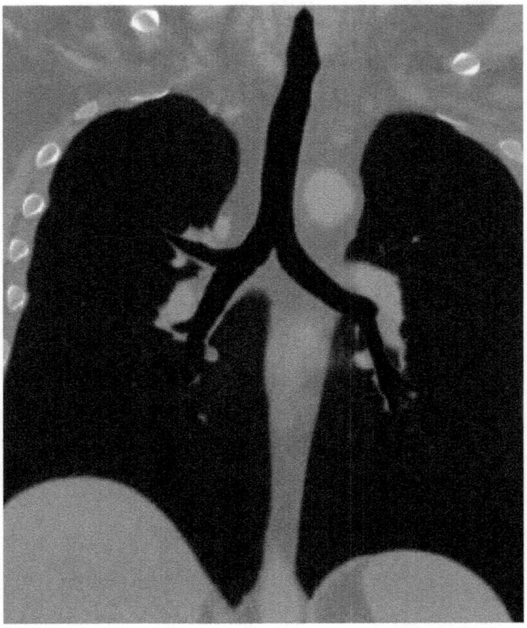

Fig. 9.10 Image reconstructed using minimum intensity projection. Note the relatively lower density of the air column in the trachea as compared to the lung parenchyma, which appears greyish. This is because the density of the lung parenchyma is a combination of air and several soft tissues making the lung parenchyma

The negative density of the air within the tracheal lumen is more than that of the lung parenchyma. This is because the tracheal lumen has only air within it, while the lung parenchyma has a mixture of air and soft tissues (Fig. 9.10). This discrepancy in lucency between the trachea and lung parenchyma can be used to detect predominantly air-containing parenchymal lesions (cysts/bulla, obstructive emphysematous areas) and to distinguish them from the normal lung parenchyma.

9.2 Mediastinal and Hilar Nodes

Normal mediastinal and hilar nodes are not visible in chest X-rays. This is because most nodes are located in the visceral compartment, are small in size and blend with the density of other soft tissues in the mediastinum. Normal nodes are always seen in a CT scan of the chest. They are small in size (less than 1 cm) and few. Their transverse diameter is constant in size as compared to the longitudinal measurements, which can vary between 10 and 25 mm [7]. The transverse diameter of the normal nodes in the carinal region can be up to 1.2 mm. The rest of the nodes are normally smaller than this measurement. Pathological nodes may remain normal in size or enlarge and widen the mediastinum. They may increase the density of the hilum or calcify and become visible even in a chest X-ray. The nodal calcification may be dense, popcorn-type, eggshell-like, diffuse or speckled. Usually, the trachea and bronchi do not show compressive effect due to nodes, unless the nodes are very large, confluent and of solid consistency. Nodes with low central density (so called necrotic nodes), even when large, generally do not compress the major airways They may completely liquefy and form a mediastinal abscess. Hilar nodes and masses may occasionally be confused with the pulmonary vascular shadows. A clue in the X-rays is the "hilum overlay sign" which implies that pulmonary vessels do not end at the edge of the enlarged hilar shadow but can be seen traversing through it to meet the main pulmonary artery lying within the hilar shadow. A hilum overlay sign signifies the presence of an enlarged node or a hilar mass, which is overlying the hilar vessels. When pulmonary vessels terminate in a hilar shadow, the shadow is that of the pulmonary artery and the sign is called the "hilum convergence sign". A dilated pulmonary artery will be seen coursing distally from the hilum into the lung parenchyma, whereas a hilar mass will not! When in doubt about the presence or absence of a hilar lesion, the issues can be resolved by a CT scan. Diseases which can lead to lymph nodal pathology include TB, sarcoidosis, fungal infections, enlarged nodes reactive to any chest disease and malignancies such as lymphomas, bronchogenic carcinomas, and metastasis. Granulomatous lesions, especially sarcoidosis, may take a long time to calcify. Usually, about 20% of sarcoidosis nodes calcify by 10 years [8].

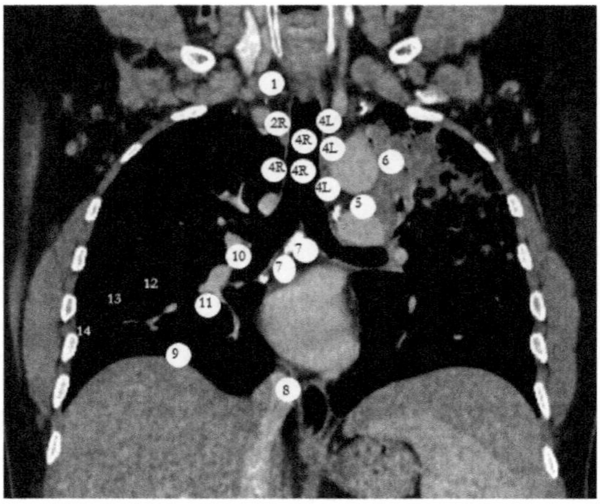

Fig. 9.11 Image demonstrating lymph node stations

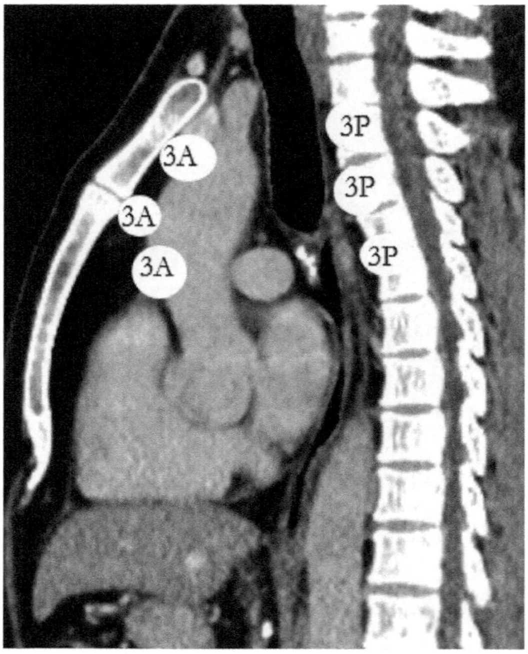

Fig. 9.12 Image demonstrating the position of station 3 nodes, best appreciated in the sagittal plane

9.3 Lymph node Stations (Figs. 9.11, 9.12, 9.13, 9.14, 9.15, 9.16, 9.17, and 9.18)

The International Association for the study of lung cancer (IASLC) has defined the stations in which the mediastinal and hilar nodes reside [9]. These stations are numbered from 1 to 14 (Fig. 9.12).

Station 1 nodes are lower neck nodes.
Stations 2–4 are superior mediastinal nodes.
Station 3A nodes are anterior to the superior mediastinal vessels and 3P are posterior to the trachea in the superior mediastinum.
Stations 5 and 6 are aortic nodes, 5 nodes are AP window nodes and 6 nodes are left paraaortic nodes.
Stations 7–9 are inferior mediastinal nodes, 7 being carinal, 8 paraesophageal and 9 being inferior pulmonary ligament node stations.

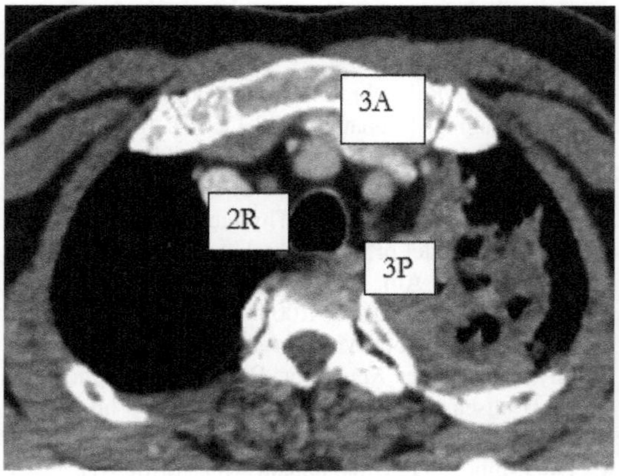

Fig. 9.13 Axial scan showing right upper paratracheal (2A), anterior (3A) and posterior (3B) prevascular nodes

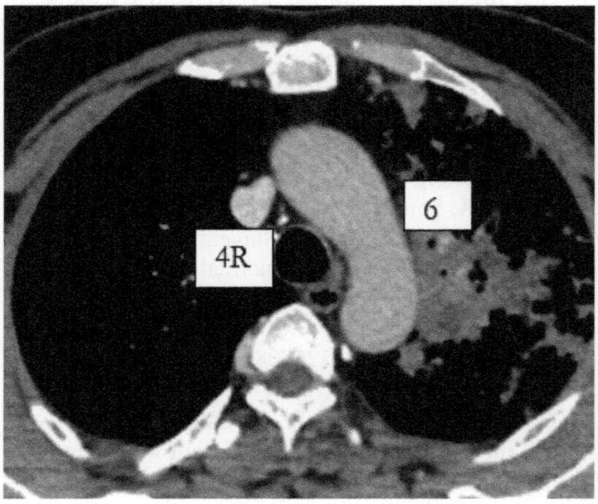

Fig. 9.14 Axial scan showing location of right lower paratracheal nodes (4R) and left paraaortic nodes (6)

Stations 10–14 nodes are, in descending order, -hilar, lobar, segmental as well as subsegmental nodes.

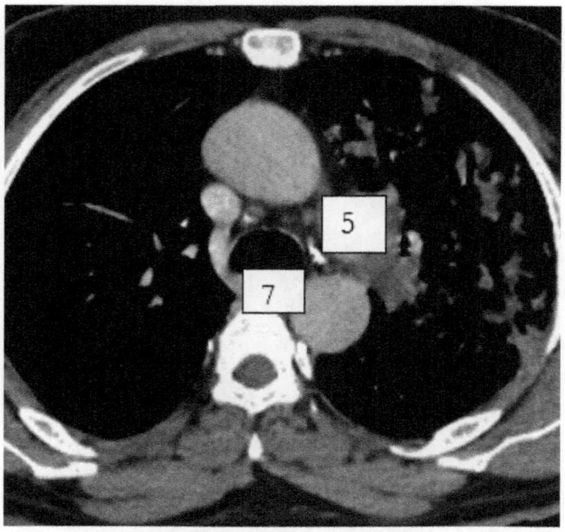

Fig. 9.15 Axial scan showing AP window (5) and carinal nodes (7)

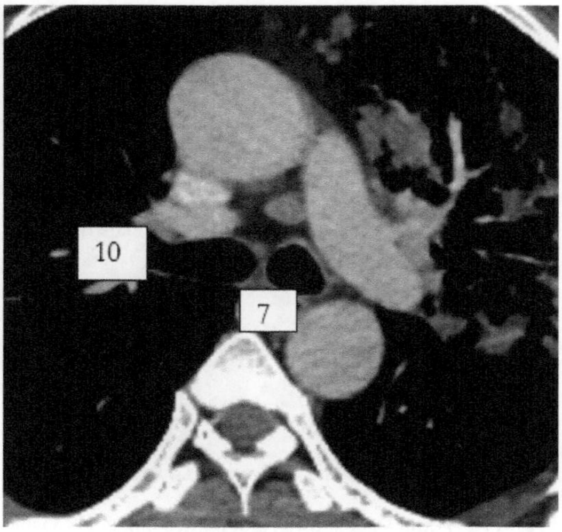

Fig. 9.16 Axial scan showing right hilar (10) and carinal nodes (7)

The anatomy of the mediastinum is distinct from the pulmonary anatomy, by way of the presence of not only cardiac but many more structures. All these structures are prone to disease and can show variations which may mimic disease. Hence, understanding the anatomy of the mediastinum is essential for the correct interpretation of chest diseases.

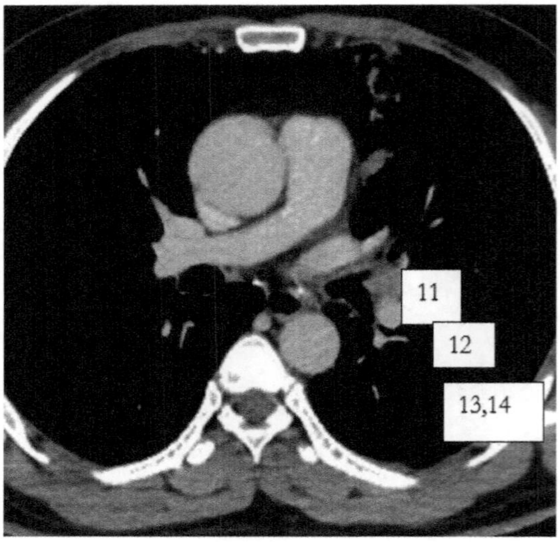

Fig. 9.17 Axial scan showing segmental, subsegmental and peripheral nodes (11–14)

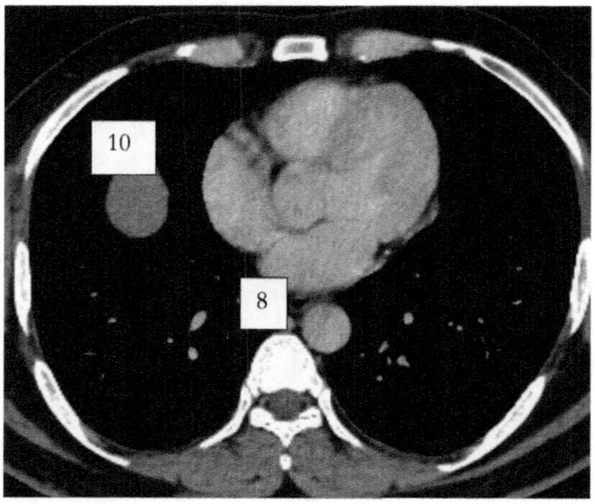

Fig. 9.18 Axial scan shows right paraesophageal (8) and inferior pulmonary ligament node (10)

References

1. Parekh M, Balasubramanya R. Chest and mediastinal imaging. [Updated 2022 Oct 3]. In: StatPearls. Treasure Island, FL: StatPearls Publishing; 2024. https://www.ncbi.nlm.nih.gov/books/NBK559145/.
2. Carter BW. International Thymic malignancy interest group model of mediastinal compartments. Radiol Clin North Am. 2021;59(2):149–53. https://doi.org/10.1016/j.rcl.2020.11.007. PMID: 33551077.
3. Westra D, Sperber M. Conventional chest radiography. In: Sperber M, editor. Radiologic diagnosis of chest disease. London: Springer; 2001. https://doi.org/10.1007/978-1-4471-0693-7_3.
4. Esien-umo EO, Chiaghanam NO, Erim AE, et al. Compliance to radiography practice of high-kilovoltage technique for chest radiography in South Nigeria. Bull Natl Res Cent. 2022;46:229. https://doi.org/10.1186/s42269-022-00907-9.
5. Goo JM, Im J-G, Kim JH, Seo JB, Kim TS, Shine SJ, Lee W. Digital chest radiography with a selenium-based flat-panel detector versus a storage phosphor system. AJR Am J Roentgenol. 2000;175(4):1013–8.
6. Furlow PW, Mathisen DJ. Surgical anatomy of the trachea. Ann Cardiothorac Surg. 2018;7(2):255–60. https://doi.org/10.21037/acs.2018.03.01.
7. Kiyono K, Sone S, Sakai F, Imai Y, Watanabe T, Izuno I, Oguchi M, Kawai T, Shigematsu H, Watanabe M. The number and size of normal mediastinal lymph nodes: a postmortem study. AJR Am J Roentgenol. 1988;150(4):771–6. https://doi.org/10.2214/ajr.150.4.771. PMID: 3258087.
8. Nunes H, Uzunhan Y, Gille T, Lamberto C, Valeyre D, Brillet P-Y. Imaging of sarcoidosis of the airways and lung parenchyma and correlation with lung function. Eur Respir J. 2012;40(3):750–65. https://doi.org/10.1183/09031936.00025212.
9. Ahmed H, et al. International Association for the Study of Lung Cancer (IASLC) lymph node map: radiologic review with CT illustration. Radio Graphics. 2014;34(6):1680–91.

10 Plain X-Ray of the Abdomen

Abstract

Despite the availability of ultrasound, CT scans, and MRI, plain X-rays of the abdomen are still routinely performed. Plain films are a basic investigation which can provide a direction to the thought process. Before the availability of ultrasound and CT, plain films of the abdomen were highly rated and many times sufficient enough to prompt surgical intervention, especially in patients of perforation with free intraperitoneal air. Radiologists who could interpret the plain films correctly were held in high esteem. Plain film interpretation is like solving a jigsaw puzzle. Correctly interpreted X-rays save time and costs to the patient. However, not every disease can be diagnosed by plain films alone. If it were so, then other techniques would not have been necessary. Therefore, a realistic approach has to be adopted and one should make the best possible use of X-rays before reaching out to other investigations.

Keywords

Plain X-rays abdomen · Perforation · Intraperitoneal air

The approach to plain films must begin by obtaining a good-quality X-ray

What makes an X-ray a good quality one?

- The X-ray should have adequate contrast and brightness. The latitude of the film should be such that both soft tissues, as well as bony structures, are adequately represented in the radiograph.
- The area included in the film, should extend from the lung bases to below the pubic symphysis.
- There should be no motion artefact or any other type of artefact.

If all these criteria are met, then the X-ray can be considered to be of good quality. If the quality is suboptimal, do not rush to repeat the film. There might be several reasons for not being able to obtain a good film. Discuss the issue with the radiologist or an associate. If the film serves the purpose, then do not repeat it.

R. Gothi, *Radiographic and Imaging Techniques for Radiology Residents and Technologists*,
https://doi.org/10.1007/978-981-96-4816-0_10

10.1 What to Look for in a Plain Film

In an X-ray of the abdomen, keep a look out for the following abnormalities:

1. **Radio-opaque shadows** (Fig. 10.1).

  - Air outside the bowel loops, that is, air in the peritoneum or retroperitoneum.
  - Air-fluid levels.
  - Look at the outlines of the normal solid structures, such as kidneys, liver, spleen, uterus and urinary bladder.
  - Do not forget the bones, that is, the spine, pelvis, and lower ribs.
  - When suspecting perforation of the gut, always ask for a chest X-ray in the erect position. This is because the spreading out of the X-ray beam brings about a good contrast between the free peritoneal gas shadow and the soft tissue density of the adjoining liver shadow. Therefore, gas under the diaphragms is best seen in a chest X-ray taken in a standing position (Fig. 10.2).

    In patients suspected to have intestinal obstruction, ask for films in supine and erect positions (Fig. 10.3), not just an erect X-ray film, something which happens quite often. An erect film shows fluid levels and free peritoneal air. A supine film shows both free peritoneal and retroperitoneal air as well as bowel gas patterns which not only lead to the site of obstruction but can sometimes demonstrate the cause of obstruction as well.

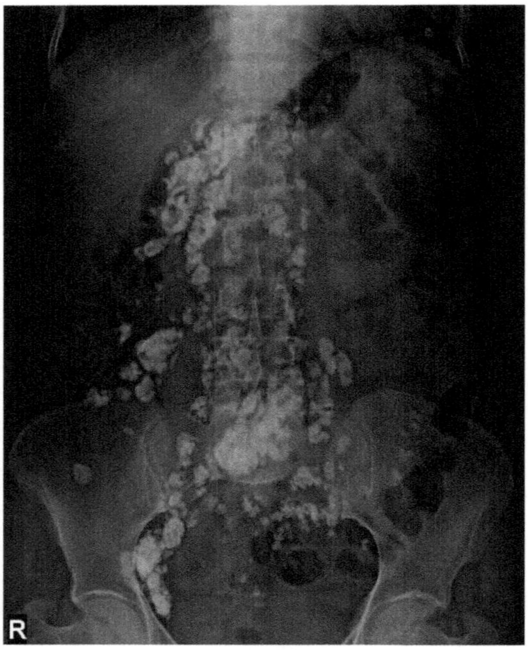

Fig. 10.1 Plain X-ray abdomen showing extensive calcified lymph nodes

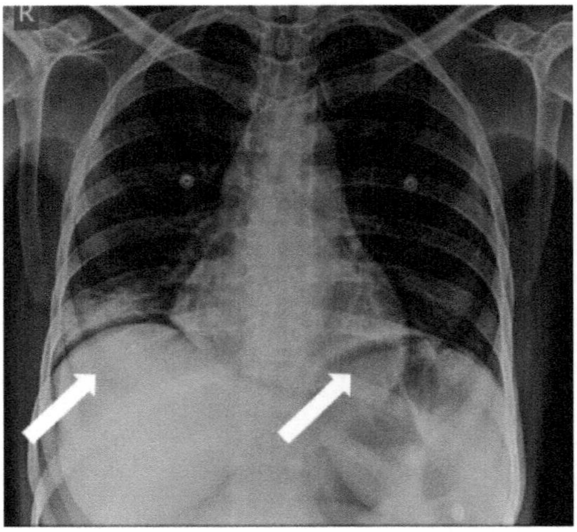

Fig. 10.2 Gas is seen beneath both domes of the diaphragm (arrows) in this X-ray chest taken in a standing position. Note the easy detection of gas on the right side brought about by the contrasting difference in density between air and the adjoining soft tissue density shadow of the liver. Gas under the left diaphragm is less easy to detect because there is no soft tissue density structure to provide contrast to the free peritoneal air. Also gas under the left diaphragm may be obscured by stomach or splenic flexure gas

  - Free fluid can also be recognized in a supine X-ray as it leads to increased haziness of the abdomen and obscures the fat planes around the urinary bladder, uterine fundus (Fig. 10.4) and flanks.
  - **Radio-opaque densities**: Certain lesions have a high-density chemical composition. They absorb the incoming X-ray photons, which results in a white shadow in the X-ray film. Barium sulphate, high-density stones containing calcium and other substances such as mercury and lead are some examples which absorb X-rays, and cast a white shadow.

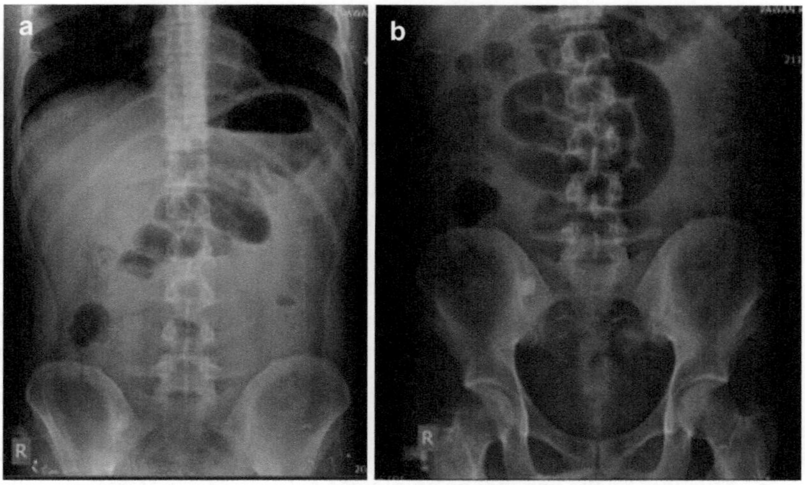

Fig. 10.3 Plain X-ray of the abdomen, erect (**a**) and supine (**b**). The supine film (**b**) shows the distension of the gas-filled small bowel loops, much better than the erect view

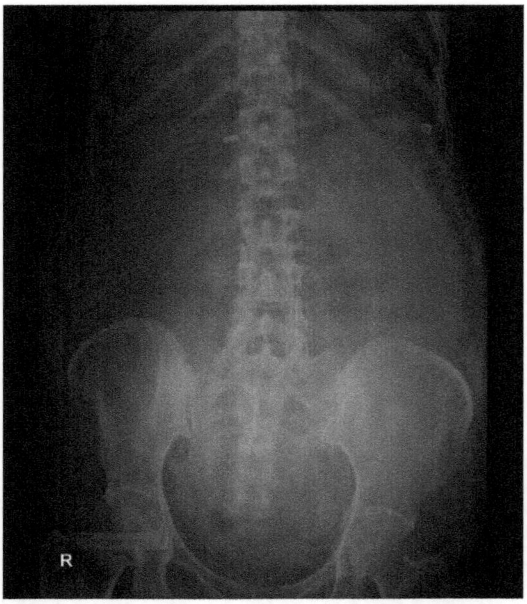

Fig. 10.4 Diffuse abdominal haze can be produced both by abundant fat or free fluid. This patient had extensive ascites which is associated with bulging flanks

- **Stones** (calculus) may be found in the gall bladder, kidneys, ureters, and urinary bladder or form in a blind loop of the intestine including in the appendix. They are normally seen in the anatomical location of the affected organ but can shift in position, especially when inside a hollow viscus or tubular structure like the ureter. A ureteric calculus, for example, can slide down the ureter in a short period. A vesical calculus can roll within the urinary bladder, can relocate in a bladder diverticulum, (if there is one), can drop into the urethra and can even be ejected spontaneously. Renal calculus can move about between dilated calyces and the pelvis. A gall bladder (GB) calculus can move within the gall bladder lumen, enter the common bile duct (CBD), or disappear into the intestines through fistulous communication with the gut. A small 1–3 mm calculus can pass out spontaneously through a normal calibre CBD [1]. In fact, stones as large as 1.5 cm have also been reported to have passed out spontaneously [2].
- Minerals deposited on a nidus in the small bowel loops, constitute what are called "enteroliths". Occasionally retained seeds are the nidus and appear as enteroliths. Enteroliths are usually found inside dilated bowel loops, especially those which have been obstructed by a long-standing distal stricture. They can also be found in blind-ending pouches such as diverticula or blind loops. Generally multilayered, they can change position due to ongoing peristaltic activity of the bowel loops.
- Other radio-opaque densities, seen in plain films are calcified nodes, which have a popcorn configuration. They do not disappear in follow-up radiographs and can

change position, with the movement of the mesenteric folds.

- Pancreatic calcification is seen in the upper abdomen, in the region of the pancreas at T12-L1 level. They are oriented along the length and direction of the pancreas, being more commonly seen in the region of the head.

  Pancreatic calculi can be found within the main pancreatic duct or in its branches.
- A calcified appendicolith, located in the right iliac fossa, makes it easy to consider the possibility of acute appendicitis.
- Occasionally, a psoas abscess may calcify and appear as a paraspinal bulge.
- Sometimes, the appendage epiploicae calcifies on undergoing torsion and loss of blood supply. These can then slough off from the colon and drop into the peritoneal cavity, which provides free space for them to move anywhere in the abdomen.
- Arteries can also calcify. The aorta and iliac arteries usually calcify secondary to atherosclerosis. If the calcified aorta is more than 3 cm in width, it is considered mildly dilated and if over 5 cm, the dilation is aneurysmal. Always check the underlying lumbar spine for any erosion of the anterior margins, caused by pulsations of a dilated aorta. Smaller vessels, namely, the splenic artery often calcify in the elderly population and may show focal aneurysmal dilatations.
- Veins, especially small pelvic veins, can show focal calcification which are called phleboliths. These look like small rings with a calcified outer border and a lucent centre. They may be mistaken for ureteric calculus, or in females, as tubal rings. When in doubt, do consider doing an intravenous urography (IVU) or a CT scan of the kidney ureter and bladder region (KUB) to resolve the issue.
- In females, fallopian tubal rings can be found in the pelvis. They appear as round radio-opaque shadows with a lucent centre and are found on either side of the uterus.
- Other radio-opaque densities seen in plain films of the abdomen include barium sulphate, used for contrast studies of the intestines, oral iodinated contrast material used in CT scans of the abdomen, ingested lead, mercury and barium carbonate. Some poisons such as rat poisons, may also appear radio-opaque. Swallowed foreign bodies such as coins (Fig. 10.5), needles, and safety

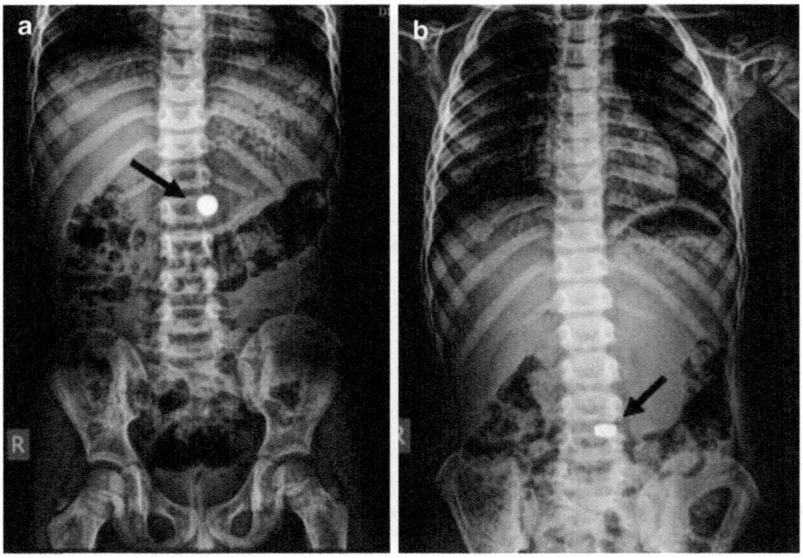

Fig. 10.5 Foreign body (lithium battery) in the stomach, seen in the supine (**a**) and standing positions (**b**)

pins may also be visible on X-ray. Whenever an X-ray is being done to locate a foreign body, make sure that the entire chest and abdomen is included in the film.

- Occasionally, the foreign body may be stuck in the oesophagus or a diverticular pouch. It may also have been passed out without the patient being aware of it. Radio-opaque foreign bodies can be seen in unusual places such as the urinary bladder, vagina and rectum, so be aware of them!
  - Both benign and malignant tumours including metastatic deposits may show faint calcification [3]. Also, look at the shape of the calcification and see if it resembles a tooth. The presence of tooth/teeth is diagnostic of a dermoid cyst or an ingested dental prosthesis.
  - Do not forget that a foetus in a pregnant woman may also be visible on the X- ray, taken inadvertently for some other reason. A small foetus overlying the sacral spine may be overlooked if the X-ray is not carefully examined.

2. **Radiolucent shadows** are produced because they are unable to obstruct the passage of X-rays through them. They are recorded as gray to black shadows. The degree of blackness depends upon the extent to which the X-ray beam has been attenuated. If all the X-ray photons pass through, then the shadow will be dark and must be due to free peritoneal air or gas within bowel loops. Gray shadows could be due to fat or gas mixed with fluid.

Bowel Gas shadows Gas is usually present in the stomach. It is rarely seen in the duodenum, except possibly in the first part of the duodenum (duodenal cap). It may be seen in the small bowel loops in neonates, infants, small children and older patients. The presence of gas in the elderly patients is due to reduced peristaltic activity. Infants and children show plenty of bowel gas shadows due to aerophagy. The colon always shows a small amount of gas as well as small air-fluid levels, caused by entrapment of air and fluid within the haustral folds. Air is normally never seen in the gall bladder and kidney. If seen in these organs, it is referred to as emphysematous cholecystitis and emphysematous pyelonephritis respectively. The bile ducts, uterus and peritoneal cavity also do not have air except under certain circumstances. The presence of air in bile ducts is called "pneumobilia" (air can enter the bile ducts following instrumentation, surgical procedure or through a patulous sphincter of Oddi). Air in the vagina and uterus could be following a surgical procedure, after a vaginal examination or following a recent sexual activity. The presence of air outside the confines of the bowel loops is made out by noting the absence of haustral or mucosal pattern in the collection of air, by demonstration of both sides of the bowel walls (Rigler's sign) abnormal location of gas, or by demonstrating free mobility of the gas with change in position. Free peritoneal air is normally seen as a crescent-shaped shadow below the diaphragms in the erect position. It outlines the borders of the ligamentum teres as well as other intraperitoneal organs, if large in quantity. An intra-abdominal abscess may show a large air-fluid level in the subphrenic space or pelvis.

Retroperitoneal gas usually outlines the psoas' shadows. Gas, both in the retroperitoneum and parietal wall presents as air bubbles, which do not change position. Fluid level is generally not seen associated with retroperitoneal air unless there is a superadded infection.

Small gas bubbles can be entrapped between bowel loops, in the bowel walls (Pneumatosis intestinalis), in various crevices in the abdomen and within abscesses.

The intestinal air helps recognize the bowel loops they occupy. Air in the jejunum shows valvulae conniventes. The ileum appears featureless. The large intestinal air has a haustral or bubbly pattern (when it is mixed with faecal matter). The calibre of the small intestines is always less than 3 cm while the large intestinal calibre can be large, depending upon the quantity of air and faecal content. The diameter of the caecum normally does not exceed 9 cm. The rest of the colon is usually up to 6 cm in diameter.

Normal air levels are visible in the left upper quadrant in the fundus of the stomach. People who are non-ambulatory or elderly may show a few air-fluid levels in the small bowel loops. The calibre of these loops, however, will be normal. When seen, they are usually in the mid-abdomen. Small air-fluid levels in the colon can be seen in the flanks and below the liver shadow, especially in a constipated patient or in patients having loose motions. Air fluid levels can be seen in both obstructive and non-obstructive situations. Paralytic ileus, malabsorption syndromes, and diarrheal states can result in the accumulation of fluid and gas in the bowel loops. Intestinal obstruction is suspected by the presence of multiple air-fluid levels. In mechanical obstruction, the width of the fluid level is lesser than the height of the air column, that is the column of air takes an inverted "U" shape. Multiple air-fluid levels may be seen at different levels in the horizontal planes (step-ladder appearance) depending on the extent of ongoing peristaltic activity, duration and level of obstruction in the patient. When the mechanical obstruction is prolonged, it gives way to paralytic ileus. In this situation, the erect film will show all the air-fluid levels drop down and line up to form a single level in the horizontal plane. By this time the bowel loops also distend and widen in calibre, resulting in a reduction in the height of the air column and a corresponding increase in the width of the fluid level ("C" shaped air-fluid level).

Absence of air can occur after prolonged vomiting, after nasogastric aspiration, in ischemic bowel diseases or following absorption of air with replacement by fluid. The latter leads to a "gasless abdomen", a sign of long-standing, almost complete obstruction due to a vascular or mechanical cause. Acute or partial small bowel obstruction can be associated with the presence of a small quantity of gas in the colon. As the small gut obstruction prolongs, the gas in the colon is either reduced in quantity or may be almost absent. In colonic obstruction, the segment proximal to the site of obstruction may distend with air. Impacted faecal residue or large fluid levels may also form proximally, especially if the ileocaecal valve is closed. However, if the ileocaecal valve is patulous, the gaseous distension may extend downstream into the distal small bowel loops.

When looking at the bowel gases, the supine film is used to study the pattern of the bowel gas shadows and the erect to appreciate fluid levels. Thumb printing due to ischemia, extrinsic pressure effects by adjoining masses, and filling defects due to any intraluminal soft tissue lesions are best-observed in a gas-filled bowel loop in a supine X-ray.

Intraabdominal Fat Fat appears gray and semi-translucent. It may be associated with calcific densities such as bone, tooth and cartilage. One can diagnose a dermoid cyst if there is a mixture of fat, soft tissue density, and high-density shadow such as a tooth.

Ascitic Fluid Fluid in the peritoneal cavity appears opaque and merges with the soft tissue of the abdomen. The fluid could be inflammatory (exudate), or non-inflammatory (transudate), due to a malignancy or intraperitoneal accumulation of blood or urine.

Finally

- Look at the bones for any evidence of destruction, sclerosis, lysis, osteoporosis, or osteomalacia.
- Look at the psoas shadows for any abnormal bulge.
- Look at the solid organs, for any enlargement, absence, malposition or abnormal shape.

10.2 Some More Examples of Bowel Gas Patterns

The plain films of the abdomen offer plenty of information and need careful interpretation and detailed interpretation. The radiologic technologist must ensure that the film quality is good. The radiologist must try to interpret the X-rays carefully, correlating the observations with the clinical data to arrive at a meaningful diagnosis (Figs. 10.6, 10.7, 10.8, 10.9, 10.10, and 10.11).

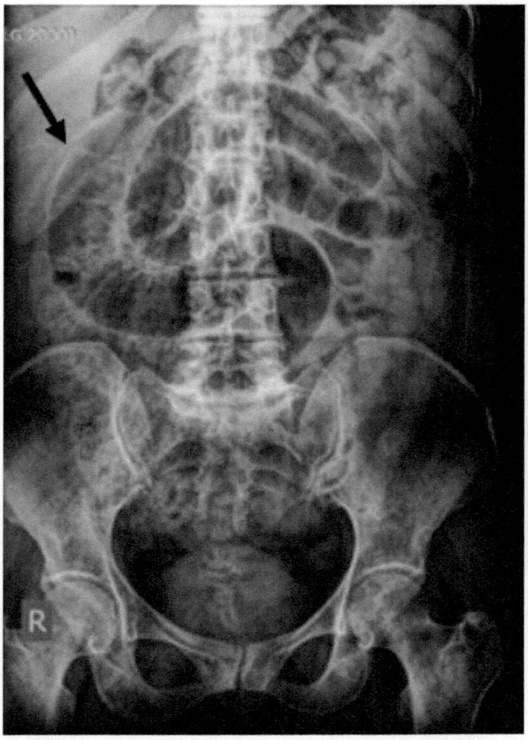

Fig. 10.6 Plain X-ray of the abdomen showing dilated gas-filled jejunal loops. These are located in the midline, and show continuity with one another. Note the stretched-out valvulae conniventes (arrow)

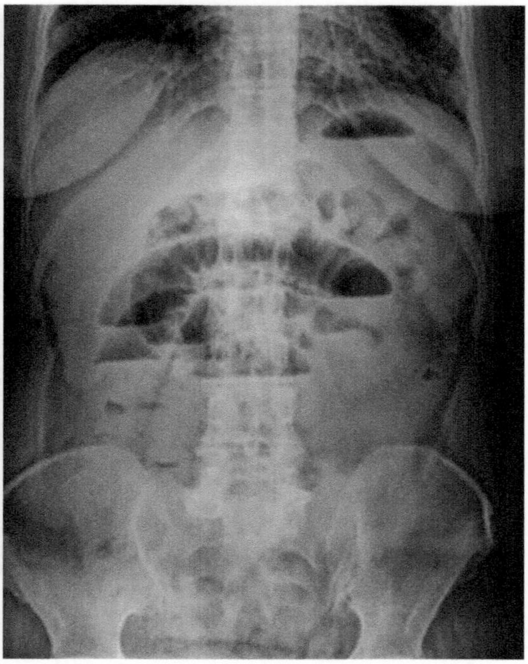

Fig. 10.7 Same patient as in Fig. 10.6. Note the fluid levels are located at different heights. This indicates obstruction. However, the air column has a "C shape". The "C shape" suggests, paralytic ileus due to prolonged duration of intestinal obstruction

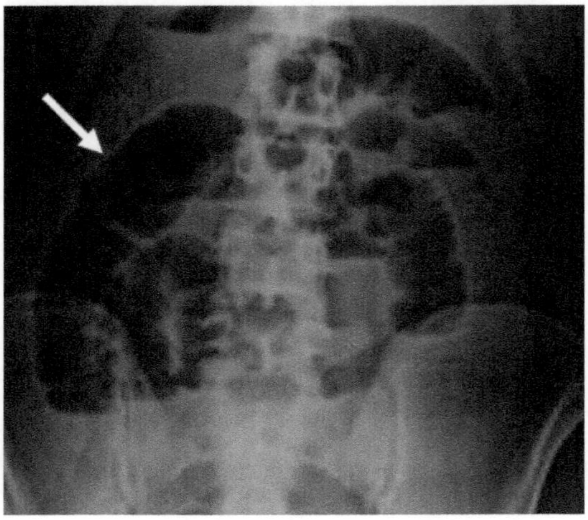

Fig. 10.8 The jejunal loops show prominent valvulae conniventes giving the appearance of spiral-binding in X-rays of the abdomen

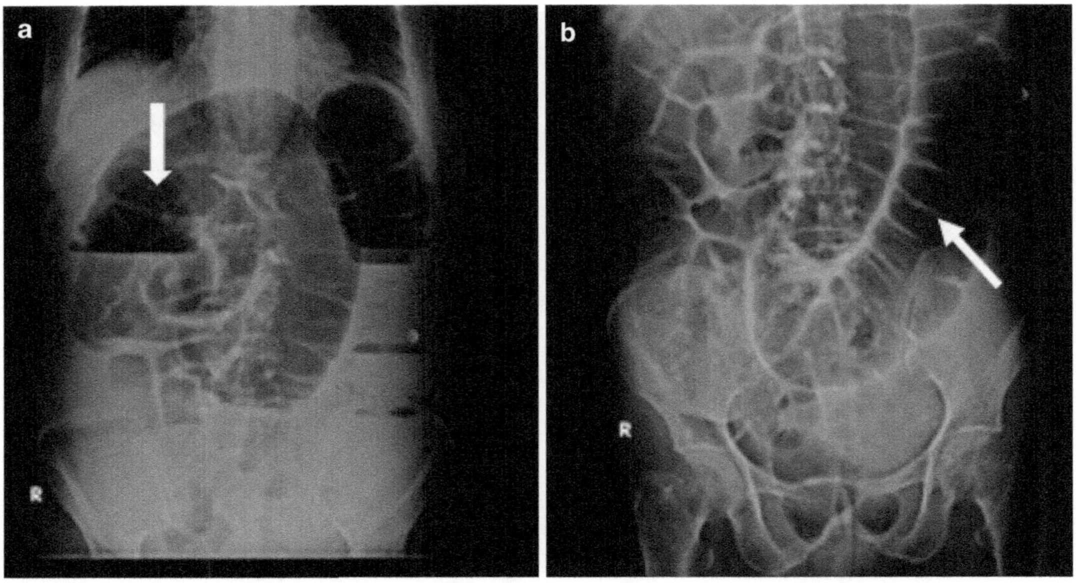

Fig. 10.9 X-rays of the abdomen show colonic distension with a large wide air fluid level in (**a**) (arrow). Figure (**b**) shows a haustral pattern (arrow)

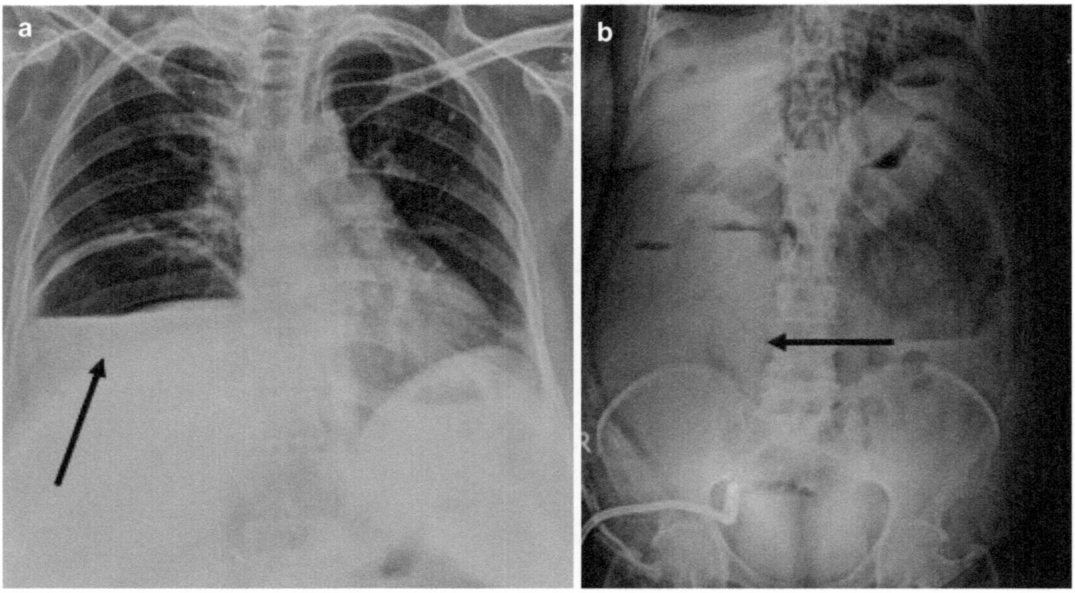

Fig. 10.10 X-ray chest posterior anterior (PA) view (**a**) and abdomen supine (**b**). The chest X-ray shows a right subphrenic air-fluid level. The abdomen X-ray shows the collection causing a soft tissue density shadow in the right flank

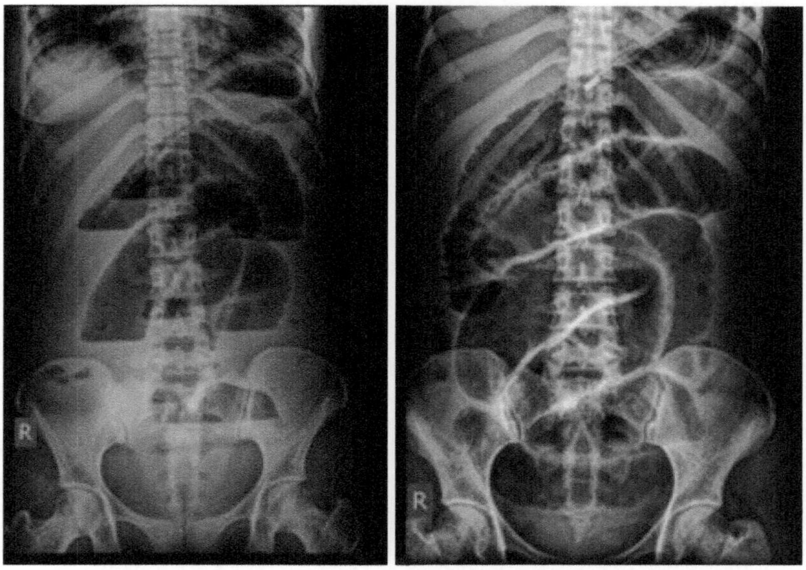

Fig. 10.11 A case of low (distal) small bowel obstruction, showing multiple air-fluid levels in the small bowel loops. These loops are in the mid-abdomen as should be the case with small bowel. They are distended and are reaching the pelvis. The findings are consistent with distal small bowel obstruction

References

1. Almadi MA, Barkun JS, Barkun AN. Management of suspected stones in the common bile duct. CMAJ. 2012;184(8):884–92. https://doi.org/10.1503/cmaj.110896.
2. Ansari MI, Pandey AS. Case report a case report of spontaneous passage of large (>1.5 cm) common bile duct calculi (4 in number) through faeces. Int Surg J. 2021;8(7):2186–9.
3. Zulfiqar M, Shetty A, Tsai R, Gagnon M-H, Balfe DM, Mellnick VM. Diagnostic approach to benign and malignant calcifications in the abdomen and pelvis. Radiographics. 2020;40(3):731–53.

11 Evaluation of the Pharynx and Oesophagus

Abstract

The pharyngoesophageal region forms the proximal part of the gastrointestinal system. The pharynx can be examined both by ENT surgeons and gastroenterologists, using the endoscope. Radiological investigations consist of barium studies and cross-sectional imaging.

In this chapter, we will consider the anatomy as well as techniques used to evaluate this region of the gastrointestinal tract.

Keywords

Pharynx · Oesophagus · Barium swallow

The pharynx and oesophagus are evaluated radiologically by barium studies. Barium, having a creamy consistency, adheres to and outlines the pharyngeal and oesophageal mucosa, thereby rendering them visible on the radiographs. Most patients present with complaints of pain or difficulty in swallowing. Occasionally, there may be a history of chest discomfort and barium swallow may be requested to exclude pharyngoesophageal pathology or gastroesophageal reflux. In the pre-echocardiography era, a barium swallow was also used to evaluate left atrial enlargement.

11.1 The Technique of Barium Swallow

- First, confirm whether the patient can swallow or not. If yes, then give a sip and watch the swallowing action. Once convinced that the patient can swallow sufficiently well, then proceed with the study. This is to avoid vomiting, choking or aspirating into the airways due to severe disturbance in the swallowing action. Depending upon the clinical status of the patient and what is required of the examination, one determines the quantity of barium that may be needed to obtain an adequate study. Usually, a few mouthfuls of barium suffice, not only to demonstrate the flow of contrast but also to coat the mucosa for assessment of mucosa-related problems. It is important to remember that barium is bland, and many patients find it unpalatable.
- Barium swallow studies can be a single contrast, using only liquid barium, which opacifies the entire lumen but renders the mucosa indistinguishable from the intraluminal barium column (Fig. 11.1). It can also be a double contrast study, in which the patient swallows a small quantity of thick barium which is given to coat the mucosa. Air, which is already present in the oesophagus, is used to provide a mucosal relief pattern.

R. Gothi, *Radiographic and Imaging Techniques for Radiology Residents and Technologists*,
https://doi.org/10.1007/978-981-96-4816-0_11

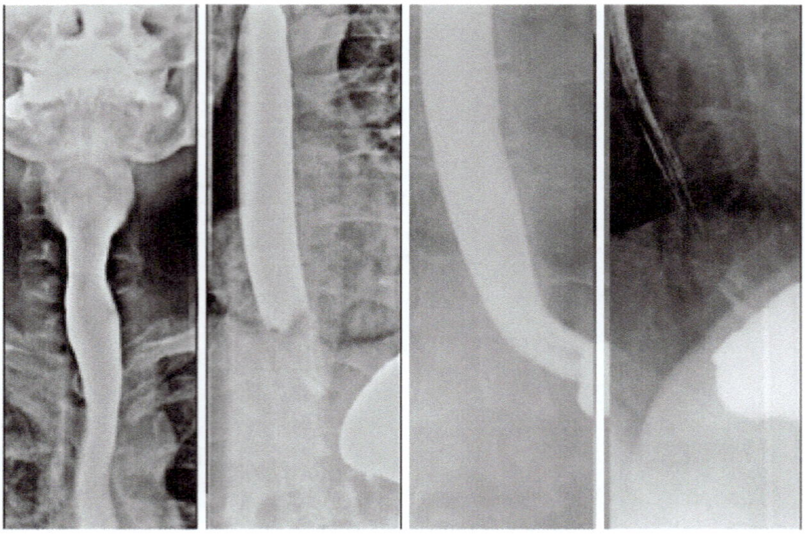

Fig. 11.1 A single contrast barium study demonstrating the pharynx, upper, middle and lower oesophagus

- The patient should be asked to swallow liquid barium in an erect position. This is to prevent inadvertent aspiration into the airways. Barium, aspirated in the lungs, may not be harmful, if the quantity is small. However, if a large quantity is aspirated, it can cause anaphylaxis, acute inflammation, and acute respiratory distress syndrome (ARDS) [1], which can lead to long-term complications such as pulmonary fibrosis.
- Mortality can also occur if the lungs are flooded with barium, especially in patients who cannot swallow it all or have a tracheo-esophageal fistula.
- The examination should be performed in the erect position under fluoroscopic guidance.
- If the patient is unable to stand or stand still but has good swallowing reflux, then the study can be performed with the patient sitting or lying in an oblique position. The head of the patient should be raised to enable drinking a mouthful of contrast and retain it in the oral cavity, till asked to swallow. When everything for exposure and fluoroscopic examination is ready, the patient is asked to swallow the barium. The flow of the barium column down the pharynx and oesophagus is captured and assessed. This also ensures that spillover, if any, into the airways is quickly recognized. Usually, patients start coughing on aspirating. However, many patients may not be able to cough despite aspirating. Should that happen, the study must be called off and the patient monitored by the clinicians.

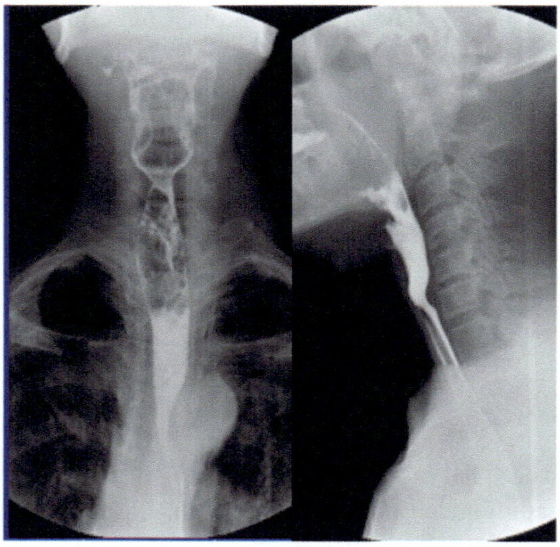

Fig. 11.2 AP and lateral views of the pharynx and upper oesophagus

- A cine study recording the entire act of swallowing is the best way of studying the oropharyngeal area. A single mouthful of barium may be enough if a cine recording is available. The cine clip can be studied and if found adequate, the examination can be terminated.
- For the pharynx and upper oesophagus, anteroposterior (AP) and lateral views are sufficient (Fig. 11.2).

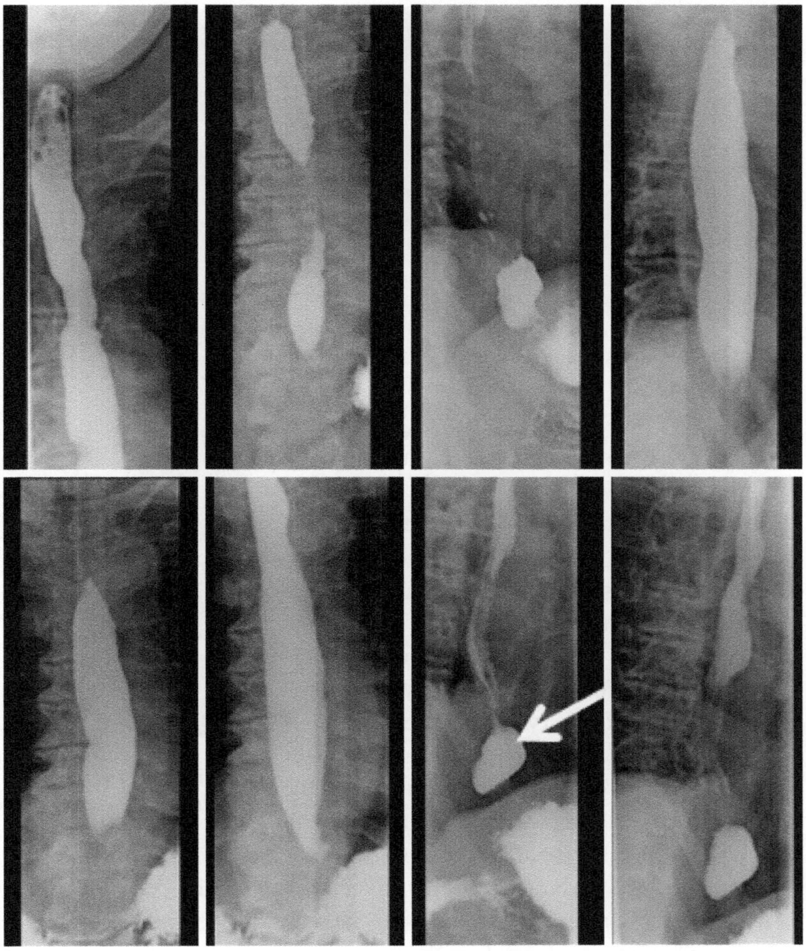

Fig. 11.3 Single contrast barium swallow study done in the supine position. Note the peristaltic contractions causing segmentation of the barium column. Also, note the presence of a physiologic phrenic ampulla (arrow)

- Images of the rest of the oesophagus are obtained in AP, right and left obliques and lateral positions (Fig. 11.3). The oblique position, especially with the left side down, eliminates the overlapping of the oesophageal and the dorsal spine shadows.
- Films for hiatus hernia are obtained in the Trendelenburg position with the images being centred on the GE junction. Alternatively, films can be acquired in the prone position with a pillow under the abdomen for pressure. However, all these manoeuvres are not physiological and tend to forcibly produce a hiatus hernia. A truly significant hiatus hernia should be visible in a supine and erect position under natural conditions.

11.2 Pathological Lesions of the Pharynx

Lesions of a hollow viscus either appear as soft tissue masses protruding into the lumen or as ulcerating mucosal lesions. A few of the lesions will be discussed here.

- **Pharyngeal web** (Fig. 11.4). A pharyngeal web is a horizontal plate-like filling defect protruding into the pharynx from its posterior wall. It is formed as a result of hypertrophy of the cricopharyngeus muscle. Similar webs may also be seen in cases of iron-deficiency anaemia.

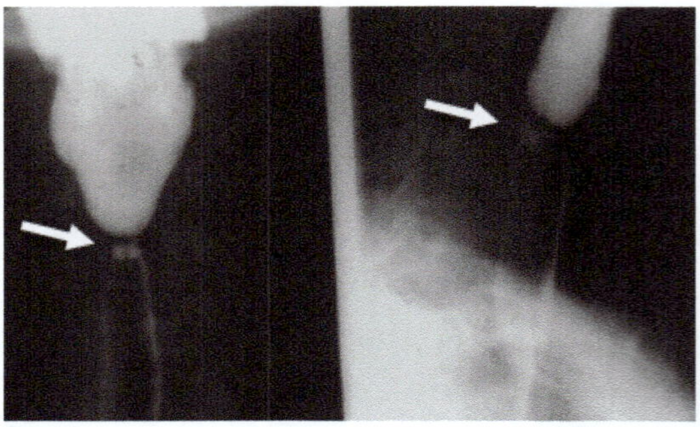

Fig. 11.4 Barium swallow showing pharyngeal web (arrow)

- **Pharyngeal diverticula**. These are mucosal outpouchings which can protrude either laterally or posteriorly about the pharyngeal lumen. The posteriorly protruding diverticulum, also called **Zenker's diverticulum** (Fig. 11.5), is a pulsion diverticulum which bulges out through a space called "Killian's space or Killian's dehiscence". The Killian's space is a spot between the cricopharyngeus muscle (which is located above the oesophagus and separates the pharynx from the oesophagus) and the superior constrictor muscle. The space is weak and allows the diverticulum to propel outwards through it. The diverticulum when filled with food particles or fluid, by compressing the posterior pharyngoesophageal wall, causes dysphagia. It can also cause halitosis, coughing due to aspiration into the airways and aspiration pneumonia.
- The upper oesophagus may be displaced anteriorly by this pouch. In a lateral plain film, it may appear as a soft tissue shadow with air bubbles or air fluid level, mimicking an abscess. A barium swallow will fill this blind ending pouch and confirm the diagnosis.

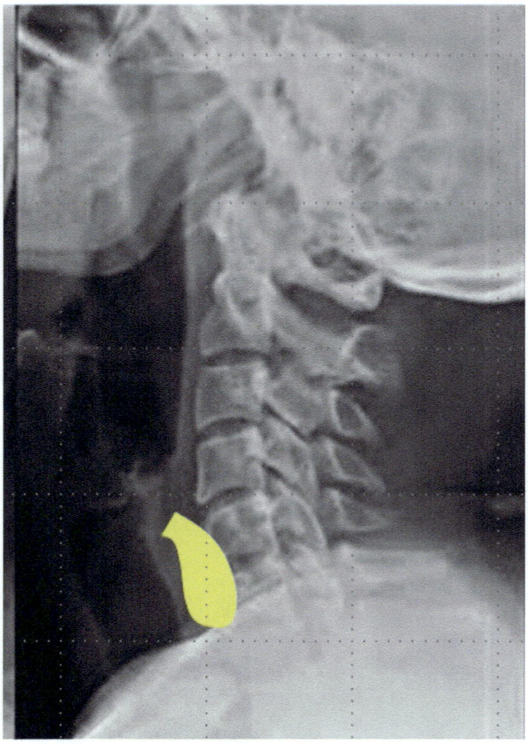

Fig. 11.5 Lateral view of the neck, showing the usual position of the Zenker's diverticulum

- The post cricoid region (Fig. 11.6) is located behind the cricoarytenoid cartilage and extends posterior to the cricoid cartilage [2]. It connects the pharynx with the upper oesophagus.
- Post cricoid carcinoma (Fig. 11.7) is a tumour, which develops at the pharyngo-oesophageal junction, just posterior to the cricoid cartilage. It appears as an irregular filling defect causing mucosal irregularity and luminal narrowing. It involves the larynx anteriorly and cervical oesophagus inferiorly.

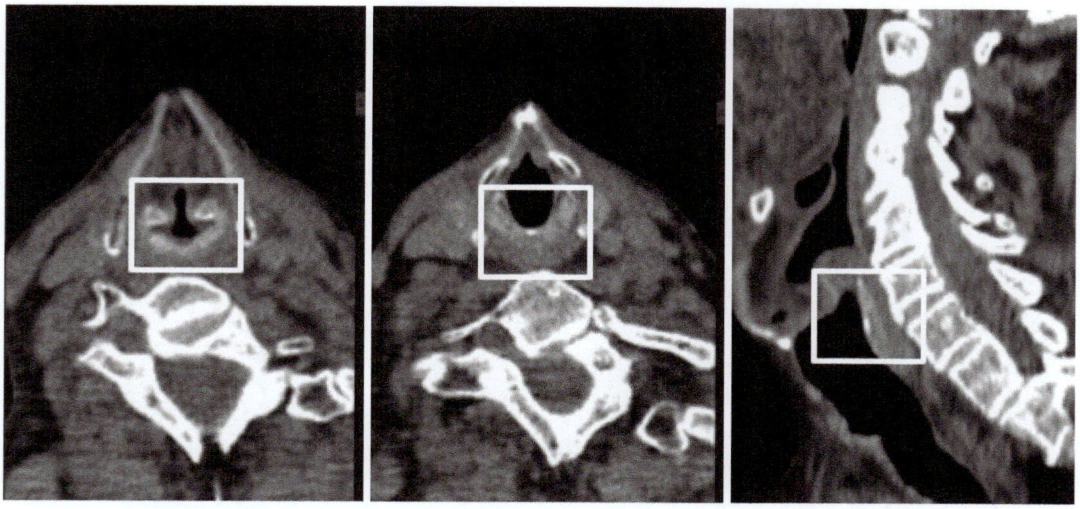

Fig. 11.6 CT scan images of the neck through the area of the post-cricoid region. Box, showing the post cricoid region, at the level of the cricoarytenoid cartilage (**a**), extending behind the cricoid cartilage (**b**) and joining the pharynx with the upper oesophagus (**c**)

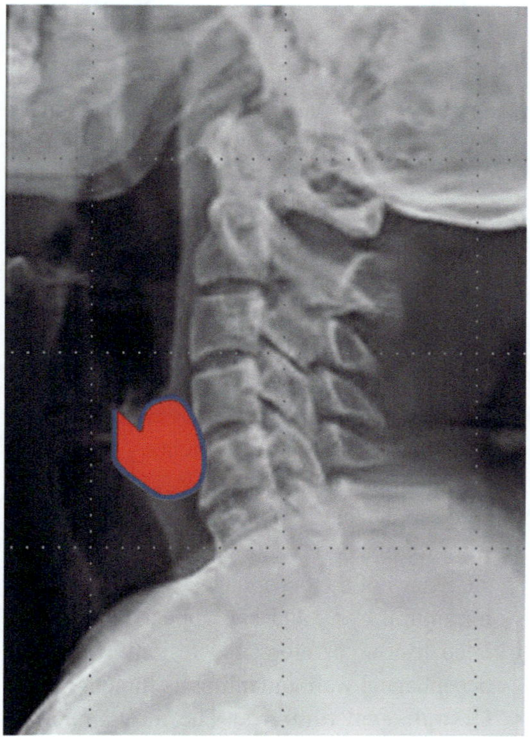

Fig. 11.7 Usual location of a post cricoid Carcinoma

11.3 Pathological Lesions of the Oesophagus

- Oesophageal atresia and trachea-oesophageal fistula (TOF) are amongst the most well-known congenital anomalies of the oesophagus. The diagnosis is easily made soon after birth. The radiographic findings include a gasless abdomen if there is no communication with the airways. This happens when the distal segment of the oesophagus is a blind pouch. The proximal oesophageal pouch may be filled with air and can be seen in a plain X-ray chest, slightly to the left of the trachea. A radio-opaque catheter, if introduced orally, will also be seen coiling into the proximal oesophageal pouch (Fig. 11.8).

  A few drops of barium, if introduced through the catheter, will outline the proximal pouch.

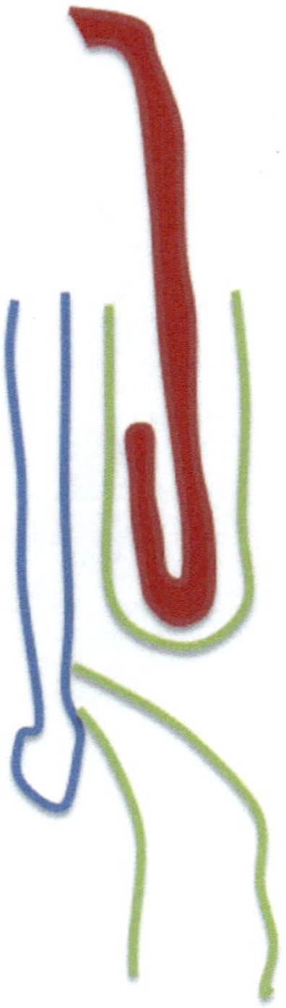

Fig. 11.8 Diagram showing the nasogastric tube (in red), coiled in the upper oesophageal pouch. The lower oesophagus communicates with the trachea above the carina. This, allows air to enter the stomach and small bowel loops

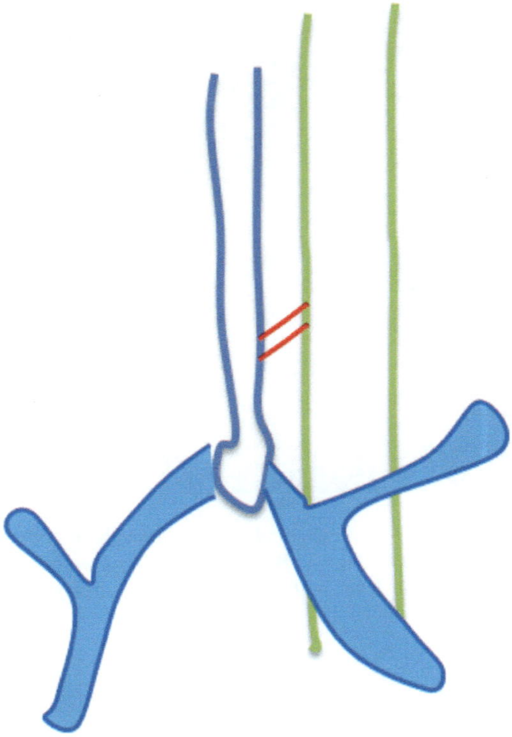

Fig. 11.9 Diagram demonstrating H type of fistulous communication between the proximal oesophageal pouch and trachea

H-types of fistula (Fig. 11.9) are difficult to demonstrate even by a barium swallow study and may need an endoscopy for diagnosis.

Patients with an "H" type of fistula may present with a history of repeated chest infections. Thin diluted barium or undiluted Gastrografin should be administered through a catheter in the prone oblique position so that it may trickle down the fistula into the trachea. The catheter should be introduced centimetre by centimetre and the oral positive contrast administered till the carina is reached. Keep looking for diminished or absent peristaltic activity in the upper and mid third of the oesophagus as well as for any spillage into the bronchi. When this is seen, stop the examination immediately. The track of the "H" type of fistula, if filled with contrast, will be seen coursing obliquely towards the trachea. A cine clip of the study is very helpful in the diagnosis of these cases as it can be played back and studied thoroughly.

- **Oesophageal duplication cysts**: Congenital cystic lesions in the posterior mediastinum can be oesophageal duplication cysts or neurenteric cysts, which are oesophageal cysts communicating with the spinal canal. The inner lining of the oesophageal duplication cyst is either that of the alimentary tract or the tracheobronchial mucosa [3].

  Oesophageal duplication cysts are formed from remnants of vacuolar spaces in the muscle planes of the oesophageal walls. These are intramural cysts and can appear both as isolated lesions or elongated lesions within the oesophageal wall, indenting its lumen.
- **Oesophageal tumours:** The most important reason for evaluating the oesophagus is dysphagia. The cause of dysphagia could be a mass, a stricture or a vascular ring, compressing it from the outside. The tumours could be both benign or malignant.

  Benign Tumours: There are several benign tumours which can affect the oesophagus. Out of these, leiomyomas (Figs. 11.10 and 11.11) are the ones most often encountered in practice.

They arise from the muscular layer of the oesophageal wall and produce a smooth impression on the barium column. They also have a propensity to ulcerate and tend to grow exophytically into mediastinum. They can be large and involve the entire oesophagus. However, their outlines usually remain smooth unless malignant degeneration sets in.

Oesophageal carcinoma. Carcinoma oesophagus is the most worrisome tumour of the gastrointestinal tract and amongst the common causes of dysphagia. The tumour may grow from the upper, middle (Fig. 11.12) or lower third of the oesophagus (Fig. 11.13).

Upper GI endoscopy is the first line of investigation in the evaluation of obstructive oesophageal growths. Barium swallow examinations are performed less frequently but are useful in determining the length of the tumours, (especially if the endoscope is unable to determine the entire length of the tumour) for planning radiotherapy. Barium studies also give an idea of the exact location of the tumour vis-a-vis the adjoining mediastinal structures. The findings on barium swallow are those of a mass lesion involving a short or long segment of the oesophagus causing mucosal irregularity, luminal narrowing and shouldering at the ends, especially the proximal end. The study must be performed with care, as there is a risk of regurgitation leading to aspiration and spillage of the orally administered contrast into the trachea.

Tumours involving the lower third of the oesophagus may extend into the fundus of the stomach, resulting in onstruction, mucosal irregularity and thickening of the gastric fundus. An erect single or double contrast study may show the lesion clearly as compared to the supine barium swallow study. Do remember that while squamous cell carcinoma is the most common oesophageal tumour, it may not be possible to radiologically distinguish one malignant tumour from another. Adenocarcinoma of the lower third of the oesophagus may develop in cases of long-standing gastroesophageal reflux. Large oesophageal masses may be seen in carcino-sarcomas and leiomyosarcoma (Fig. 11.11).

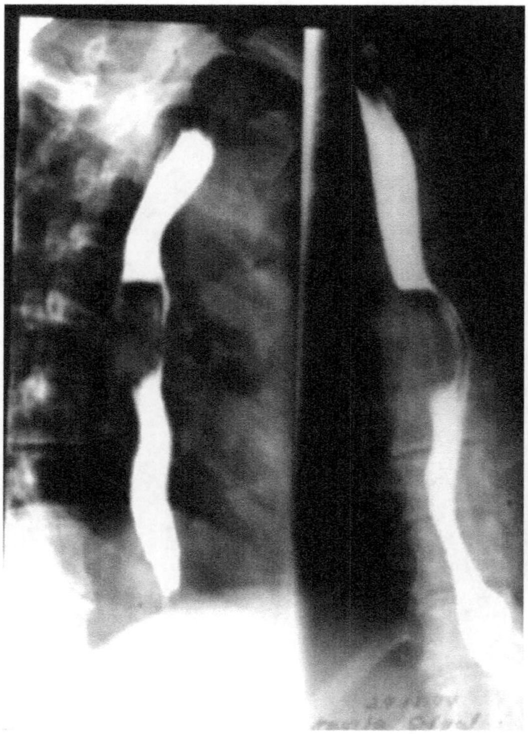

Fig. 11.10 Case of an oesophageal leiomyoma. Note that "shouldering" can be seen even in benign masses

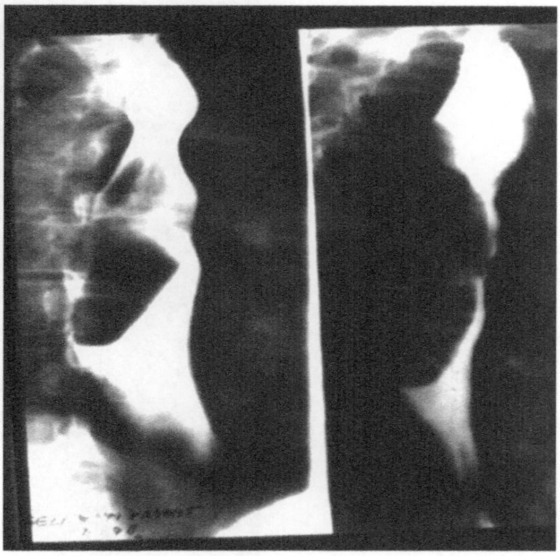

Fig. 11.11 Case of leiomyosarcoma of the oesophagus, appearing as a large multilobulated mass and causing distension of the oesophageal lumen

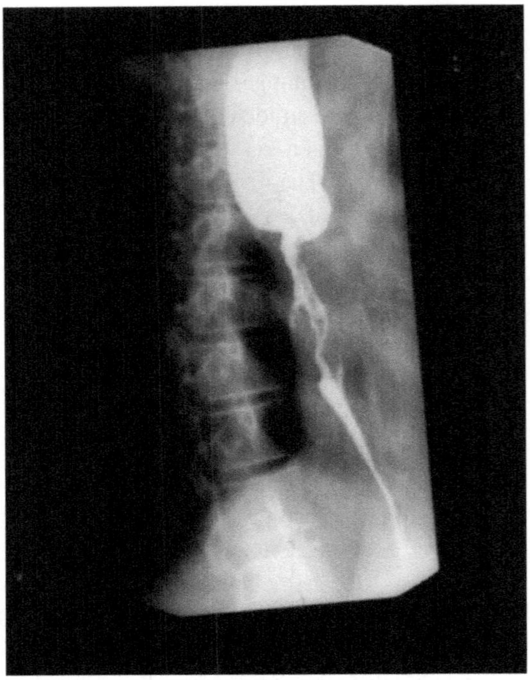

Fig. 11.12 Barium swallow of a case of carcinoma oesophagus showing a mass below the carina causing luminal narrowing and distortion with associated shouldering at its proximal end

- *Benign strictures*

  These are generally smooth. They can be short or long, (Fig. 11.14) without any associated mass and do not show any evidence of shouldering. They may develop as a result of corrosive poisoning. A short stricture at the lower end of the oesophagus may be a functional disturbance called cardiospasm/achalasia cardia (Fig. 11.15). Achalasia cardia leads to gross dilatation and tortuosity of the oesophagus over a period of time. The dilated oesophagus is located in the right paraspinal region and may show an air-fluid level or a food-residue level in the erect position.
- *Oesophageal dilatation*

  Besides achalasia cardia, strictures and other obstructive lesions, and cases of scleroderma can also cause a diffusely dilated oesophagus. There is slow transit of barium in the supine position. On the contrary, when barium is given in the erect position, the transit is rapid. Hardly any peristaltic wave is seen indenting the barium column which looks tubular.

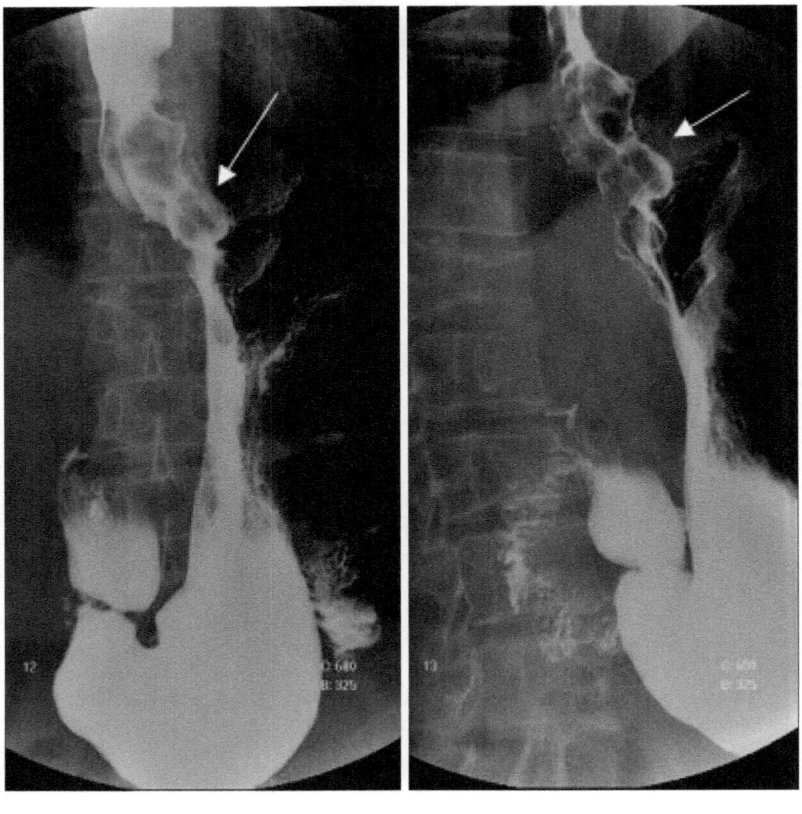

Fig. 11.13 Growth at the lower end of the oesophagus, involving the fundus of the stomach

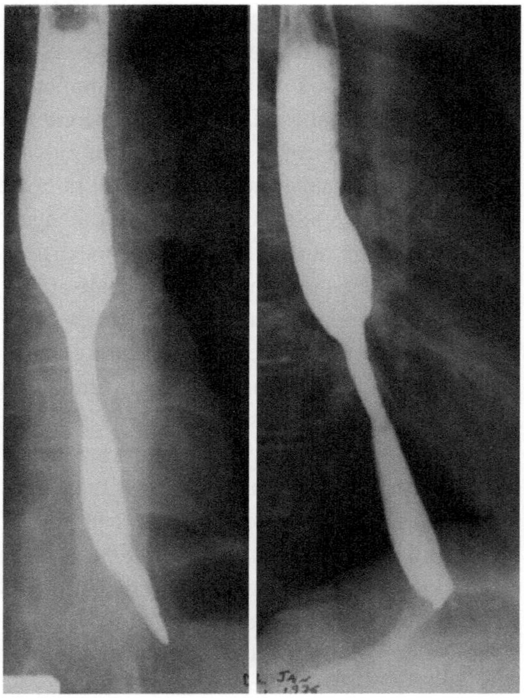

Fig. 11.14 Long smooth benign stricture of the oesophagus

Oesophageal dilatation and deformity can also result from traction caused by mediastinal and pulmonary fibrosis—mostly induced by tuberculosis or any other fibrosing disease affecting the mediastinum.

- **Oesophagitis.** Mucosal irregularity without mass effect could be due to oesophagitis (Fig. 11.16). Oesophageal inflammation can be localized to the lower third of the oesophagus as in cases of gastroesophageal reflux or it may be diffuse when the cause is moniliasis—a fungal infection seen in immuno-compromised or diabetic patients. Other fungal infections and tuberculosis may also involve diabetic and immunocompromisied patients.
- **Corkscrew oesophagus** (Fig. 11.17). When there is muscular incoordination, it results in non-propulsive contractions and the oesophagus assumes a corkscrew shape. This condition is often seen in elderly patients and is also called presbyesophagus.

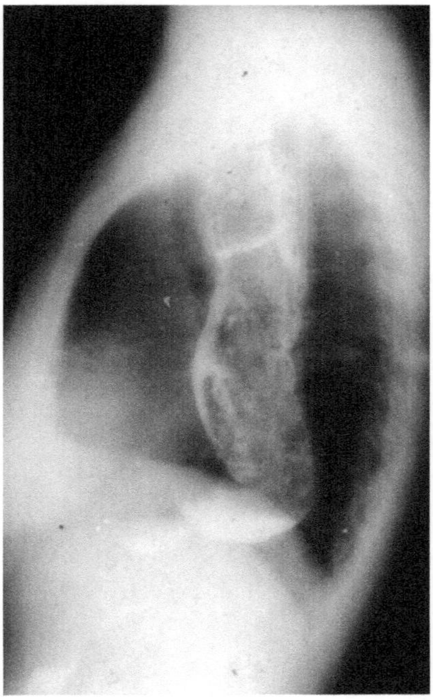

Fig. 11.15 Barium swallow of a case of achalasia cardia shows the presence of food residue in the distended oesophagus

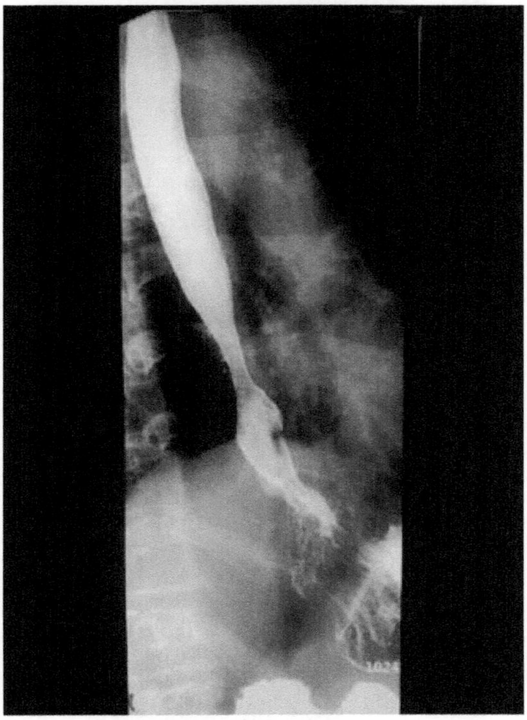

Fig. 11.16 Barium swallow showing fine mucosal ulcerations along the lower end of the oesophagus

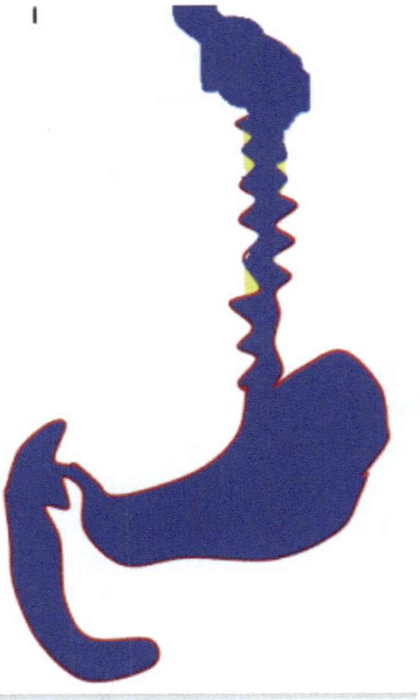

Fig. 11.17 Diagram showing a corkscrew oesophagus due to physiological disturbance of peristaltic activity

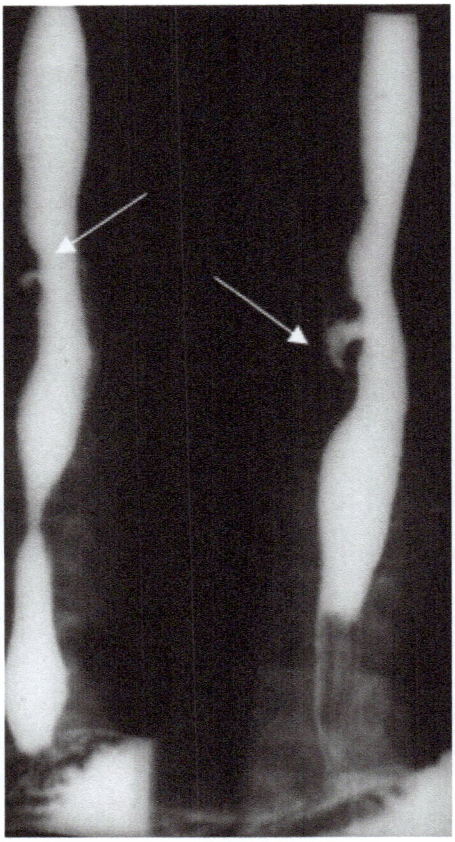

Fig. 11.18 Traction diverticulum in the middle third of the oesophagus (arrows) caused by adherence to a necrotic tubercular lymph node

- **Oesophageal diverticulum**
  Oesophageal diverticula can be due to traction caused by adjoining inflammatory pathologies, especially nodal tuberculosis (Fig. 11.18). It could also be due to pulsion caused by muscular incoordination or rarely it could be congenital. Congenital oesophageal diverticula are rare and appear as a pouch arising from anywhere in the oesophagus. They have been reported in preterm babies, neonates and small children. An interesting condition known as intramural pseudodiverticulosis may infrequently be seen in elderly patients, especially those having gastroesophageal reflux disease, malignancies and candidiasis. Traction diverticula are usually seen around the mid oesophagus at the level of the carina.
- Pulsion diverticula develop in the mid and lower third of the oesophagus (Fig. 11.19). A congenital oesophageal diverticulum may look similar. It is a rare condition and may be associated with other oesophageal deformities or any intrauterine insult [4].

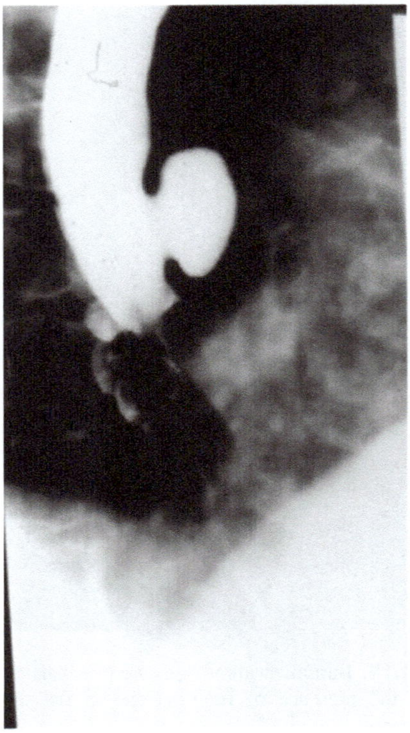

Fig. 11.19 Pulsion diverticulum with a wide neck, seen arising from the middle third of the oesophagus

Traction diverticula usually show adjoining fibrosis or nodes, whereas no such thing is seen with pulsion diverticulum. Traction diverticula are generally triangular and are associated with distortion of the oesophagus. Pulsion diverticula possess a neck and are globular in shape. A pulsion diverticulum above the oesophageal hiatus is called the epiphrenic diverticulum.

Barium swallow shows dilated oesophageal mucosal glands, appearing as barium-filled diverticula (Fig. 11.20), which are seen within the oesophageal wall, often involving it diffusely. They are caused by propulsion of the mucosa through the muscles by increased intraluminal pressure or weakening of the muscle wall—hence the name pulsion diverticula. These are normally acquired and seen in the mid and distal oesophagus.

- **Extraneous Impression on the Oesophagus**

Extraneous impression on the oesophagus can be caused by the left main bronchus (Fig. 11.21), left atrium, vessel traversing between the trachea and oesophagus (e.g., aberrant left subclavian artery), prominent aortic knuckle, a dilated descending aorta, an anomalous left or right subclavian artery and nodes/masses in the posterior mediastinum abutting the oesophagus. Other conditions which can cause an extraneous impression include adjoining large nodes, oesophageal duplication and other posterior mediastinal masses.

Nodes, usually tubercular, which are located in the carinal region below the tracheal bifurcation can abut and may burrow into the oesophageal wall, resulting in ulceration, fistula formation and narrowing.

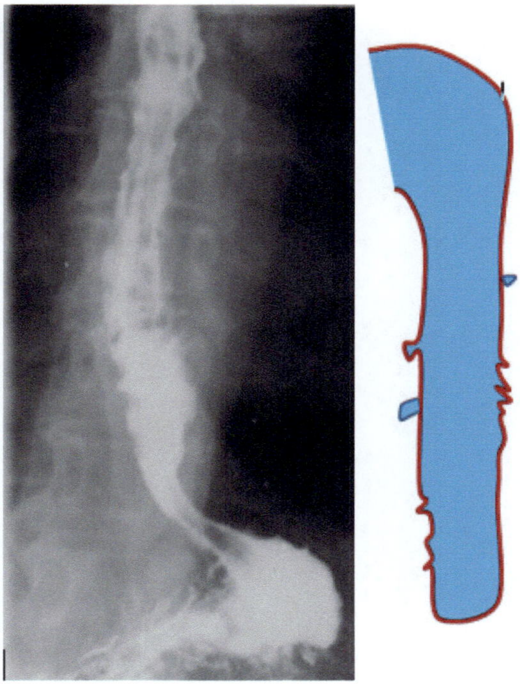

Fig. 11.20 Barium swallow and a pictorial diagram showing the presence of pseudodiverticula

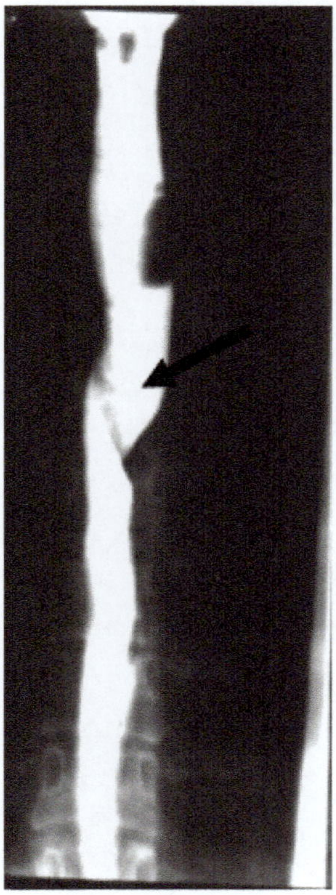

Fig. 11.21 Extraneous impression (arrow) on the oesophagus caused by the left main bronchus

The pharynx and oesophagus are important parts of the digestive tract and their lesions usually cause dysphagia or odynophagia (painful swallowing). The imaging findings demonstrated by barium studies may provide an answer to the cause of these symptoms.

References

1. Yadav S. A clinical and radiographic paradox in a case of barium aspiration. Cureus. 2022;14(8):e28370. https://doi.org/10.7759/cureus.28370.
2. Schmalfuss IM, Mancuso AA, Tart RP. Postcricoid region and cervical esophagus: normal appearance at CT and MR imaging. Radiology. 2000;214(1):237–46.
3. Wahi JE, Safdie FM. Esophageal duplication cysts: a clinical practice review. Mediastinum. 2023;25(7):1. https://doi.org/10.21037/med-22-33.
4. Lindholm EB, Hansbourgh F, Upp JR Jr, Cilloniz R, Lopoo J. Congenital esophageal diverticulum—a case report and review of literature. J Pediatr Surg. 2013;48(3):665–8. https://doi.org/10.1016/j.jpedsurg.2012.12.037. PMID: 23480930.

Stomach and Duodenum

12

Abstract

With the availability of upper GI endoscopy and CT scans, the indications for barium meal upper gastrointestinal (GI) study of the stomach and duodenum have declined. To a large extent, barium studies have been replaced by "Upper GI" (UGI) endoscopy and CT scans.

However, they are still requested by paediatric surgeons and sometimes by GI and bariatric surgeons. Therefore, it is important to know how to perform it well, as well as know the appearance of the structures seen in an upper gastrointestinal series and what diseases as well as post-operative sequelae look like.

Keywords

Barium studies · Upper GI series

Barium meal upper GI series are requested to study the gastroesophageal junction, the stomach, duodenal and proximal jejunal pathologies.

Barium studies help in evaluating post-surgical complications such as occurring after bariatric surgery, gastrojejunostomies, and to determine causes of gastric outflow obstruction, duodenal pathology, both congenital and acquired, as well as any other post-surgical situation. Very fine gastric mucosal lesions were picked up by the once popular a high-quality double contrast study of the stomach. In cases of post-operative leaks instead of barium, water soluble contrast medium should be used as barium may obscure the findings, if surgery is to be performed.

12.1 Techniques

Patients should be fasting for 4–6 h prior to barium studies in order to have an empty, residue-free stomach. This helps in proper evaluation of gastric mucosa. There is generally no restriction on drinking sips of clear water, especially in hot weather, except when examining cases presenting with gastric outlet pathology.

12.2 Upper GI Studies

There are two ways of performing barium studies of the stomach—a single and double contrast study.

In a single contrast study, initially, a small quantity, about 75 ccs of barium 15–25% weight by volume is given to the patient. The patient swallows a mouthful, which is observed under fluoroscopy, as it flows down the oral cavity through the pharynx and oesophagus into the stomach and duodenum. Thereafter more barium is given, if required. In a double-contrast barium study, a small quantity of high-density barium (150% weight by volume) is given. Air is intro-

R. Gothi, *Radiographic and Imaging Techniques for Radiology Residents and Technologists*,
https://doi.org/10.1007/978-981-96-4816-0_12

duced by using effervescent agents available in the form of granules or tablets. To prevent air bubbles from distorting the images, surfactant agents are also given. A well-performed study shows gastric mucosa in great detail and even subtle mucosal lesions, including early gastric cancers, can be detected. The positions in which the images are obtained are the same as in the single contrast study.

12.3 The Technique as Well as Some of the Positions Are Described as Under

Barium studies should always be done under fluoroscopic screening.

Screening commences as soon as the patient swallows one or two mouthfuls of barium. The flow of contrast is followed from the pharynx to the stomach. The stomach is evaluated in the supine and erect position, obtaining multiple images in right anterior oblique (RAO), AP, PA and lateral positions. The gastric fundus, body and pylorus are carefully examined for any abnormality.

Thereafter, the duodenum is examined in the anteroposterior (AP), posteroanterior (PA) and both oblique positions. This allows examination of the all parts of the duodenum. The study is continued till the proximal jejunal loops are filled and can be terminated at this point. If a small bowel follow-through study is also needed, then an additional 200 ml of barium is administered.

A single contrast study of the upper GI is a basic study. It may miss mucosal and small intraluminal lesions. If large volumes of barium are given, then even large intraluminal lesions may be obscured (Fig. 12.1). For this reason, the study must always be performed using a small quantity of barium and should preferably be a double contrast examination.

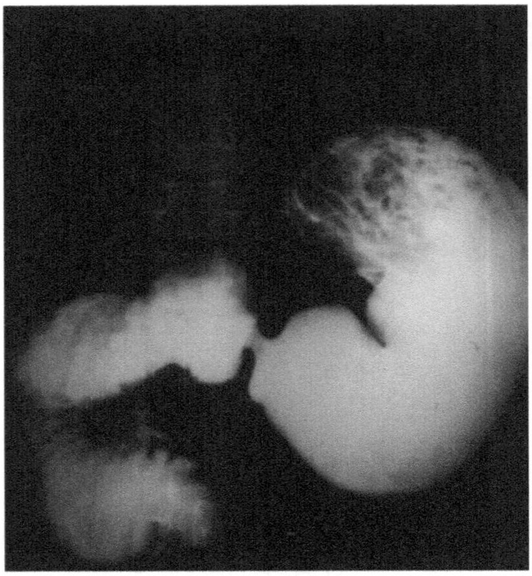

Fig. 12.1 A single contrast study of the upper GI. The barium administered is excessive and can mask both luminal and mural lesions

12.4 Some Cases of Barium Meal Upper GI Are Presented to Demonstrate the Value of This Technique

- **A case of gastric volvulus**: Gastric volvulus is malrotation of the stomach about its axis. The stomach can rotate about its short axis, which is called the mesenteric volvulus. It can also flip around its long axis, which is also known as organo-axial volvulus (Fig. 12.2). The patient, especially those having mesenterioaxial volvulus [1] may be asymptomatic. The common presentation is with symptoms such as abdominal pain and vomiting, especially if the rotation exceeds 180°. Plain X-rays of the abdomen, may show a distended single gas-filled stomach bubble in the organo-axial volvulus and two air fluid levels in mes-

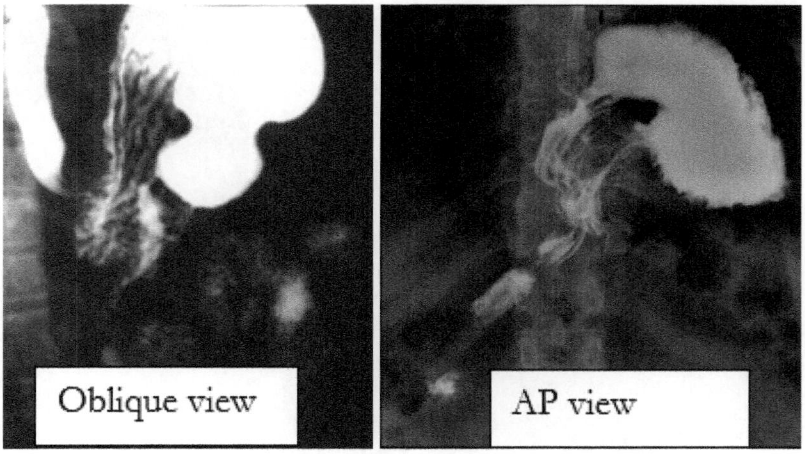

Fig. 12.2 An upper GI study demonstrating a mesentericoaxial gastric volvulus

entericoaxial volvulus. An upper GI endoscopy may suspect a volvulus. However, barium or CT findings are confirmatory. In the barium study, in patients having a mesentericoaxial volvulus, the pyloric antrum will be located above the gastric fundus [1]. In organoaxial volvulus, the stomach lies horizontal with the greater curvature lying superior to the lesser curvature.

- **A case of trichobezoar**: Bezoars, are ingested food materials, which stay in the stomach, causing distension and formation of a lump in long-standing cases. The common materials ingested are hairs, fruit and vegetable fibres [2]. A single contrast barium meal upper GI study using a small quantity of barium can easily and convincingly show the bezoar. Bezoars can also be easily suspected in a CT scan [2]. Ultrasonography will show an echogenic shadow in the upper abdomen, which may be mobile, depending upon its size. In this patient (Fig. 12.3) a single contrast study was performed, which shows the stomach filled with a mixed density soft tissue. On questioning the patient, a history of consistent trichobezoar was elicited.
- **A case of corrosive stricture of the stomach** (Fig. 12.4): The diagnosis of corrosive poisoning is based on the history of swallowing corrosives. These patients can develop strictures in the oesophagus and stomach. The purpose of performing a contrast study of the upper GI study is to demonstrate the extent of damage caused by the corrosive, to observe residual distensibility of the gastric lumen, obstruction, if any to the flow of the contrast and to demonstrate any fistula formation [3]. A sin-

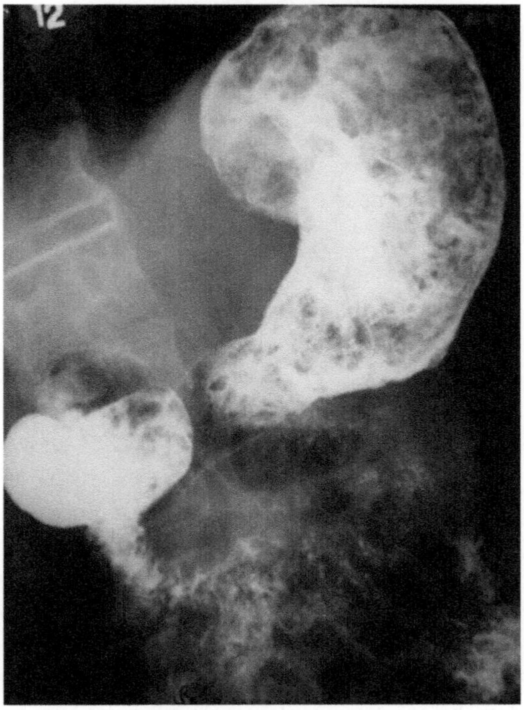

Fig. 12.3 Case of trichobezoar filling the stomach

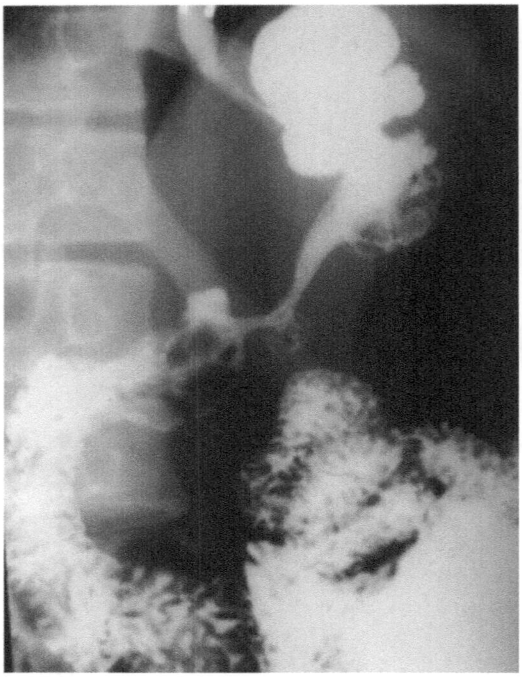

Fig. 12.4 A case of corrosive poisoning showing deformity of the stomach

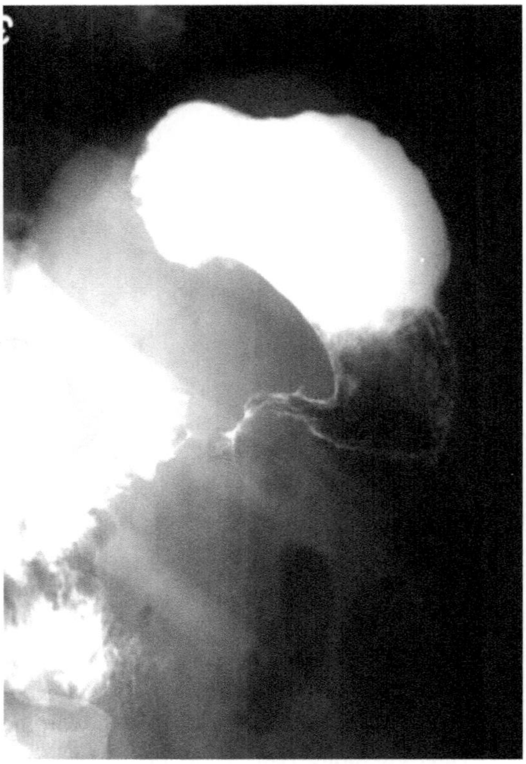

Fig. 12.5 A case of carcinoma pyloric region of the stomach

gle contrast barium study is sufficient to show narrowing and altered appearance of the distal stomach.

- **A case of carcinoma pyloric antrum.** The distal end of the stomach (Fig. 12.5) shows narrowing with ulcerations. In such an advanced case, a double contrast does not appear necessary. A single contrast study, performed after gastric lavage, enables easy visualization of the antral mass (Fig. 12.5).

The upper GI series are rarely performed these days having been replaced by other modalities. However, they are still needed in paediatric patients, post-operative cases and for the reasons demonstrated in this chapter. The technologist as well as the radiologist must learn the art of performing and interpreting this study.

References

1. Chin JZ, DeLappe E, McCarthy PA. Asymptomatic mesenteroaxial gastric volvulus and midgut malrotation in a 84 year old man; 2007. https://doi.org/10.1594/EURORAD/CASE.61042.
2. Ripollés T, García-Aguayo J, Martínez M-J, Gil P. Gastrointestinal bezoars: sonographic and CT characteristics. Am J Roentgenol. 2001;177(1):65–9.
3. Agarwal A, Srivastava DN, Madhusudhan KS. Corrosive injury of the upper gastrointestinal tract: the evolving role of a radiologist. Br J Radiol. 2020;93(1114):20200528. https://doi.org/10.1259/bjr.20200528.

The Small Bowel

13

Abstract

The small intestine forms the longest segment of the gastrointestinal (GI) tract. It elongates with age, reaching a length of approximately 22 feet in an adult. In this chapter, the reader will be introduced to the anatomy and conventional radiologic techniques for the evaluation of the small bowel loops. The reader will also be introduced to common pathological conditions affecting the small bowel using images from barium studies and CT scans.

Keywords

Jejunum · Ileum · Small bowel · Barium studies · CT scan · MRI

13.1 Brief Anatomy

The small bowel begins at the duodenojejunal junction (Fig. 13.1), which is located to the left of the pedicle of the L2 vertebral body. It lies anterior to the aorta and behind the body of the stomach.

The proximal small bowel loops, also known as the jejunal loops, are approximately 3 cm in width. Their mucosal folds, called "valvulae conniventes" have a herringbone appearance, which is seen when the loops are filled with air or positive contrast (barium or iodinated positive contrast). The distal small bowel loops are called "the ileal loop". They are smaller in calibre as compared to the jejunal loops and are featureless.

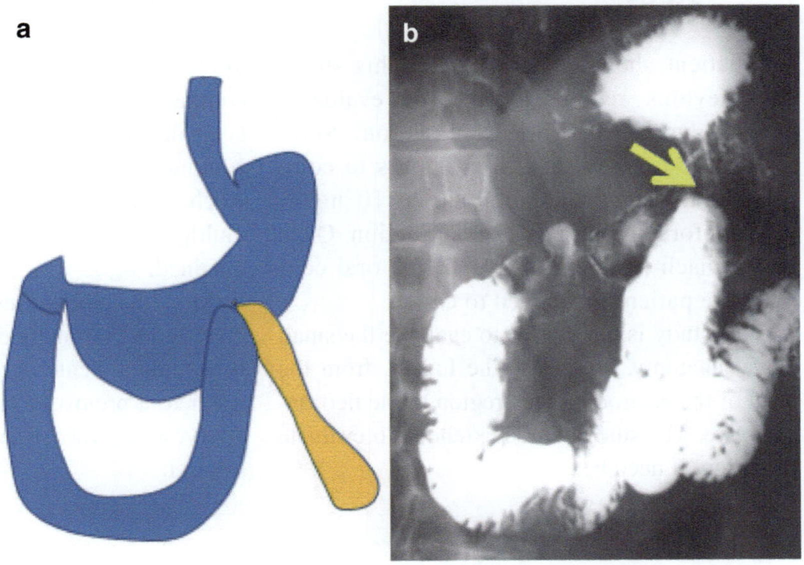

Fig. 13.1 Drawing (**a**) and oblique view of the barium meal study (**b**) showing the location of the duodenojejunal (DJ) junction

R. Gothi, *Radiographic and Imaging Techniques for Radiology Residents and Technologists*,
https://doi.org/10.1007/978-981-96-4816-0_13

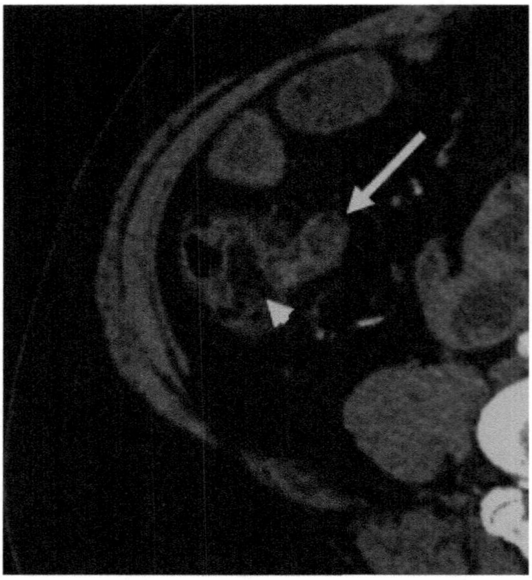

Fig. 13.2 A CT scan image of the abdomen, showing the ileocaecal junction (arrow). Note the fat surrounding the ileocaecal valve (arrowhead)

They terminate into the medial wall of the caecum, through an opening which is guarded by a valve called the ileocaecal valve (Fig. 13.2). This valve is surrounded by fat, which helps in recognizing the ileocaecal junction.

13.2 Barium Meal Follow-Through Study

The patient should be fasting for this study. All previous records should be evaluated before commencing the examination. Since the procedure may take a few hours to complete, a tablet of Metoclopramide 10 mg is given before beginning the examination. Once the stomach is almost empty of the oral contrast, the patient is allowed to eat.

This study is performed to evaluate the small bowel anatomy, especially the lumen, from the level of the gastroduodenal region to the ileocaecal valve. The study can be extended to evaluate the colon, if need be.

Usually, about one to two cups or a glass of about 250 ml of barium suspension is needed for the study. The patient is asked to drink it slowly in order not to feel sick.

The study should be performed under fluoroscopy. The flow of barium down the oesophagus should be observed. A film of the stomach and duodenum may be obtained. Thereafter, serial films of the small bowel are obtained with the patient lying in the prone position. The prone position helps in maintaining an uninterrupted column of barium throughout the small bowel. In the supine position, barium is squirted out intermittently by gastric contractions. The continuity of the barium column is not maintained and it appears segmented.

Barium studies of the small bowel are commonly a single contrast study, where only barium is administered. Small bowel enterography is another method of evaluating the intestines. This can be either a single or a double contrast study (also called "Double Contrast Barium enteroclysis (DCBE)". Both studies are performed by introducing an enteroclysis tube, also called a "Bilbao Dotter tube" (Fig. 13.3). This tube is inserted through the nose and negotiated under fluoroscopic control till its tip crosses the DJ junction, which is the site of attachment of the Ligament of Treitz. Positioning the tip of the tube beyond this level prevents contrast from refluxing into the stomach. In a single contrast study, only diluted barium is introduced while in a double contrast study, performed under fluoroscopic control, a mixture of diluted barium and air are continuously administered, till the ileum is reached. As the barium goes down the intestine, multiple films of the jejunum and ileum are obtained.

Since the tube causes discomfort to the patient, there is another method which can be performed. It is called "enterography". It entails adding water to a premixed composition of barium and effervescent powder and quickly swallowing the solution.

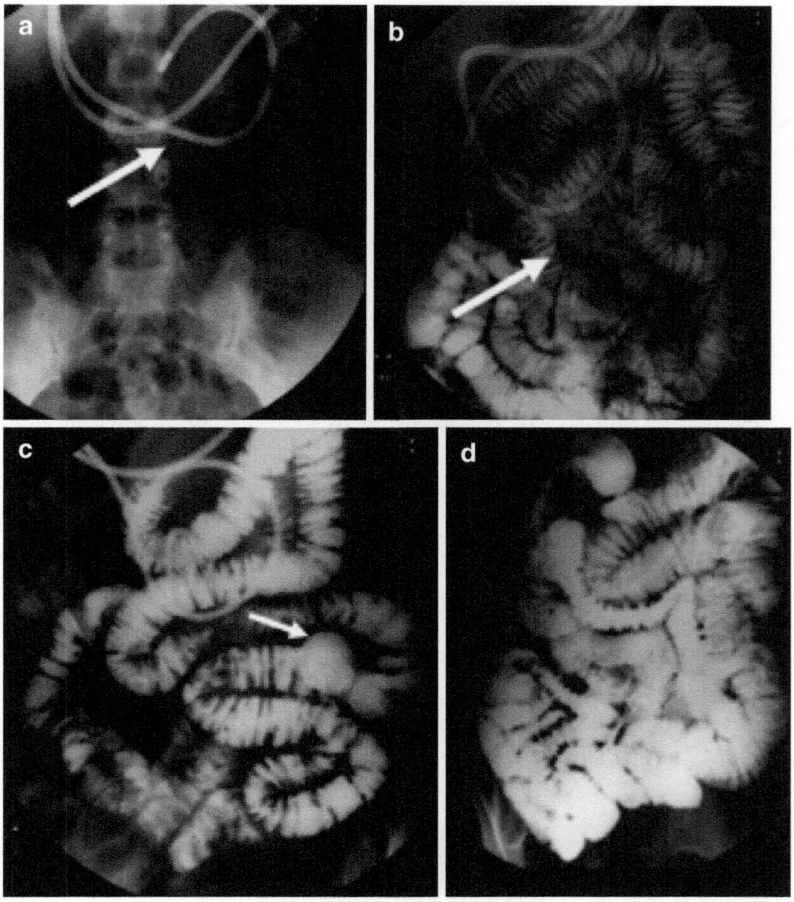

Fig. 13.3 Single contrast enterography using Bilbao Dotter tube (**a**, **b**). The tube has crossed the area of the ligamentum Treitz (**a**). This reduces the chances of barium refluxing into the stomach. Figure (**b**) shows adequate distension of the jejunal loops with a nice demonstration of the valvulae conniventes. Note the presence of jejunal diverticulum (arrow in "**c**"). Image "**d**" is a case of eosinophilic enteritis showing thickened mucosal folds

13.3 How to Evaluate the Small Bowel in a Barium Meal Follow-Through

- **Start by examining the position of the bowel loops**. Most proximal jejunal loops will lie to the left of the mid-line. The rest of the jejunal loops and the proximal ileal loop will spread on either side of the spine in the mid-abdomen. The distal ileal loops will extend from the umbilical region downwards into the pelvis. The terminal ileum will rise from the pelvis, reach the right iliac fossa and open into the caecum through the ileo-caecal valve.
- **Look for the relationship of the bowel loops with one another.** Most small bowel loops will be close to or parallel to one another with their lumen being separated by the intervening walls. The bowel loops can also be separated from one another by the intervening peritoneal fat. If the gap between the bowel loops is unusually wide, it could be due to an abnormally thickened bowel wall, exuberant fat interposed between the bowel loops, the presence of masses, enlarged nodes or fluid collection. This observation will need further evaluation by cross-sectional imaging.
- **Make a note of the transit time of barium** from the stomach to the caecum. It should not exceed 4 h. Too rapid a transit could either be due to intestinal hurry or a fistulous communication with other small bowel loops or the large bowel. In the latter case, some small bowel segments may escape opacification, barium having entered the distal segments of the small bowel or the colon through the fistulous communication. This is why a barium

study should be performed under supervision, especially in cases of Crohn's disease, where fistulas are known to occur.

- **Examine the calibre of the small bowel loops.** The calibre of the jejunum should not be more than 3 cm and the ileum 2 cm [1]. In fact, the 3-6-9 rule is a good way to remember the maximum normal diameter of the bowel loops [2]. 3 cm is the small bowel calibre, 6 cm is the large bowel calibre, 6 mm is the calibre of the appendix and 9 cm is the maximum calibre of the caecum. An increase in calibre, especially, if persisting in several images obtained during the course of the study, is abnormal. An abnormally dilated loop suggests likelihood of an obstructive lesion just beyond the dilated segment. This segment (and not the dilated proximal segment) is the real problem. It should be carefully searched for in every case of abnormal intestinal dilatation.
- **After the calibre, look at the mucosal pattern.** The jejunum will show valvulae conniventes (Fig. 13.4), while the ileum will normally be featureless. If the ileum shows mucosal folds, it is called jejunization of the ileum, which is seen in Celiac disease. Examine the folds of the jejunum carefully. They should be long and sharp. If they are short, thick (> 3 mm) and blunted, see if the thickening is generalized or localized. Generalized thickening can be due to any condition causing fluid accumulation in the bowel wall. These could be vascular, oedema, protein deficiency, or lymphedema. Localized thickening could be due to infections, infestations, infiltrations and invasions by malignancies. In such cases, the mucosal pattern will be irregular in appearance.
- **Finally, evaluate the lumen for any abnormal shadow within it**. These shadows could be due to food bolus in transit, held-up bolus due to a distal obstruction, calculus dropped from the gall bladder into the intestine through a fistulous communication, radio-opaque tablets, enteroliths, foreign bodies, lipomas, polyps or masses (both benign and malignant). These intraluminal lesions may be asymptomatic or cause pain and obstruction, which is especially true if it is intussusception, a congenital intraluminal obstructive lesion such as a web, a drug-induced membrane (NSAID-related ulcerations and membranes in the small bowel), polyps or a bunch of roundworms.

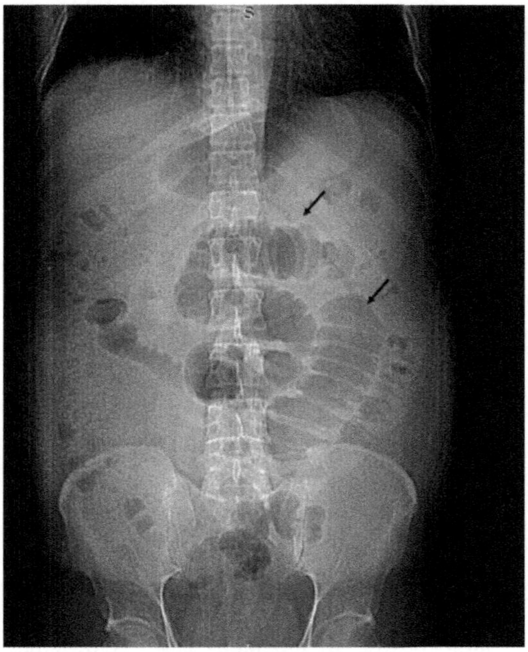

Fig. 13.4 Scanogram of a CT scan showing prominent thick valvulae conniventes of a distended gas filled jejunal loops (arrow)

13.4 Small Bowel Pathology

13.4.1 Positional Anomalies

The small bowel can be malrotated or non-rotated (Fig. 13.5).

In a normal situation, when the small bowel returns to the abdomen during the 10–12-week foetal age, it normally completes a 270° counterclockwise rotation around the axis formed by the superior mesenteric vessels and occupies its normal position inside the abdomen. The proximal or arterial midgut (small bowel loops) lies to the left of the midline, and the distal or post-arterial midgut (caecum and rest of the large intestine) is to the right.

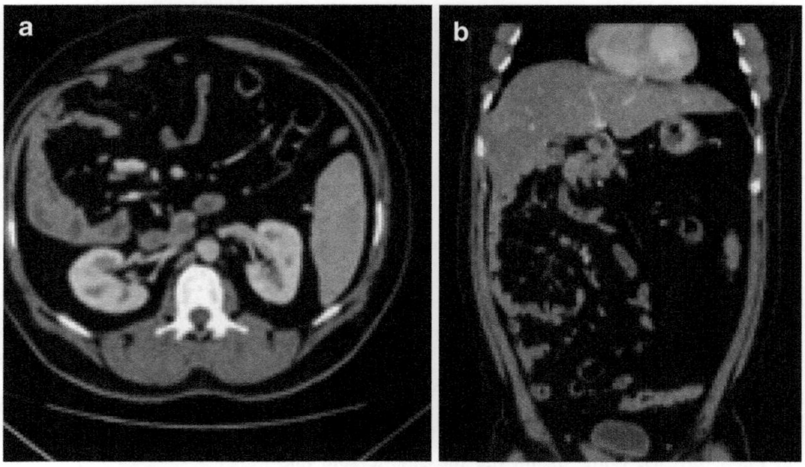

Fig. 13.5 Axial (**a**) and coronal scans (**b**) scans of the abdomen show small bowel loops located to the right of the midline, a feature compatible with malrotation

In malrotation, the small bowel loops do not rotate beyond 180° [3]. In this position, the duodenojejunal junction (DJ junction) and small bowel loops are to the right and the large gut including the caecum are to the left of the midline, the latter being found in the upper abdomen to the left of the DJ junction.

In non-rotation, the midgut rotates until about 90° [4]. Therefore, the DJ junction and proximal midgut lie anterior and to the right of the superior mesenteric vessels, and the distal midgut lies anterior and to the left of the axis formed by the mesenteric vessels. The caecum is located in the mid-abdomen.

The relationship of the superior mesenteric vessels can be observed in a CT scan or by ultrasound and is important to identify suspected cases of intestinal malrotation. Normally, the superior mesenteric artery (SMA) lies to the left of the Superior Mesenteric Vein (SMV). In malrotation, this relationship alters, with the SMA now lying to the right of the SMV.

Intestinal malrotation can be accompanied by volvulus and the presence of abnormal mesenteric bands, which can cause obstruction. One of these bands is a Ladd's band, which, in cases of malrotation, attaches the caecal pole, located to the left of the DJ junction, to the peritoneal fat planes in the right subphrenic area. This can cause upper GI obstruction.

Intestinal position anomalies can be easily seen in barium meal upper GI and small bowel studies. In the upper GI series, the position of the DJ junction can be ascertained. If the third and fourth parts of the duodenum turn back towards the right flank, it is malrotation. The follow-through study can show the location of the rest of the small bowel loops as well as the position of the caecum. A barium enema can also tell the position of the caecum, which will be abnormal in case of malrotation and non rotation.

13.4.2 Bowel Wall Lesions

Lesions of the small bowel could be extramural, mural, mucosal or intraluminal. Extramural lesions are those that invade the small bowel wall from outside (Fig. 13.6).

- Extramural lesions can be lymphangiomas, lymphomatous or peritoneal deposits and rarely gastrointestinal stomal tumours. These can involve the serosal surface of the bowel loops.
- Mural lesions are those which arise from the wall of the bowel loops. Mural lesions could be present as mass-forming lesions such as gastrointestinal stromal tumours, a carcinoma or lymphoma (Fig. 13.7).

Mural lesions can also be non-malignant involving the bowel loops diffusely or focally and causing luminal narrowing.

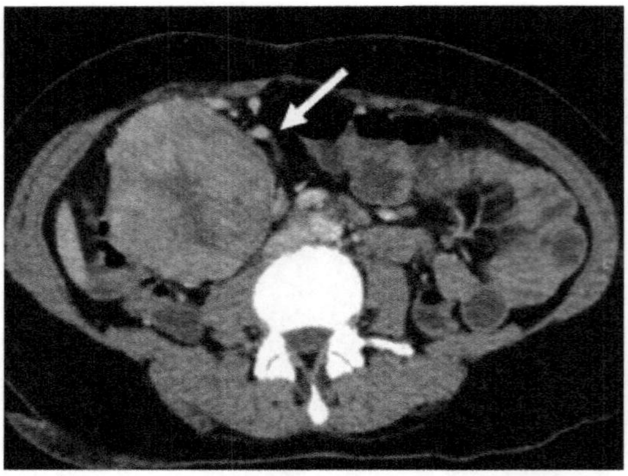

Fig. 13.6 CT scan of the abdomen, showing an extramural mass (arrow), lying within the mesenteric fold and compressing the adjoining small bowel loops

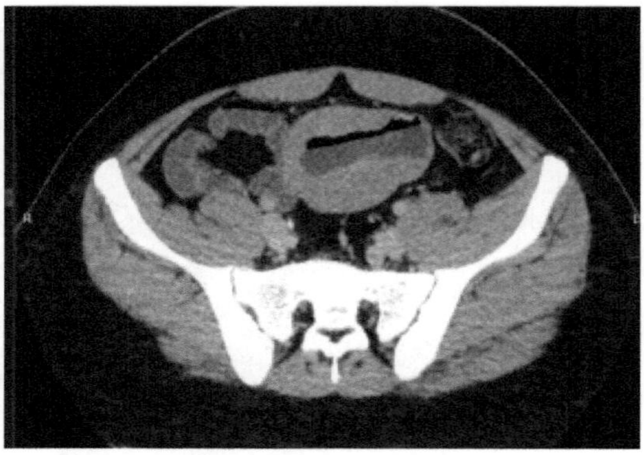

Fig. 13.7 A case of non-Hodgkin's lymphoma causing circumferential bowel wall (mural) thickening

- Long segment mural thickening is usually seen in a patient having exudative ascites, allergic angioedema (Fig. 13.8), venous occlusion, following radiation as well as autoimmune and inflammatory disorders [5].

Short segment thickening could be due to focal inflammatory or infective lesions or malignancies.

Mucosal pathologies such as celiac disease, polyps, post-inflammatory/post-infiltrative diseases and fat-depositing conditions can result in changes ranging from atrophy to hypertrophy to distortion of valvulae conniventes of the jejunum, (the ileal mucosa is normally featureless, hence may not show much change. However, jejunization of the ileum can happen, if the jejunum, for some reason, is short or there is evidence of celiac disease.

Intraluminal lesions could range from masses to foreign bodies. The gut lumen, therefore, must be carefully evaluated. The location of the foreign body must be mentioned in the radiology report (Fig. 13.9).

Fluid collection within the small bowel loops due to paralytic ileus can cause distension of both the small bowel loops and large bowel loops. These loops show air-fluid levels. The fluid levels in cases of the ileus are almost in the same horizontal plane in an erect X-ray of the abdomen or an axial CT scan. In those patients where there is an obstructive lesion, the loops, just proximal to the site of obstruction, are distended with fluid and retained food residue, producing what is called as the "positive fecal matter" sign in a CT scan.

The small bowel mucosa can also prolapse and protrude outside through the bowel wall forming a diverticula. These can be single or multiple and are most commonly seen in the duodenum and jejunum (Fig. 13.10). A congenital diverticulum called Meckel's diverticulum may also be seen in a barium study or a CT scan of the abdomen. These diverticula can have heterotrophic gastric mucosa and pancreatic tissue. Meckel's diverticula follows the rule of 2, that is, it is seen in 2% of the population, is 2 inches in length and is 2 feet away from the ileocaecal junction (Fig. 13.11).

Amongst the various causes of obstructive lesions of the small bowel, is intussusception. This can be transient or fixed. Usually, it is the fixed type like an ileocolic or ileoileal intussusception, which causes acute obstruction.

Transient, non-obstructive intussusceptions are often seen in the jejunum. Fixed obstructive intussusceptions can be due to prominent Peyer's patches, roundworm infestations and mucosal tumours such as lipoma (Fig. 13.12).

Amongst stricture/stenosis forming lesions, granulomatous diseases (Fig. 13.13), especially tuberculosis is one of the most common aetiologies. A stricture should be suspected in patients presenting with intestinal obstruction. Most tubercular strictures are longstanding and cause

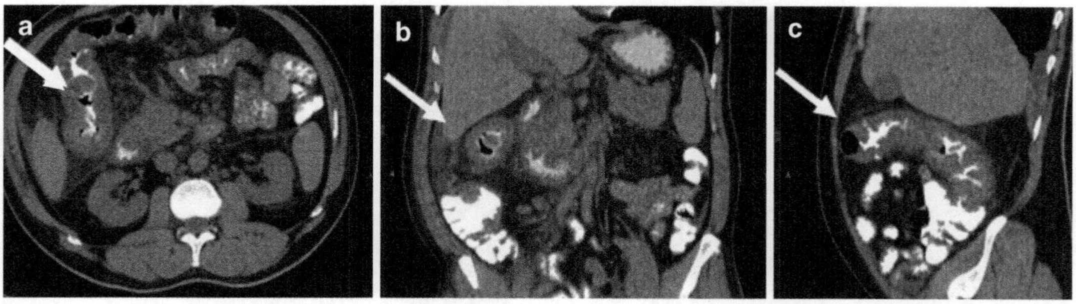

Fig. 13.8 Axial (**a**), coronal (**b**) and sagittal (**c**) sections of abdominal CT. There is diffuse inflammatory small bowel disease causing concentric mural thickening with mucosal irregularity and luminal narrowing (arrow)

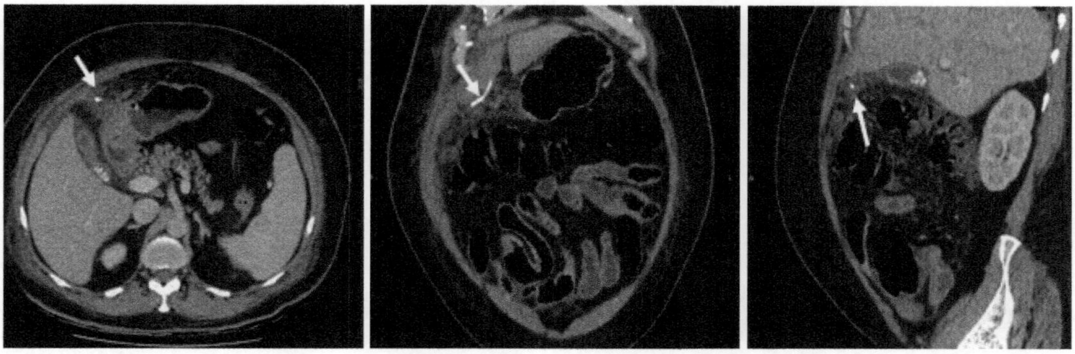

Fig. 13.9 Axial, coronal and sagittal sections of a case of fishbone perforation (arrow) from the stomach wall into the subhepatic space

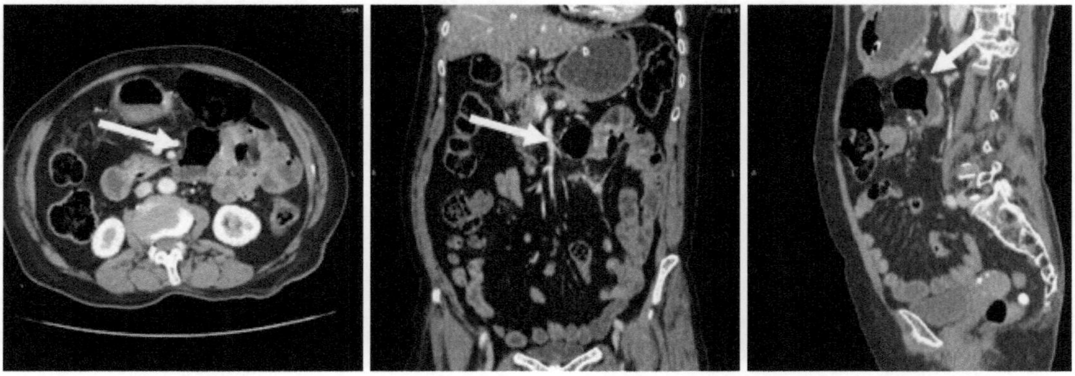

Fig. 13.10 Axial, coronal and sagittal sections show a thin-walled air containing jejunal diverticulum, protruding through the bowel wall (arrow)

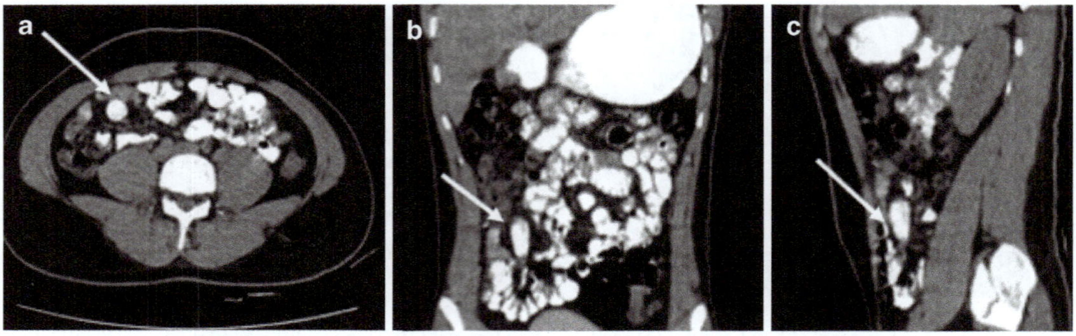

Fig. 13.11 A CT scan of the abdomen, shows a Meckel's diverticulum (arrow), in axial (**a**), coronal (**b**) and sagittal planes (**c**)

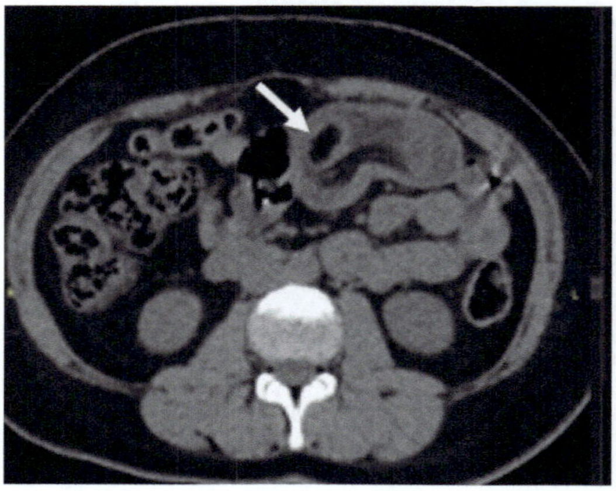

Fig. 13.12 An axial section of the abdomen showing a lipoma (arrow), associated with a jejunojejunal intussusception

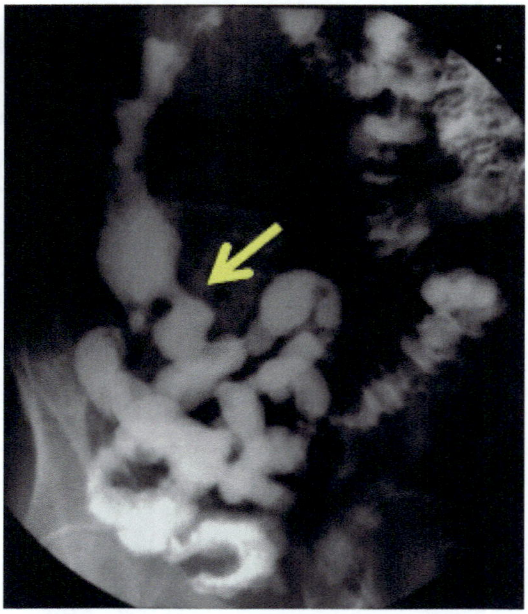

Fig. 13.13 A case of ileocaecal Kochs show in a barium meal follow through study. Note the deformed IC valve and caecum (arrow)

chronic abdominal pain. However, they can present acutely if an enterolith or a gallstone occludes the stenotic segment completely. Strictures/stenosis can be single or multiple and can involve any segment of the small bowel. There may be associated mesenteric nodal enlargement.

Tuberculosis can also present as an abdominal cocoon (Fig. 13.14). This is a cluster of small bowel loops encapsulated within a chronic inflamed peritoneal sac. This condition is also known as sclerosing mesenteritis and may be non-tubercular in aetiology. A cocoon can also form if the bowel loops enter into an internal hernial sac.

It is quite obvious that the small bowel is a difficult area to investigate by conventional methods. Often a CT scan is needed to evaluate it. Orally administered contrast may be required in some cases, especially in those who have been recently operated and are suspected to have an anastomotic leak. However, pathological small bowel loops are almost always recognizable in a CT scan even without the use of oral contrast. Routine use of oral contrast is, therefore not necessary unless, there is a specific indication.

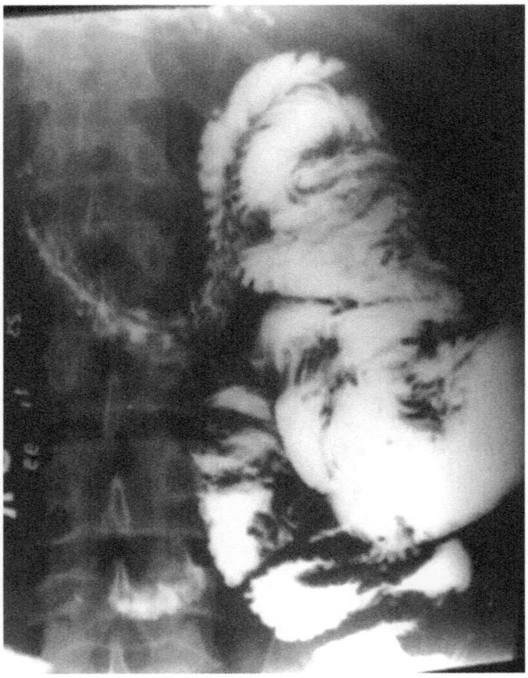

Fig. 13.14 Barium meal follow-through showing clumped small bowel loops forming a cocoon

References

1. Cronin CG, Delappe E, Lohan DG, Roche C, Murphy JM. Normal small bowel wall characteristics on MR enterography. Eur J Radiol. 2010;75(2):207–11. https://doi.org/10.1016/j.ejrad.2009.04.066.
2. Hacking C, Iqbal S, Saber M, et al. 3-6-9 rule (bowel). Radiopaedia.org. https://doi.org/10.53347/rID-66259.
3. Pickhardt PJ, Bhalla S. Intestinal malrotation in adolescents and adults: spectrum of clinical and imaging features. Am J Roentgenol. 2002;179(6):1429–35.
4. Gaillard F, Sharma R, Murphy A, et al. Intestinal malrotation. Radiopaedia.org. https://doi.org/10.53347/rID-1643.
5. Macari M, Megibow AJ, Balthazar EJ. A pattern approach to the abnormal small bowel: observations at MDCT and CT enterography. AJR Am J Roentgenol. 2007;188(5):1344–55. https://doi.org/10.2214/AJR.06.0712.

The Large Bowel

14

Abstract

The large bowel includes the caecum, the ascending colon, the hepatic flexure, the transverse colon, the splenic flexure, descending colon, the sigmoid, the rectum and the anal canal. It can be affected by several illnesses ranging from infectious disorders to inflammatory and vascular pathologies, granulomatous diseases and malignancies. Diseases of the large bowel are also more common than those affecting the rest of the gastrointestinal tract. Many large intestinal pathologies are visible in the conventional radiograph of the abdomen, barium studies as well as in CT and MRI of the abdomen. Pathological changes affecting the large bowel walls can also be visualized by ultrasonography.

This chapter will explore the large bowel using both conventional barium studies as well as images from other modalities to provide the readers with basic information about this very important region of the alimentary tract.

Keywords

Large bowel · Caecum · Colon · Rectum · Anal canal · Barium enema · CT · MRI · USG

We will first discuss the anatomy, followed by ways of investigating the large bowel using different imaging techniques, then look at the normal appearance and examine some of the common pathologies, affecting the large gut.

- **The caecum**: This is the widest part of the large intestine, and can reach a maximum diameter of 9 cm [1]. It extends from the ileocaecal (IC) junction downwards over a depth of 6 cm, ending as a pouch (Fig. 14.1) The appendix arises from its posteromedial wall and is located 2 cm below the ileocaecal junction [2].

  It is a large structure which acts as a reservoir or a sump, meant for temporarily holding faecal contents, till they are moved out and evacuated.

  The appendix, arising from the caecal pole, is a blind-ending tubular, aperistaltic structure, approximately 6–8 mm in diameter and of varying length. It can be retrocaecal, paracolic, abdominal or pelvic in location. It may contain a calcified or non-calcified appendicolith, may show air within and is generally not opacified with barium.
- **The colon**: Beyond the IC junction, the caecum continues upwards as the ascending colon. The ascending colon, on reaching the liver,

R. Gothi, *Radiographic and Imaging Techniques for Radiology Residents and Technologists*,
https://doi.org/10.1007/978-981-96-4816-0_14

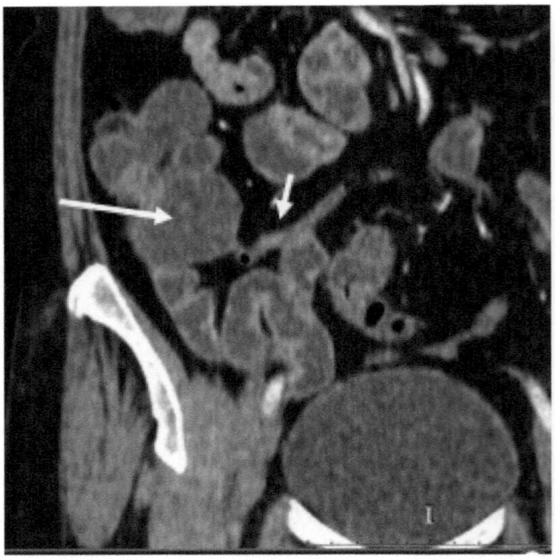

Fig. 14.1 The caecum (long arrow) and appendix (short arrow)

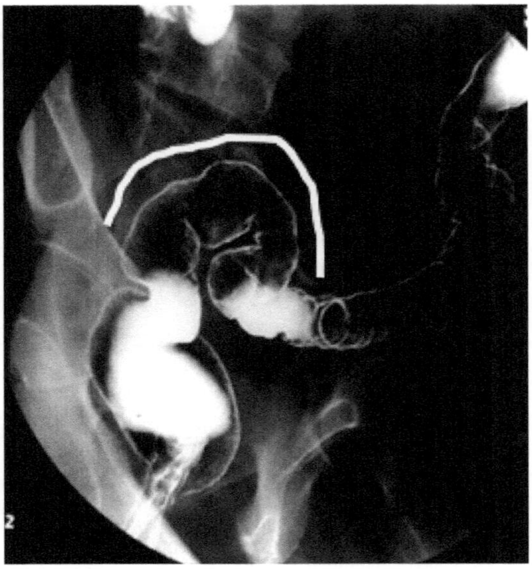

Fig. 14.2 A double contrast study showing the pelvic colon curve backwards towards the sacrum to form the signed colon (curved line)

folds beneath it to form the hepatic flexure which leads to the transverse colon. This is an anteriorly located loop, extending across the abdomen, strung between the hepatic and splenic flexures of the colon. It can be located (suspended) anywhere from the level of the diaphragm to the pelvis. It has a mesentery, which provides it with mobility. The flexure at the distal end of the transverse colon called the splenic flexure, lies below the spleen and is suspended by the phrenicocolic ligament. From here begins the descending colon, which reaches the pelvis.

- **Sigmoid colon**: In the pelvis, the colon turns backwards towards the sacrum to form the sigmoid colon (Fig. 14.2). The sigmoid colon is suspended by its mesentery and leads to the rectum. The rectum lies in the concavity of the sacrum and joins the anal canal. The anal canal opens in the perineal region behind the perineal body at the anal verge. It remains contracted most of the time due to the sphincteric action of the anal canal, opening during the act of defecation.
- The colon is surrounded by three muscle ribbons, which are called the taenia coli and are responsible for the formation of folds, called the haustral folds. These haustral folds help in storing fecal contents, absorption of fluid from the faecal residue and in controlling the forward propulsion of the faecal contents. They differ from the valvulae conniventes of the small bowel. They are large and blind-ending pouches forming an extension of the colonic lumen while the valvulae conniventes are sharp closely approximated mucosal folds protruding into the jejunal lumen. They increase the surface area of the small bowel for absorption of nutrients in the ingested food. Unlike colonic haustra, which merge with the colonic lumen and may not be well seen when the colon is distended, valvulae conniventes are always seen.

  At this point, it is important to note that the appendix, transverse colon, sigmoid colon and superior part of the rectum, which is close to the sacrum and is just beyond the sigmoid colon, are intraperitoneal structures. The caecum, right and left colon, as well as the inferior part of the rectum and anal canal, are retroperitoneal structures.
- **The ano-rectum**:

  The anatomy of the anorectal region needs to be recounted in some detail.

  The sigmoid colon curves backwards from the pelvic colon towards the sacral spine to form the rectosigmoid junction. The bend can also be appreciated in the AP view and better still in the oblique and lateral views (Fig. 14.3).

The rectum is located within the concavity of the sacrum (Fig. 14.4) and has an approximate length between 10 and 15 cm. The rectum has multiple side-ways bends (Fig. 14.5), which increases its capacity.

- **Parts of the rectum:**

  The rectum consists of three parts (Fig. 14.6).

  The upper pelvic part of the rectum is intraperitoneal and located approximately 10 cm above the anal verge. It lies above the pelvic diaphragm (levator ani muscles) and bends forward to join the sigmoid colon.

  The middle and distal parts are extraperitoneal in location. The distal part, which leads into the anal canal, is less than 6 cm above the anal verge [3]. It first curves forward, then angulates slightly backwards, forming the anorectal angle and enters the anal canal which opens behind the central perineal tendon to terminate at the anal verge.

  The rectum is surrounded by fat on all sides. The uppermost intraperitoneal part is surrounded by the mesorectal fat which contains blood vessels, lymphatics and nodes. Here the peritoneal reflection [4] turns forward and arches over the bladder dome. This results in making the remaining segments of the rectum, extraperitoneal. The fat surrounding the anorectum below the pelvic diaphragm (formed by the levator ani muscles) is in the ischiorectal fossa proximally and ischioanal fossa distally. Posteriorly, is the presacral fat (Fig. 14.7).

  The anal canal is approximately 4 cm in length and is thicker than the rectum. This is because it has an internal sphincter, which is a continuation of the inner circular and outer longitudinal muscles of the anorectal wall, and an external sphincter, which is the downward continuation of the puborectalis muscle of the pelvic diaphragm. It opens externally through the anal verge in the perineum in front of the coccyx. The anal canal is normally closed under the action of the internal and external sphincters. During the act of defecation, these sphincters relax, thereby allowing the anal canal to expand and let the faecal contents pass out.

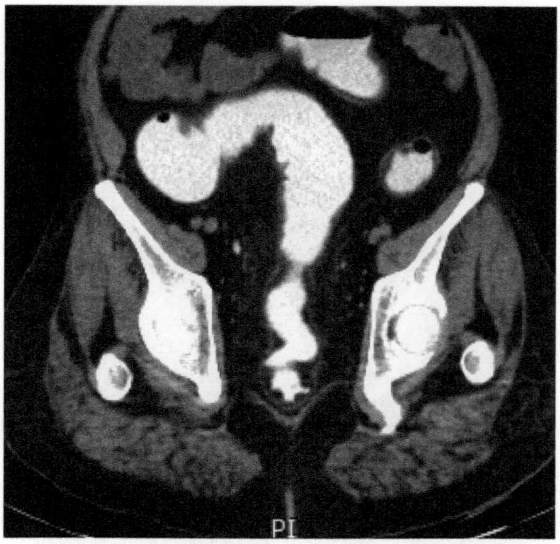

Fig. 14.3 Reconstructed CT image. The rectosigmoid region. The rectum lies in front of the sacrum while the sigmoid curves anteriorly away from the sacrum

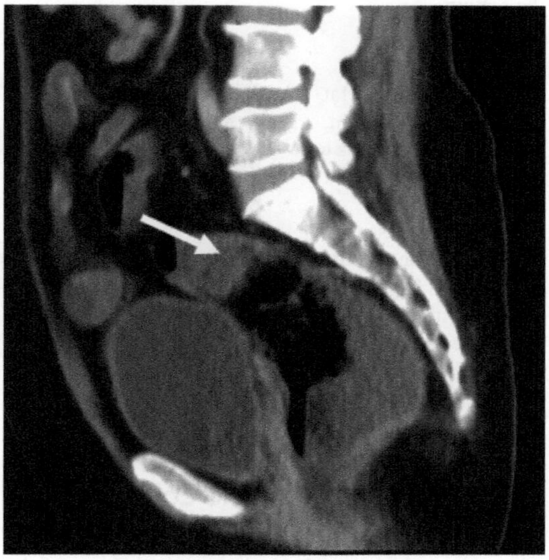

Fig. 14.4 Sagittal reconstruction of CT scan of the pelvis, showing how the rectum lies within the concavity of the sacrum. Above the urinary bladder, it is seen bending forward to meet the sigmoid colon (not shown in this image)

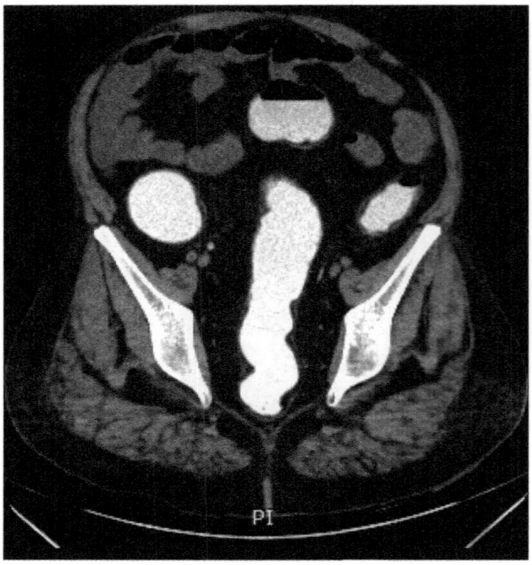

Fig. 14.5 Reconstructed image of CT scan of the pelvis with rectal contrast. Note the multiple sideways bends of the rectum

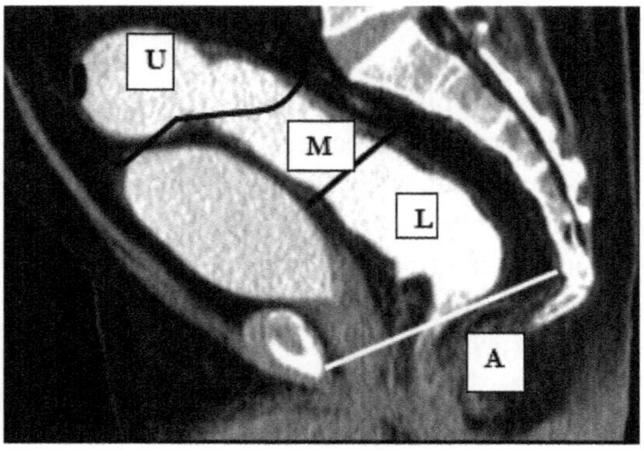

Fig. 14.6 Parts of the rectum are shown in the sagittal reformatted image of CT pelvis. Upper rectum (U) is enclosed by the perineum. Middle rectum (M) and lower rectum (L) are extraperitoneal. Below the straight line between the pubic symphysis and the sacrococcygeal region, is the anorectal region, which shows a bend, leading into the anal canal (A)

Fig. 14.7 Presacral fat pad (**a**) and outlined in (**b**). This region needs to be careful evaluated for the presence of any disease. It increases in width when the rectum contracts, as happens in patients with chronic ulcerative colitis

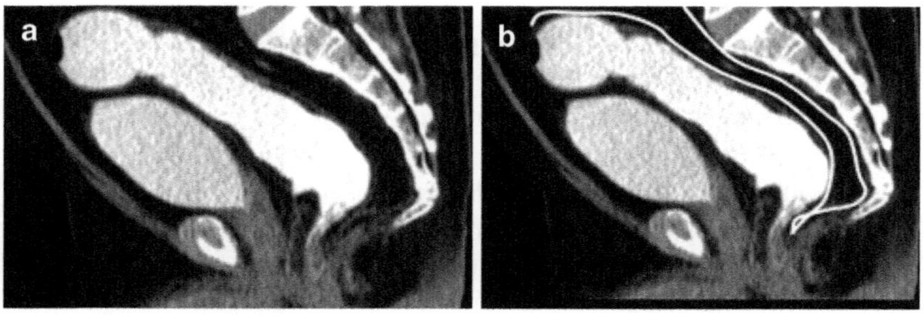

14.1 Evaluation of the Colon

The colon can be evaluated as a continuum of the barium meal follow-through study. The orally administered barium enters the colon through the ileocaecal valve and gradually reaches the anorectal region. However, this study does not distend the colon and is unable to provide adequate information about luminal and mucosal pathology. Hence, although it works well for evaluating the ileocaecal region and sometimes the colon, but by itself, it is not a complete or recommended study for the evaluation of the large bowel. A barium meal follow-through should also not be performed if there is suspicion of or a known colonic obstruction. Barium will accumulate proximal to the obstruction, thereby causing further obstruction. It is also likely to spill into the peritoneal cavity during surgical resection.

The colon should be evaluated by a barium enema study. The study can be a single-contrast or a double-contrast examination (Fig. 14.8).

Ideally, a double contrast barium enema should be performed after a thorough cleansing of the colon. In a single contrast barium study, diluted barium is introduced per-rectally through an enema tube. Thereafter, by turning the patient around in various positions, on the X-ray table itself, barium is maneuvered into different parts of the colon till it reaches the ileocaecal (IC)

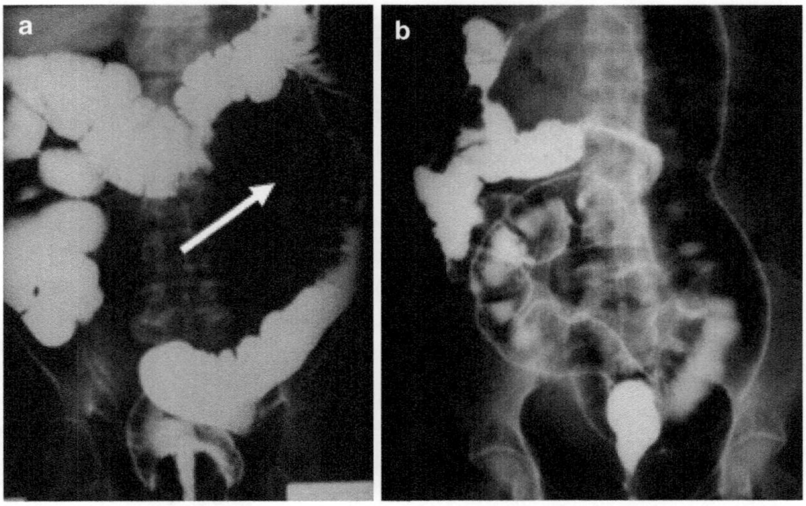

Fig. 14.8 A single (**a**) and double contrast barium enema (**b**) of two different patients. The single contrast study shows an impression on the descending colon (arrow) caused by a mass in the left flank. The double contrast study of another patient shows a normal appearance of the gas-filled left colon with a contrast-outlined mucosal layer

junction. The quantity of contrast introduced is determined by the patient's capacity to retain barium without evacuating and without undue discomfort. This method allows visualization of large lesions but obscures smaller mucosal or intraluminal lesions.

In a double contrast barium enema (Fig. 14.9), the quantity of barium used is small and it is pushed onward by air insufflation. The contrast coats the bowel mucosa and the infused air, produces a double contrast study, which allows adequate visualization of small ulcers and polyps, which would otherwise be obscured in a single contrast study.

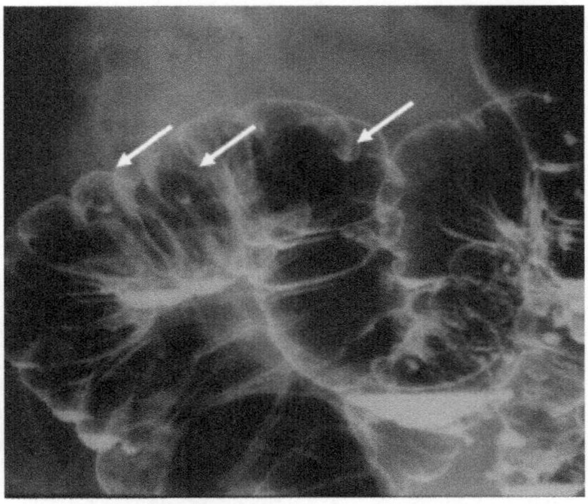

Fig. 14.9 A double contrast barium enema demonstrating colonic polyp (arrows)

The other ways to evaluate the colon are CT scans with rectally administered neutral, negative (air) or positive contrast. MRI can also be used to evaluate the colon. The colon being located along the flanks and in the pelvis can also be examined by ultrasound. The rectum and anal canal can be examined both by transabdominal and transrectal ultrasound.

The colon is vulnerable to various diseases, both benign as well as malignant. We shall discuss some common diseases, which can affect the colon.

These include infective and inflammatory disorders such as amoebiasis, bacterial infections, granulomatous pathology, especially tuberculosis, and inflammatory bowel diseases including both Crohn's disease and ulcerative colitis. Other benign pathologies include Hirschsprung's disease, anorectal malformation, intussusception, intestinal polyps, post-surgical causes and diverticular diseases.

14.2 Colonic Malignancies

Colonic cancers are a common cause of hospital admissions. Patients may present with altered bowel habits, abdomen pain, loss of weight, presence of a mass, rectal bleeding or features of intestinal obstruction. These lesions can be detected by ultrasound, barium enema and CT (Figs. 14.10, 14.11, and 14.12) scans. Once detected, they are subjected to histopathological evaluation, usually through sigmoidoscopy or colonoscopy biopsy. Large lesions can be detected in a single contrast study. Smaller lesions may need a double contrast barium enema or CT colonography/conventional colonoscopy. The advantage of the latter is the ability to obtain tissue for histopathological evaluation.

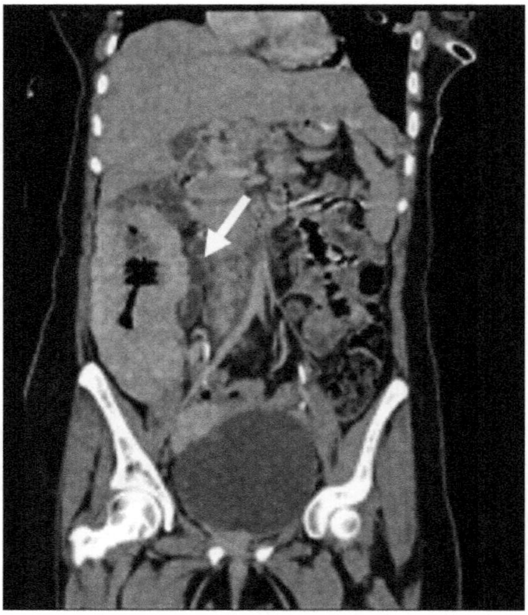

Fig. 14.10 Coronal CT scan showing a large soft tissue right colonic mass (arrow). This mass is compatible with a malignancy. It would be difficult to decide which type of malignancy it is based only on imaging findings

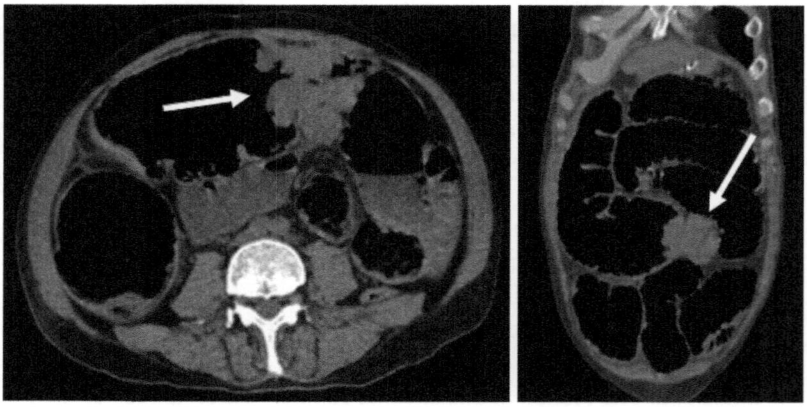

Fig. 14.11 Axial and coronal non-contrast CT scan of the abdomen showing a lobulated solid mass in the distal transverse colon, obstructing and causing proximal colonic distension (arrows)

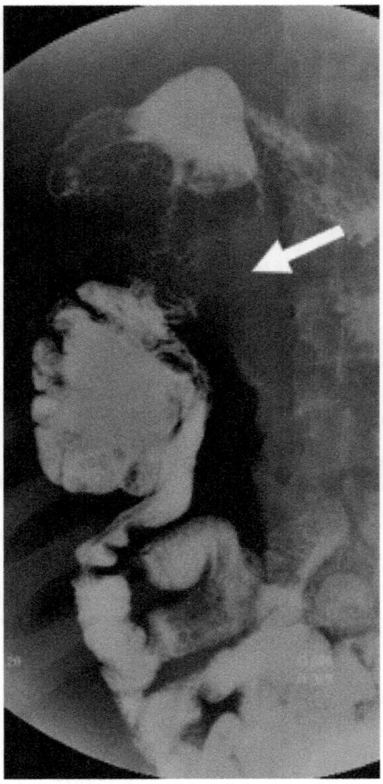

Fig. 14.12 A barium meal follow-through study was performed. It shows a mass (arrow) involving the ascending colon and causing luminal narrowing and irregularity. This appearance of the mass is also called "apple core" appearance. The mass is just distal to the ileocolic junction and indenting the contrast column distally, produces a "shouldering" effect. A word of caution! Instead of a barium meal follow-through study, a barium enema should have been performed. Barium given orally can complete a partial obstruction. In this case, the clinical data did not mention any large bowel pathology

14.3 A Case of Ileocolic Intussusception (Fig. 14.13)

Intussusceptions can be diagnosed by ultrasound. It is the investigation of choice in children. A barium enema study as well as a CT scan can also demonstrate intussusception. The advantage of the CT scan is that often the cause of intussusception can also be identified.

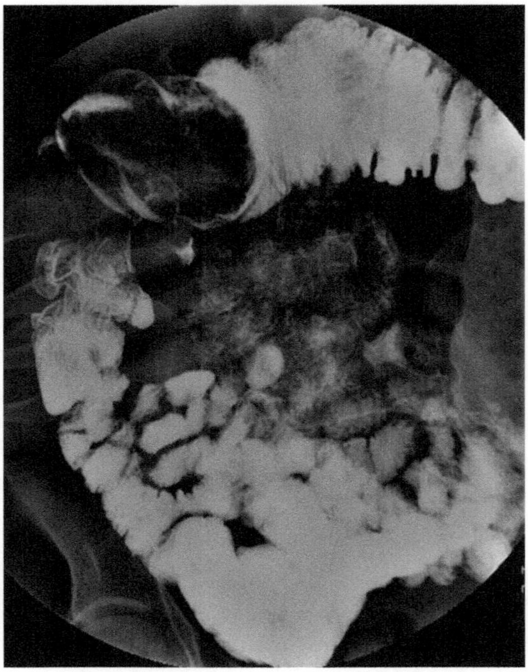

Fig. 14.13 A barium meal follow-through demonstrating an ileocolic intussusception. The orally administered barium is blocked by the obstruction. The appearance of the obstruction can also be spring-coil or cobra head type. An contrast enema was therefore carried out at the same sitting to try and reduce the intussusception

14.4 Diverticular Disease of the Colon

These are mucosal outpouchings, through areas of weakness in the walls of the large and small intestines. Faecal contents, food particles, tablets and barium collect in these sacs which can lead to inflammation, called diverticulitis. They are easily seen in both single and double barium contrast studies (Figs. 14.14 and 14.15) as well as in CT scans (Fig. 14.16).

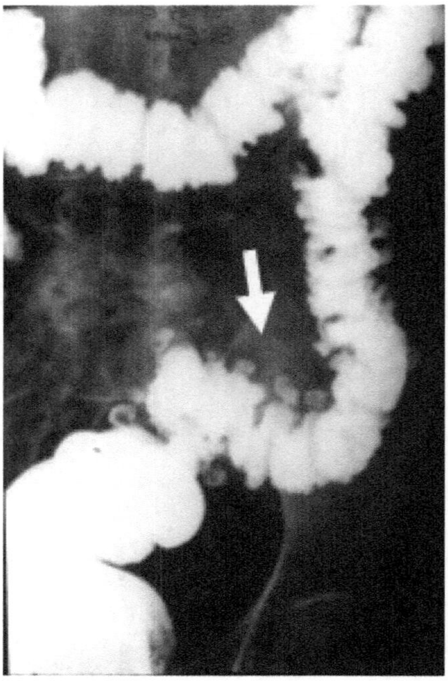

Fig. 14.14 Single contrast barium study showing barium filled sigmoid diverticula

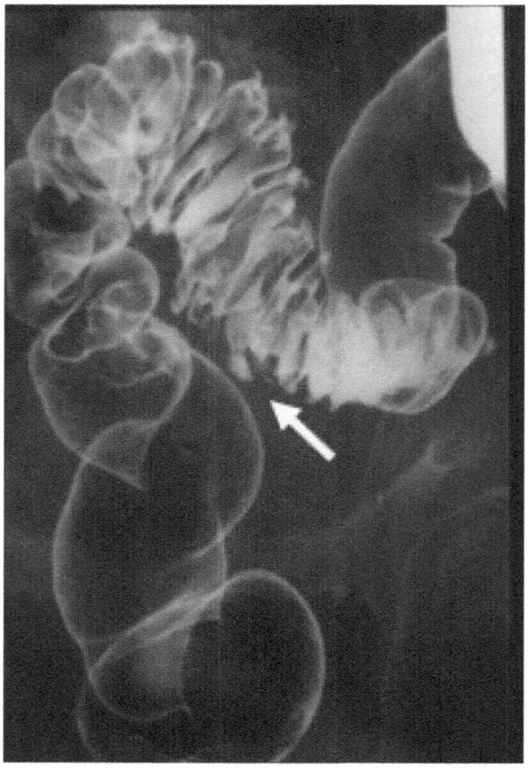

Fig. 14.15 A double contrast barium enema using a small quantity of barium along with air infused through a tube in the rectum. Note also the demonstration of small colonic diverticula by this method also (arrow)

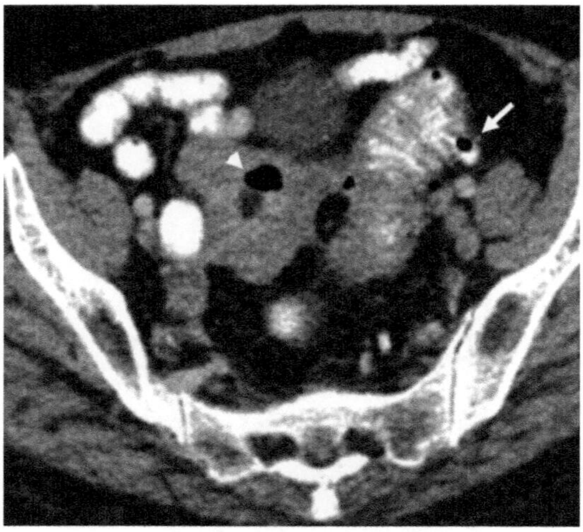

Fig. 14.16 A CT scan of the abdomen, performed with orally administered positive contrast, which has reached the colon. The presence of a colonic diverticulum filled with air and contrast medium is visible in this image (arrow). Also, note (arrowhead) the formation of a pelvic abscess, which was secondary to diverticular perforation, a complication of diverticulitis

14.5 Infective Diseases of the Large Bowel

The large bowel is prone to numerous infections and inflammatory disorders. In these cases, an ultrasound or a CT scan is the preferred investigation. Ultrasound does not require any preparation and can provide excellent details of the affected bowel loop (Fig. 14.17). The inflamed or infected bowel loop demonstrates what is called the "gut signature" which is the thickening with relatively preserved layers of the bowel wall (Fig. 14.18). Additional findings such as inflammatory changes in the surrounding fat planes and enlarged regional nodes can also be detected by sonography. Intravenous contrast-enhanced CT scans with or without oral contrast, can also show diffuse colonic thickening (Fig. 14.19) as well as surrounding inflammatory changes.

A barium meal follow-through study can also be performed, especially if a granulomatous disease such as tuberculosis is suspected. It may show ileocaecal (IC) involvement, with

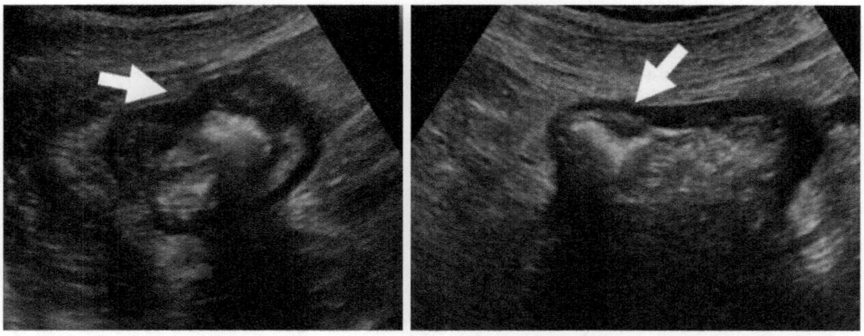

Fig. 14.17 Ultrasonography showing a typical "gut signature". This is a segment of the right colon which shows thick walls (arrows), the layers of which appear preserved. A case of amoebic colitis

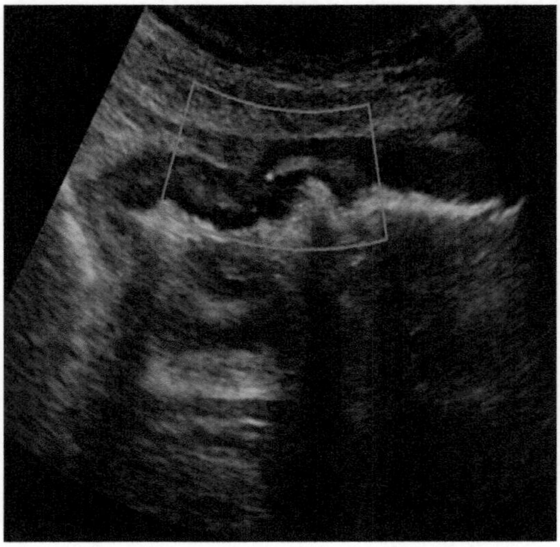

Fig. 14.18 Same case. The colon is demonstrated in the longitudinal plane. Note the preserved layers of the colonic wall with vascularity demonstrated within it on colour Doppler

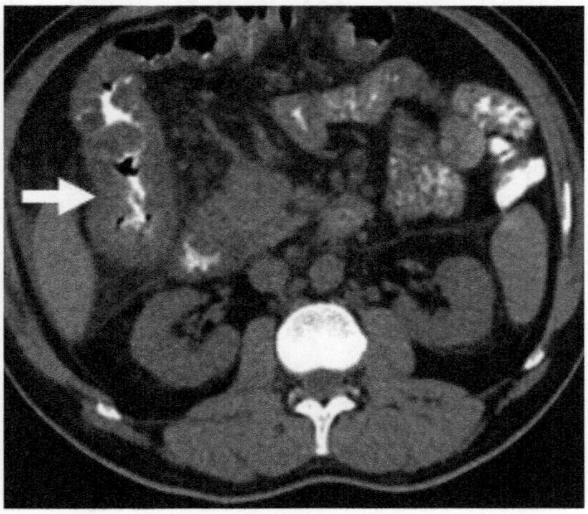

Fig. 14.19 Axial CT scan of the abdomen, showing diffuse circumferential thickening of the right colon with irregular mucosa (arrow). These findings are suggestive of inflammatory bowel disease of the colon

a patulous IC junction, caecal contraction or contraction of the ascending colon. However, barium studies are time-consuming and do not show any mural or extramural abnormality. Hence, CT scan is currently the preferred investigation for the evaluation of infective and inflammatory large bowel pathologies.

14.6 Other Lesions

Both double contrast barium enema as well as CT scans (Fig. 14.20), especially CT colonography, can demonstrate small sessile or pedunculated polyps. The double contrast study can also demonstrate mucosal ulcerations.

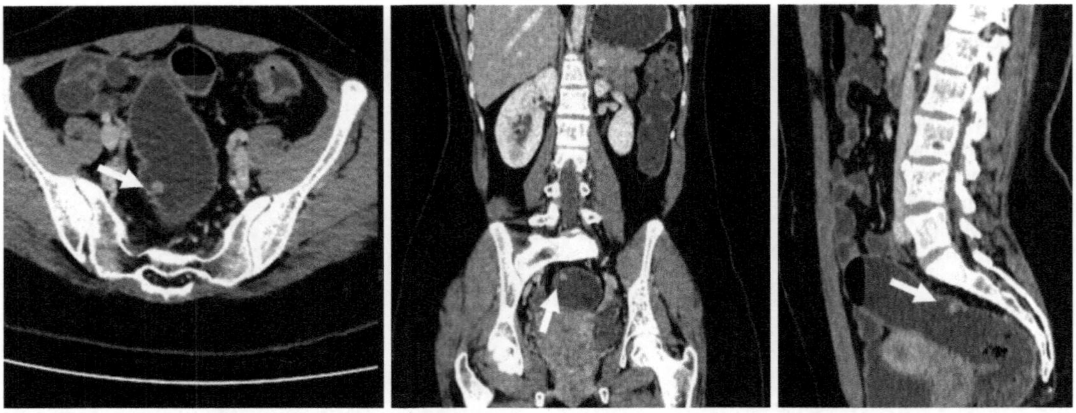

Fig. 14.20 Axial, coronal and sagittal views of CT scan of the pelvis, showing a rectal polyp

Since the colon is a seat of many diseases, every effort and available technique must be applied to identify the pathology and institute appropriate treatment.

References

1. Knipe H, Ashraf A, Worsley C, et al. Cecum. Radiopaedia.org. https://doi.org/10.53347/rID-22635.
2. Butler P, Mitchell A, Healy JC, et al. Applied radiological anatomy. Cambridge University Press; 2012.
3. Dimitriou N, Michail O, Moris D, Griniatsos J. Low rectal cancer: sphincter preserving techniques-selection of patients, techniques and outcomes. World J Gastrointest Oncol. 2015;7(7):55–70.
4. D'Souza N, Balyasnikova S, Tudyka V, et al. Variation in landmarks for the rectum: an MRI study. Color Dis. 2018;20(10):304–9.

15 The Urinary Tract

Abstract

Urinary tract pathologies are a common occurrence in daily clinical practice.

Imaging is frequently needed to elucidate the anatomical and pathological findings for the management of patients with upper and lower urinary tract problems.

The imaging study which sets the ball rolling is an ultrasound of the urinary tract. Plain X-ray of the Kidney, Ureter and Bladder region (KUB) and Intravenous Urography (IVU) are not as frequently requested as were in the previous decades. If ultrasound is unable to provide any clues or if further investigation is needed, it is usually a CT scan of the urinary tract, both without and with the intravenous administration of iodinated non-ionic contrast medium which is advised, based on the clinical suspicion. If the patient is allergic to iodinated contrast medium or if it is a pregnant woman or a child with some congnital anomaly, then MR urography can be performed. For the evaluation of the lower urinary tract, contrast studies are very much needed and their value is unlikely to diminish any time soon.

In this chapter, we will consider all investigations which are in use in the evaluation of the various regions of the urinary tract.

Keywords

Urinary tract · KUB · Ultrasound · CT KUB · IVU · MCUG · MR urography

The urinary tract consists of the kidneys, ureters, bladder and urethra.

A patient coming in with urinary tract symptoms is first evaluated by ultrasound. In many cases such as those of calculus disease, incidentally detected hydronephrosis, cystic and solid masses, congenital anomalies, and bladder and urethral pathology, ultrasonography (USG) either provides the diagnosis or offers a lead for further investigation and management. Plain films of the urinary tract are less often requested these days but can be useful for many other reasons.

We will now discuss the various imaging procedures in some detail.

15.1 Plain X-ray of the Kidney, Ureter and Bladder Region

- **Preparation**

  Normally a single X-ray film of the abdomen is sufficient to cover the entire abdomen. In a tall patient, sometimes two films are needed to cover both the upper and lower urinary tracts. Plain films of the urinary tract region should be performed after adequate bowel preparation. Tiny calculi, especially ureteric, may be obscured by bowel gas shadows. The patient should be asked to withhold solids for about 12 h, clear the bowel before coming and not pass urine for at least 1 h before the study. There should be no restriction on drinking water, but soft drinks and juices should be avoided to prevent the accumulation of gases in

R. Gothi, *Radiographic and Imaging Techniques for Radiology Residents and Technologists*,
https://doi.org/10.1007/978-981-96-4816-0_15

the bowel lumen, which may obscure the urinary tract. A distended bladder helps displace bowel loops out of the pelvic cavity, providing a clear view of the vesicoureteric junctions. Small calculus in the distal ureters including the vesicoureteric junction (VUJ) and within the bladder are more liable to be detected when the bladder lumen is distended than if it is either partially filled or empty. The X-ray KUB should include the external genitalia in male patients to avoid missing a urethral calculus.

- **Why are plain films still be considered useful**

  Plain films of the abdomen are usually requested to confirm/exclude/locate a calculus. They help in determining the size, shape and number of calculi. Sometimes even after an ultrasound of the urinary tract, where there is some uncertainty about the presence of a calculus, a plain X-ray KUB, after good preparation, can be offered. This does not mean that plain X-ray KUB can replace CT KUB, which is more sensitive in detecting calculus disease of the urinary tract than an X-ray.

  Plain films are required following DJ stent placement to rule out slippage of stent and the presence of any calculus along the stent.

  Plain films give an idea about bones, bowel loops and the presence of gas in the urinary tract (emphysematous pyelonephritis).

  Plain films are unable to detect many abnormalities of the urinary tract including radiolucent or low-density calculi, hydronephrosis, congenital renal abnormalities, a small renal mass and urinary tract infections. Often phleboliths near the vesicoureteric junction may be mistaken for ureteric calculi.

  For these reasons, an IVU or CT scan of the urinary tract, which is currently the most preferred investigation, is performed.

15.2 Intravenous Urography (IVU)

Intravenous urography or intravenous pyelography is a study meant to evaluate the pelvicalyceal system, ureters, and urinary bladder. It also gives an idea about the function of the kidneys. The renal outlines and parenchyma are visible in the early phases of the study. However, IVU is not particularly efficient in detecting parenchymal abnormalities confined within the normal reniform outlines of the kidney.

Earlier on, ionic contrast such as Urografin 76% or Conray 420 was used. However, because of the increased risk of both minor and serious side effects with these contrasts, they have now been replaced by non-ionic contrast media.

Before the study, the renal parameters such as blood urea, serum creatine level and eGFR need to be checked. The use of iodinated contrast media is not advisable in patients with extremely low eGFR.

The study is performed after preparation of the abdomen so that gas and faecal shadows do not overlap on the images of the urinary tract. The patient needs to be off solid food for 6–8 h before the investigation. The patient can have water as per need. The reason for not allowing solids is to reduce the risk of feeling sick following injection of iodinated contrast. Laxatives for clearing the bowel loops are not of much help.

- A plain X-ray KUB is initially obtained to look for abnormalities such as calcification, calculus, abnormalities in the renal outlines, and other soft tissue or bony lesions which might be a cause of concern and also explain the patient's symptoms. The lung bases which are invariably included in the study, are also examined for any suspicious lesion. In a male patient, the study should also include the penile urethra so as not to miss any urethral calculus. The plain X-ray KUB helps in positioning the image plate correctly to record images of the kidneys as well as the rest of the urinary tract.
- IV contrast is then administered slowly using an appropriate-sized needle. The dose can vary from 0.5 to 1.5 cc/kg of body weight.
- An abdominal binder is used to compress the abdomen during the initial part of the study. It should be applied over the mid-abdomen. This reduces the abdominal thickness thereby reducing the exposure dose and improving the quality of the films. It also compresses the mid ureters, which helps in further distending the upper renal tract.

- A nephrographic phase between 1 and 3 min (60–120s) is first obtained. The focus in the nephrographic phase is on the renal parenchyma.
- This is followed by an early pyelographic phase of around 5 min.
- Once the pyelographic phase is acquired, then, after another 7–10 min of waiting, the abdominal binder is relaxed. The contrast held up in the upper collecting system flows down into the bladder, and a film of the entire KUB area is obtained immediately. This very often, but not always, helps in capturing the image of the entire length of the contrast-filled ureters.
- In cases showing hydronephrosis, sometimes delayed and prone films of the urinary tract are needed. This is because in the supine position, contrast pools into the posteriorly located calyces. On turning the patient prone or reevaluating after ambulation, the iodinated contrast-laden urine flows into the more anteriorly located calyces, pelvis and ureters opacifying them.
- Thereafter, a full urinary bladder film (cystogram) is taken. The patient may have to wait for the bladder to fill up before the film is taken.
- The urinary bladder is filmed again after micturition.
- Delayed X-rays of the renal tract are needed to establish any functional delay in a diseased/hydronephrotic kidney. However, an isotope scan is a better way of identifying functioning renal tissue.

15.3 Non-contrast CT of the Kidney, Ureters and Bladder (NCCT)

There are many limitations of IVU. The study needs bowel preparation, takes more time to complete and is often compromised by overlying gas shadows. Above all, there is a higher risk of contrast reaction probably because the patient has to be fasting for a longer time for the test.

Hence, instead of an IVU, a non-contrast CT scan of the urinary tract (CT KUB) is preferred, especially for confirming the presence of a small ureteric calculus which may not be evident in X-rays and even in an ultrasound examination of the urinary tract..

NCCT KUB does not require any preparation. It can be performed at anytime and provides immediate results. It can give the size, number, location and attenuation value (that is, the density) of calculus, thereby enabling the surgeon to plan appropriate management. It also gives information about renal size, parenchymal thickness and outline, and the presence of any mass lesion or air. It enables evaluation of the surrounding fat planes, adjoining organs and bones, much better as compared to an IVU. Therefore, if an ultrasound examination is suboptimal, most urologists and radiologists prefer going ahead with a non-contrast CT KUB.

15.4 Intravenous Contrast-Enhanced CT Scan of the Urinary Tract

Contrast studies of the urinary tract include CT urography and multiphasic CT for evaluation of renal masses, florid haematuria and renal donor kidneys.

- CT urogram is needed in problem cases where accurate renal anatomy and probable aetiology of urological symptoms needs to be determined. It provides additional and more detailed information about the urinary tract as compared to the IVU. It is used for the detection and evaluation of masses involving the entire urinary tract including the urinary bladder, obstructive lesions involving the urinary tract and for evaluating complex renal anatomy in cases of congenital anomalies.
- Multi-phasic CT with contrast, which includes angiography in addition to urography, can be performed in patients with gross haematuria, renal and bladder tumours, or for preoperative assessment of renal donor kidneys.
- There is another technique used by surgeons and performed in the operating theatre. This technique is called retrograde urography. In this procedure, following cystoscopy, contrast is introduced through a catheter inserted into the ureter to delineate any ureteric, or renal

pelvic abnormality, which is not clearly defined by other means. The radiologist may be called upon to interpret this study and should be aware of how it is done and what it looks like.

- It appears similar to a urography images obtained during IVU or in cases of CT urogram,but will show a catheter in the ureter, introduced through the urinary bladder.

15.5 Antegrade Urography

This is a percutaneously performed procedure in which contrast is injected through a pigtail catheter into the kidney. The kidney should be large with confirmed hydronephrosis. The catheter should enter the renal pelvis. It will drain the obstructed kidney as well as enable the determination of the cause and site of obstruction.

15.6 Retrograde Urethrography (RGU) and Micturating Cystourethrography (MCUG)

These techniques are meant to evaluate the lower urinary tract.

The entire urethra is imaged in anteroposterior (AP) and both oblique planes, the latter being performed by turning the patient towards the right and left. This ensures that the shadow of the penile urethra does not overlap with on the pelvic bones and the femur and urethral lesions are not obscured.

In a female, an AP position while micturating is sufficient to evaluate the urethra.

Both RGU and MCUG should include films of the entire urethra and urinary bladder. One film during cystography should also cover the upper renal tracts to ascertain the presence and grade of vesicoureteric reflux, if present.

The RGU is done with the patient lying on the table while an MCU can be performed with the patient being either in a supine oblique or in an erect oblique position.

Both studies complement one another and therefore should always be performed together, under fluoroscopic guidance.

15.7 The Technique of Performing RGU and MCUG

The patient lies in the supine position. A control film of the KUB area and lower urinary tract is obtained.

The foreskin, if present, is retracted and the glans penis is thoroughly cleaned using saline or Savlon.

A catheter with an inflatable balloon is then inserted into the glans penis. About 1–2 cc of saline is introduced to distend the balloon. A gentle tug on the catheter ensures that it fits snugly within the glans and is unlikely to come out during the introduction of contrast medium.

The patient is now positioned obliquely with one side raised and the leg closer to the table flexed at the hip and knee. The other leg is kept exdtended over the flexed leg.

Under gentle traction, the penile shaft is straightened to remove any slack. Care should be taken that the penis does not overlap on the pelvic bones or femur or else the lesion, if any, may not be well seen.

Iodinated contrast medium, diluted with saline is injected through the catheter and images of penile urethra are obtained in the anteroposterior and oblique positions, by turning the patient from one to the other side. A slight resistance may be felt as the contrast attempts to negotiate the posterior urethra to enter into the urinary bladder. The posterior urethra is never fully distended in an RGU. The verumontanum can be seen as a filling defect within it. Since an MCUG must follow an RGU, it is advisable to have the bladder at least partially full and not empty. About 20–30 cc of iodinated contrast followed by saline (as much as the patient can tolerate) is introduced, the latter to flush the urethra as well as to distend the bladder. The iodinated contrast mixes with the urine within the bladder and opacifies it. The catheter can now be removed. The patient is asked to roll on the table for proper mixing of the contrast and the urine within the bladder. Note that it is important to achieve high contrast density within the bladder or else the density of the contrast within the urethral may be inadequate. A full bladder film in the AP position, called the cystogram, is obtained.

The patient is now prepared to void urine. For this, the position of the patient can be either supine oblique or better still, erect oblique. A urinal is provided to the patient to hold beneath the penis, during the act of micturition.

Films are obtained during micturition, in AP and both oblique positions, ensuring that the penile shaft does not overlap with the femur.

Finally, a post-evacuation film of the urinary bladder is obtained, to complete the study.

The number of films will be a plain X-ray KUB, two to three RGU films, one cystogram, a KUB film for any vesicoureteral reflux, two MCUG films and a post-void film of the urinary bladder. This will complete both RGU and MCUG.

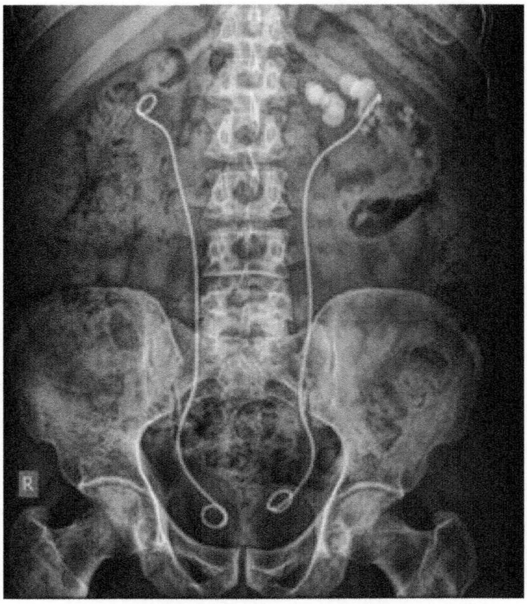

Fig. 15.1 X-Ray KUB showing bilateral double "J" (DJ) stents with multiple radio-opaque calculi in the left kidney. Note that the stents are properly positioned and have not slipped down into the ureter

15.8 Isotope Scans

When the issue of inferring renal function is considered, an isotope scan can be performed using either Tc-99m DTPA or MAG3 scan. The DTPA scan uses Tc-99m, which is bound to diethylene triamine pentaacetic acid (DTPA). In the MAG 3 (mercaptoacetyltriglycine) scan, Tc-99m is bound to MAG3 to form the radiopharmaceutical. Isotope scans can provide data about the percentage of function of individual kidneys. They can also show the time it takes for the isotope to clear from the pelvicalyceal system. They are particularly helpful in cases of management of congenital pelvic ureteric junction stenosis and in the evaluation of vesico urethral reflux.

Isotope scans used to study the renal parenchyma are different from those used to study functioning renal tissue. Technetium 99m dimercaptosuccinic acid (DMSA) and glucoheptonate (GHA) are used to perform these scans.

There are many diseases which can be diagnosed by various imaging methods.

A pictorial review of some of these diseases is provided (Figs. 15.1, 15.2, 15.3, 15.4, 15.5, 15.6, 15.7, 15.8, 15.9, 15.10, 15.11, 15.12, 15.13, 15.14, 15.15, 15.16, 15.17, 15.18, 15.19, 15.20, 15.21, 15.22, 15.23, 15.24, 15.25, 15.26, 15.27, and 15.28).

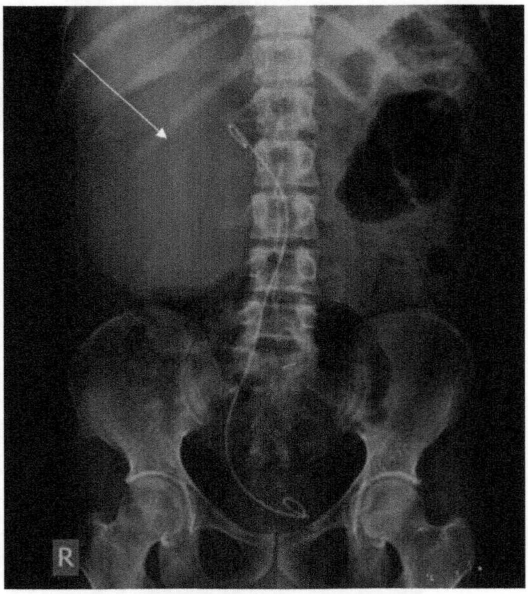

Fig. 15.2 X-Ray KUB showing a DJ stent on the right side. Note the presence of soft tissue in the right renal area (arrow). The plain X-ray does not give any idea about the nature of the mass. It could be a cystic or solid lesion. What can be deduced is the absence of fat, air or calcification in the periphery or within the lesion

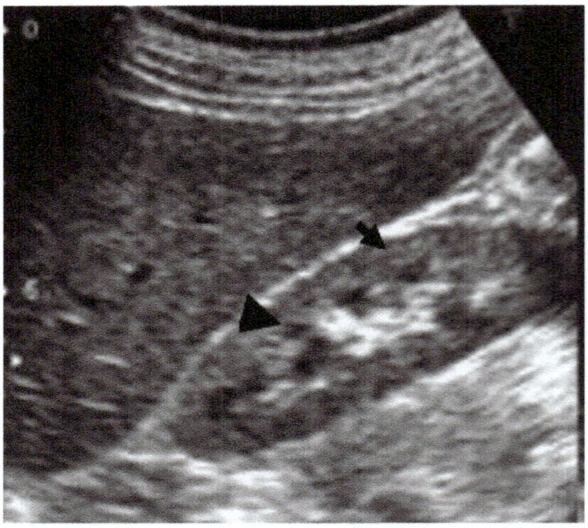

Fig. 15.3 Normal appearing kidneys on ultrasound. The echotexture of the cortex (arrow) is brighter than the medulla, which appears dark (arrowhead) [1]

As is obvious, there are several ways of identifying and demonstrating diseases affecting the urinary tract. The studies require excellent-quality images as well as a thorough knowledge of the anatomy of this region. With the availability of ultrasound and CT, the use of conventional radiology is declining. Nevertheless, the technologist and radiologist must be able to perform these studies and provide accurate information needed for the management of disorders of the urinary tract.

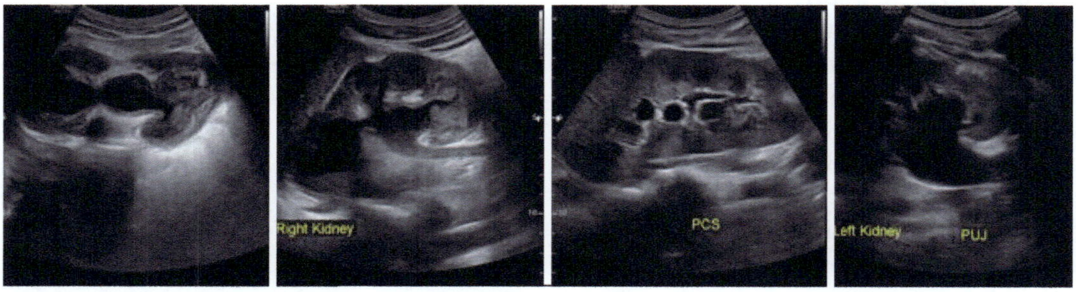

Fig. 15.4 Ultrasound showing bilateral hydronephrotic kidneys with proximal hydroureter. Ultrasonography is an excellent modality for investigating the urinary tract. It also gives a good idea about renal parenchyma. Always compare the echogenicity of the renal parenchyma with the liver. Echogenicity should be equal to or less than that of the liver parenchyma

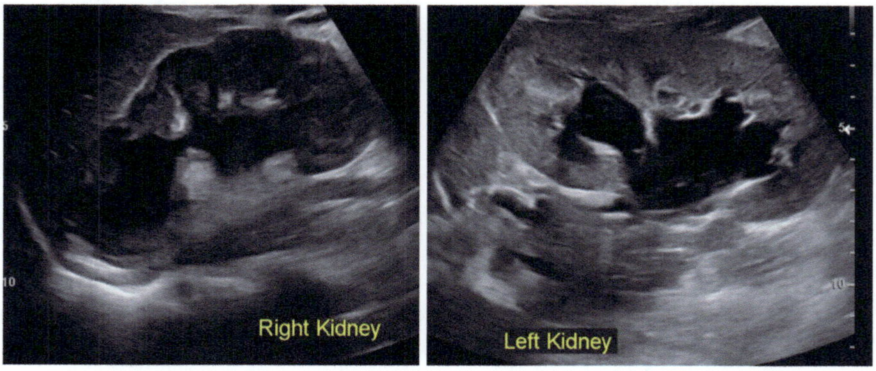

Fig. 15.5 Note the difference in the echotexture between the right and left kidneys. The parenchyma of the right kidney appears less echogenic as compared to the left. The renal pelvis shows fine internal echoes on both sides. This is a case of acute pyelonephritis of right kidney with bilateral pyonephrosis, affecting the right kidney more than the left

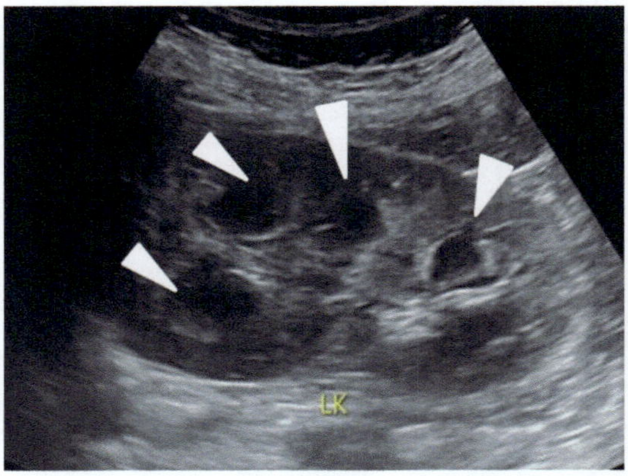

Fig. 15.6 Ultrasound of the kidney showing normal hypoechoic renal medulla which can be mistaken for dilated calyces

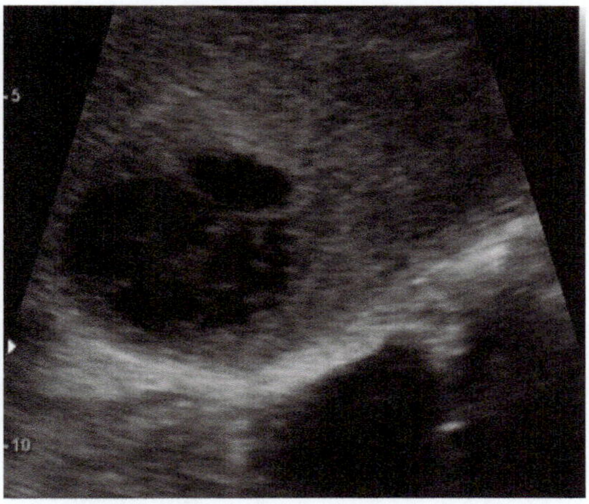

Fig. 15.7 Ultrasound of the kidney shows a multiloculated renal abscess containing fine internal echoes

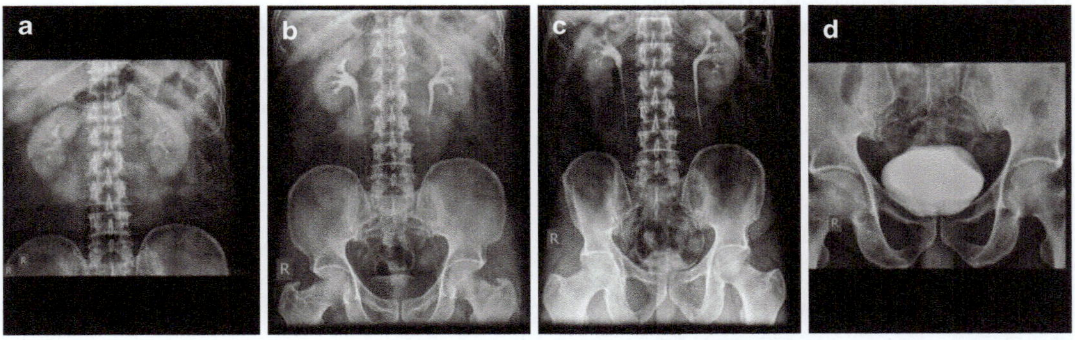

Fig. 15.8 Intravenous urography showing 1-min nephrographic phase (**a**), a pyelographic phase in supine position (**b**), a prone film attempting to fill the ureters (**c**) and cystographic phase (**d**)

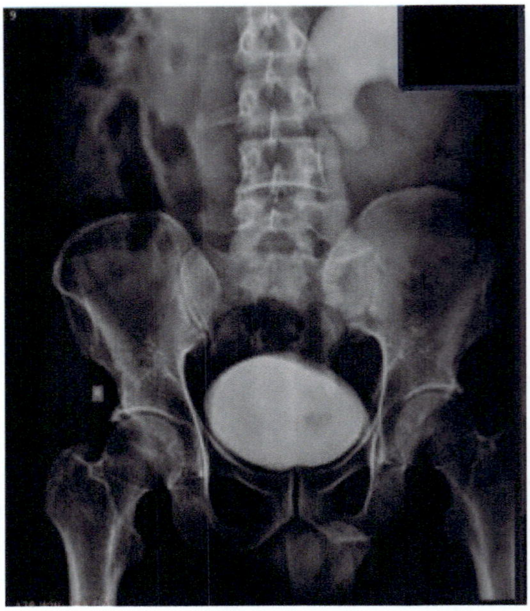

Fig. 15.9 A delayed phase of IVU, showing left-sided obstructive hydronephrosis with contrast in the urinary bladder (cystogram)

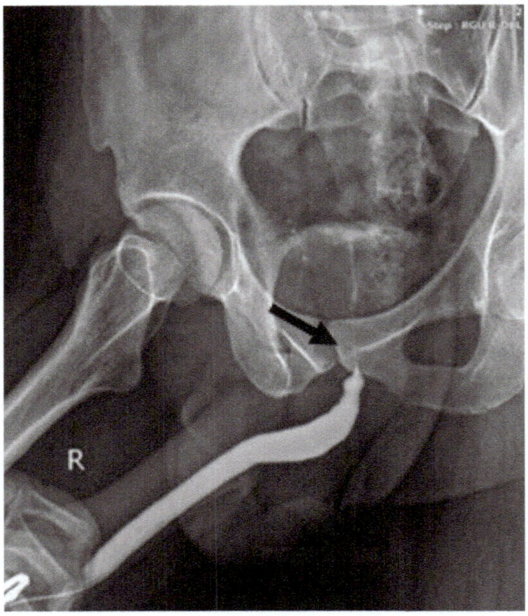

Fig. 15.10 A retrograde urethrography showing contrast being injected into the urethra. The normal posterior urethra (arrow) does not distend fully during retrograde filling

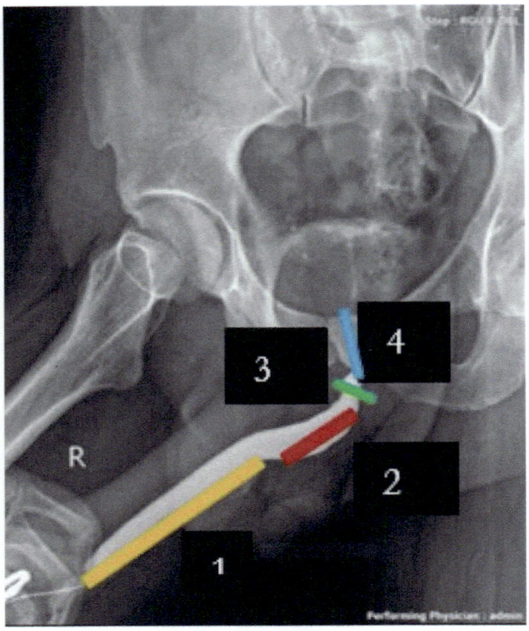

Fig. 15.11 Anatomy of the normal anterior and posterior urethra. Penile urethra (1), bulbous urethra (2), membraneous urethra (3) and posterior urethra (4)

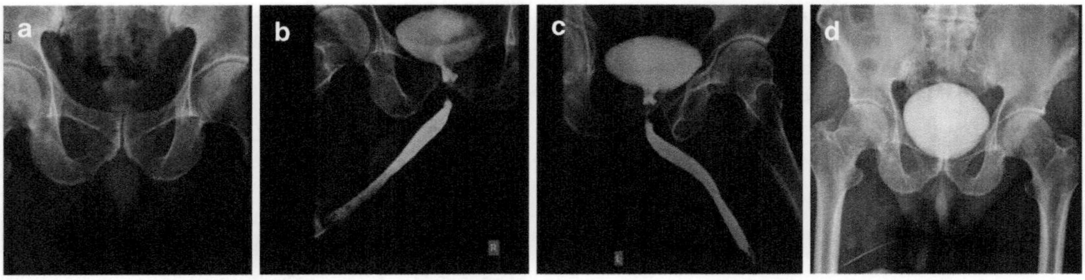

Fig. 15.12 A retrograde urethrography study showing (**a**) pre-contrast control film, (**b, c**) urethrogram and (**d**) cystogram

Fig. 15.13 Right and left oblique views of a retrograde urethrogram showing urethral stricture (arrow)

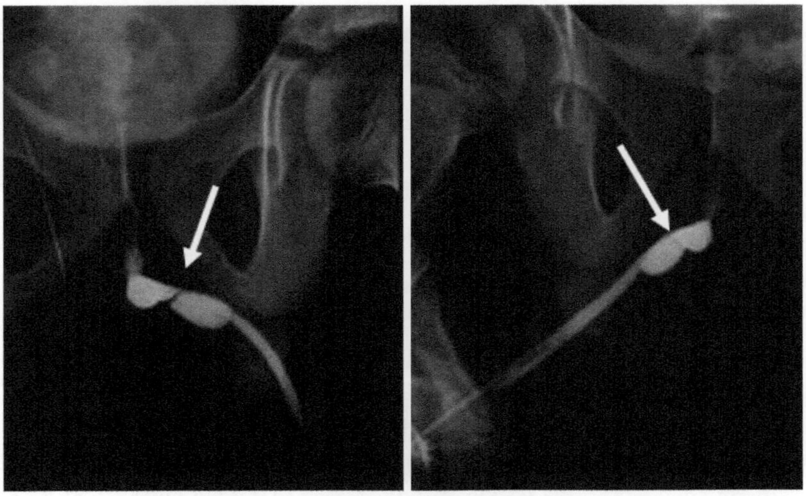

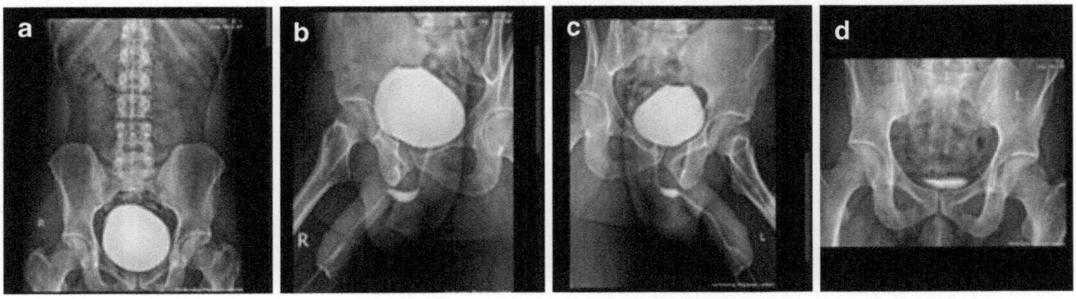

Fig. 15.14 An MCUG showing cystogram (**a**), urethrogram in right and left oblique positions (**b, c**) and post-void film (**d**)

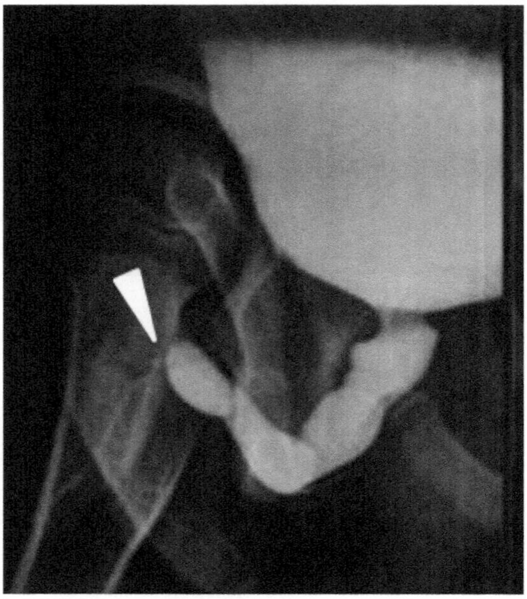

Fig. 15.15 An MCUG showing dilatation of the posterior and bulbous urethra (arrow) with a normal calibre of the penile urethra, consistent with an anterior urethral stricture

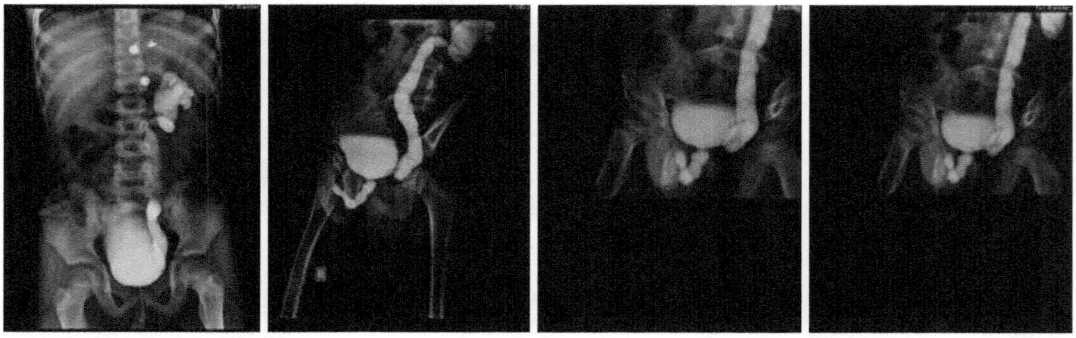

Fig. 15.16 MCUG showing left-sided vesicoureteral reflux

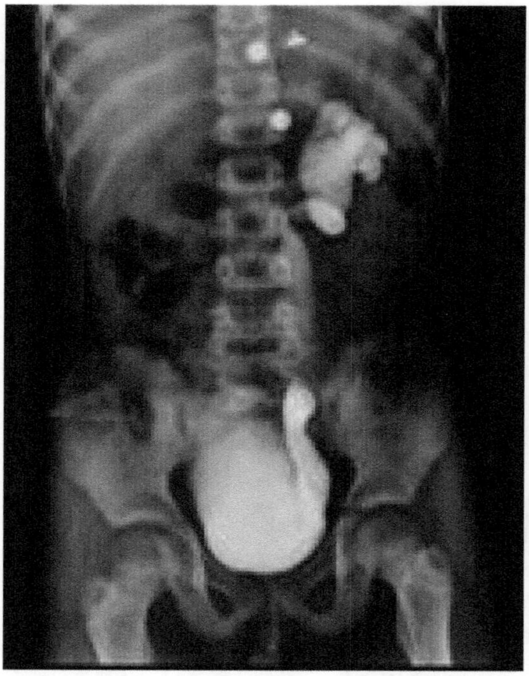

Fig. 15.17 Film showing left-sided vesicoureteric reflux. Always obtain one film of the KUB region, during straining, if vesicoureteric reflux is suspected

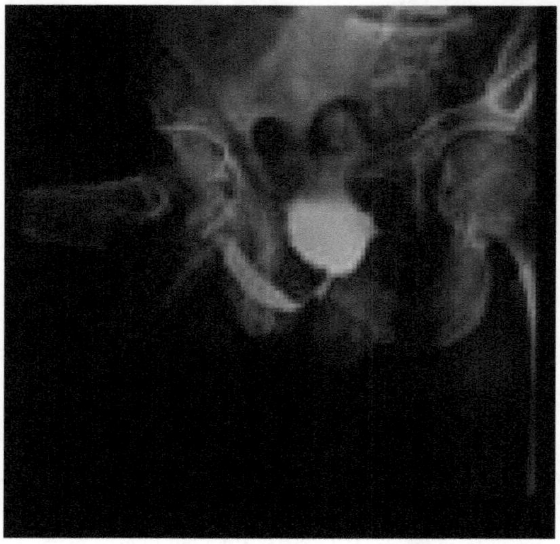

Fig. 15.18 Compare the normal posterior urethra seen in this image with Fig. 15.15 and notice the difference in the calibre

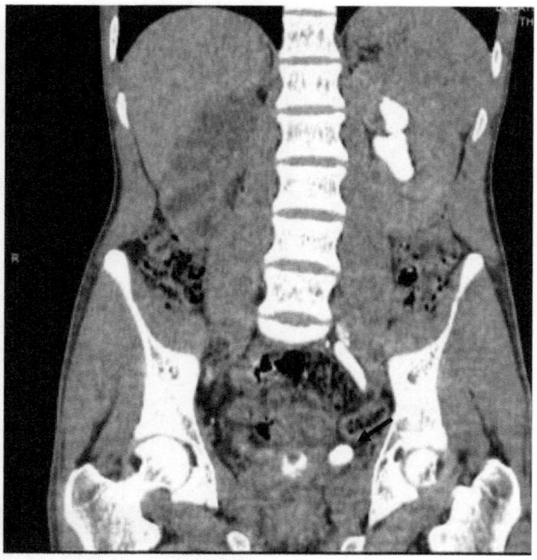

Fig. 15.19 An NCCT KUB, showing a left renal and distal ureteric calculus (arrow)

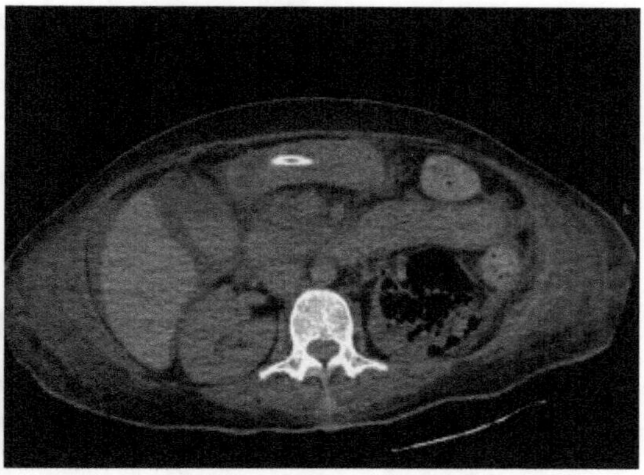

Fig. 15.20 An NCCT KUB showing air affecting the left kidney (emphysematous pyelonephritis)

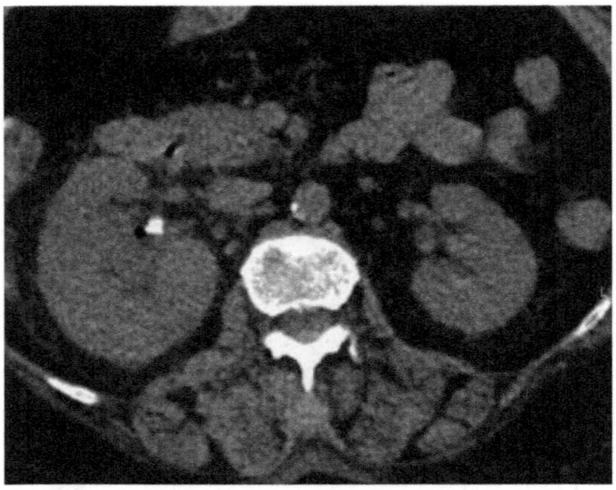

Fig. 15.21 An NCCT KUB, showing an enlarged right kidney, as compared to the left. Note the calculus (bright shadow) and an air bubble (dark shadow), suggestive of a calculus-related urinary tract infection with a gas-forming organism

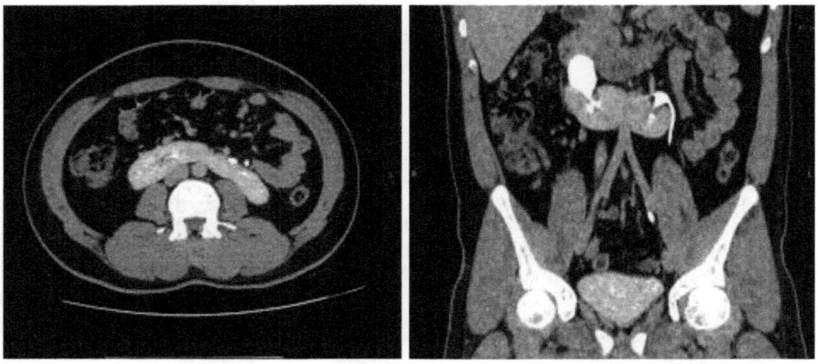

Fig. 15.22 Axial and coronal CT urogram showing a horseshoe kidney

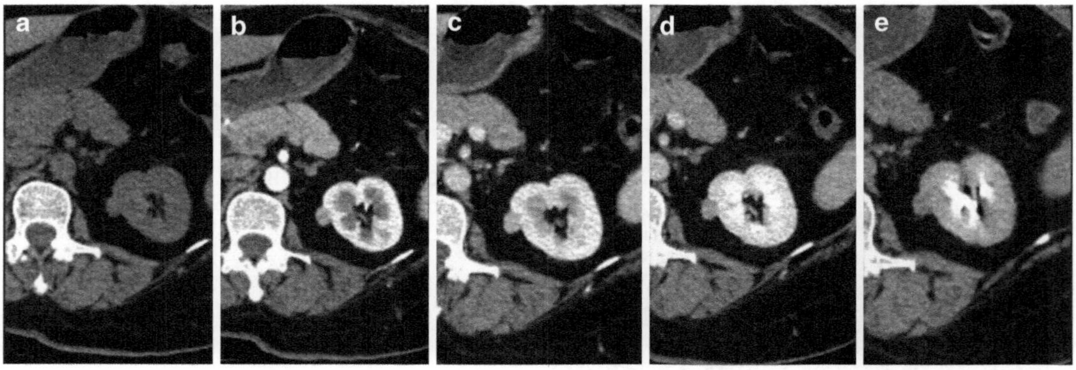

Fig. 15.23 A multiphasic CT to evaluate a small renal mass arising from the medial cortex of the left kidney. (**a**) Non-contrast phase, (**b**) angiographic phase, (**c**) delayed arterial phase, (**d**) venous phase and (**e**) pyelographic phase

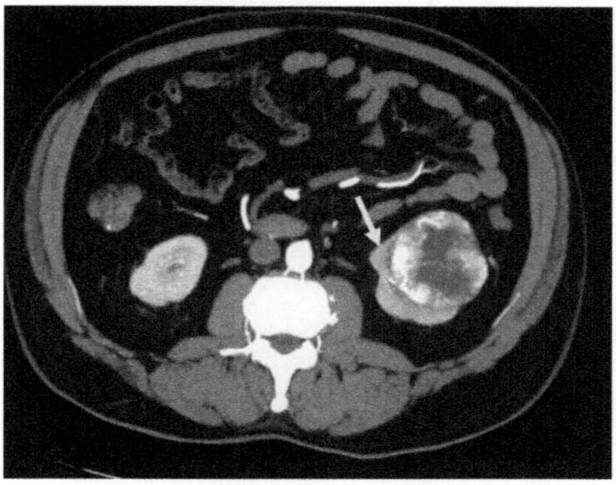

Fig. 15.24 A maximum intensity projection (MIP) showing dense contrast enhancement of the outer non-necrotic component of the left renal mass. Note the difference between the contrast density of the normal renal parenchyma (arrow) and the mass

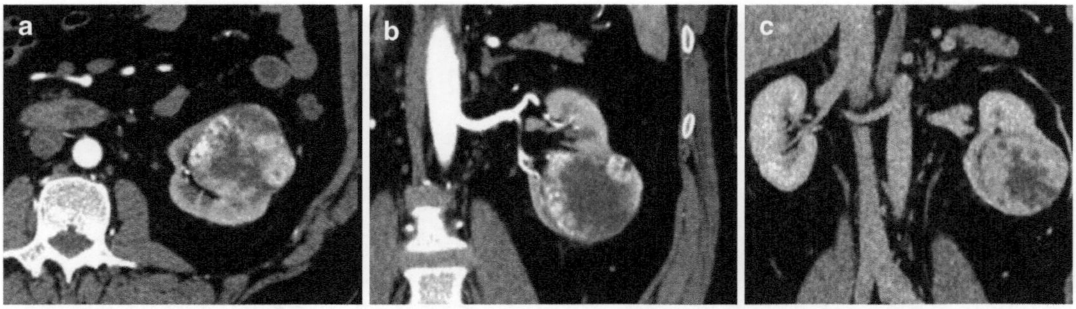

Fig. 15.25 Axial (**a**), coronal (**b**) and sagittal (**c**) projections of the left renal mass, showing the change in density between the arterial (**a, b**) and venous phase (**c**)

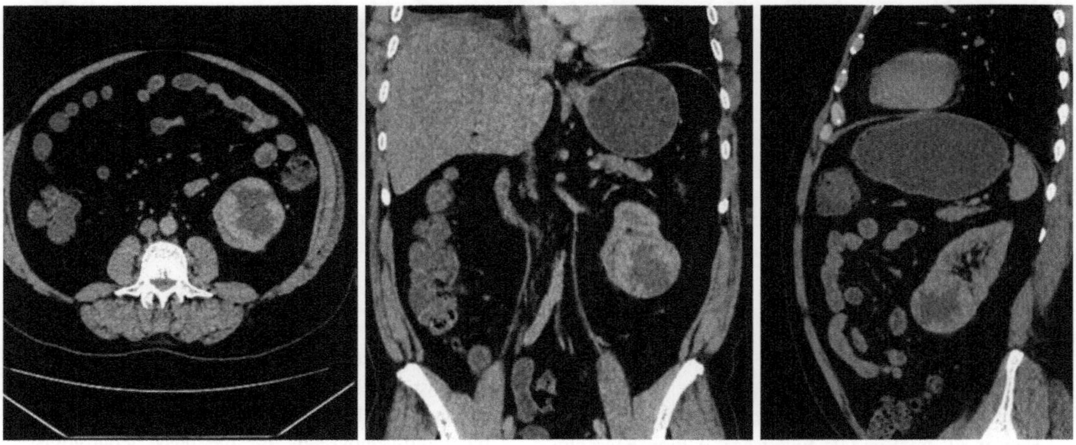

Fig. 15.26 Same case, the left renal mass in the venous phase, showing a reduction in density of the peripheral solid portion of the tumour. The central low-density portion is suggestive of necrosis within the tumour

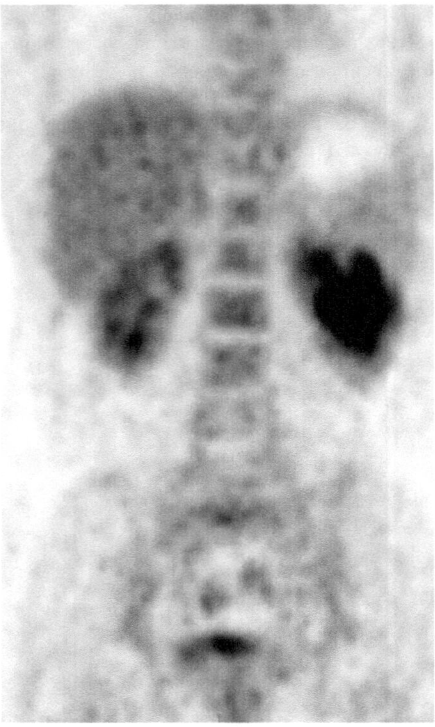

Fig. 15.27 DTPA scan showing left-sided obstructive uropathy with accumulation of the isotope in the obstructed kidney

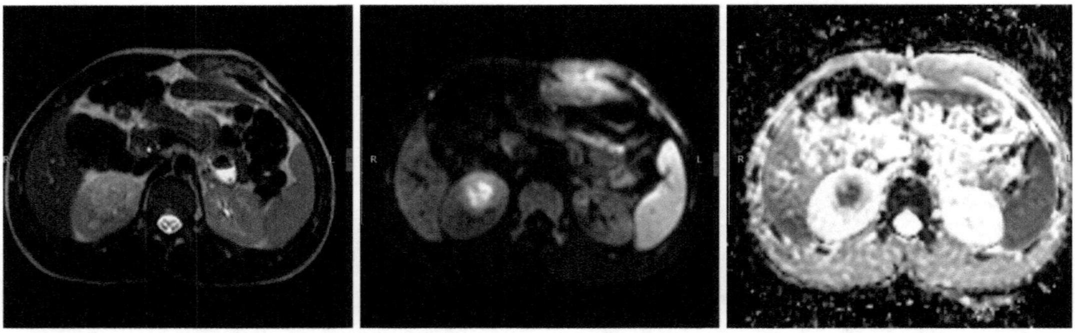

Fig. 15.28 MRI of right renal abscess in T2 W, DW I and ADC maps. MRI gives excellent information about the kidneys. MR urogram can be performed without the use of contrast. MR angiography can be performed both without and with the administration of IV Gadolinium-based contrast medium

References

1. Hansen KL, Nielsen MB, Ewertsen C. Ultrasonography of the kidney: a pictorial review. Diagnostics (Basel). 2015;6(1):2. https://doi.org/10.3390/diagnostics6010002.
2. Koratala A, Bhattacharya D, Kazory A. Point of care renal ultrasonography for the busy nephrologist: a pictorial review. World J Nephrol. 2019;8(3):44–58. https://doi.org/10.5527/wjn.v8.i3.44.

Bones and Joints

16

Abstract

Conventional radiology is still the most widely used imaging procedure by orthopaedic surgeons, rheumatologists and many other specialists. There are several conditions like trauma, pain, growth-related issues, developmental defects post operative studies and malignancies, why they are needed. Should it be necessary, the skeletal system can be further evaluated by CT scans, MRI, isotope scans, PET scans and USG. X-rays of the bony skeleton need two or sometimes multiple views. A single view may not be sufficient. Performing X-rays of the skeletal system requires a good knowledge of the anatomy and technique. Often, it requires ingenuity on the part of the technician to deliver an appropriate view. In this chapter we will look at the skeletal system, using various imaging modalities.

Keywords

Bone · Joints · Skeletal system · Techniques

16.1 Let Us Go Through Some Basic Rules

(a) Always begin by obtaining the history. Examine the area that needs to be x-rayed. Look for any deformity, fracture, dislocation, swelling, painful area, presence of sinus or anything else which is unusual. The area of complaint should always be correctly marked in the X-ray so that the radiologist can delve deeper into that region. Talk to the patient and ask relevant questions regarding the problem.

(b) Correctly positioned X-rays of the bones and joints must be obtained. Extremity X-rays should always include at least one joint near the area of interest.

(c) At least two basic views at right angles to one another should be acquired.

(d) While examining the X-ray, look at the bony cortex, medulla, joint space, articular surface and surrounding soft tissues.

(e) When unsure, ask for additional views or request further examination by some other modality.

16.2 Some Uncommonly Performed Views Asked by Orthopaedic Surgeons

There are often some views which are infrequently requested by the treating orthopaedic surgeons.

These will be discussed in the subsequent sections:

R. Gothi, *Radiographic and Imaging Techniques for Radiology Residents and Technologists*, https://doi.org/10.1007/978-981-96-4816-0_16

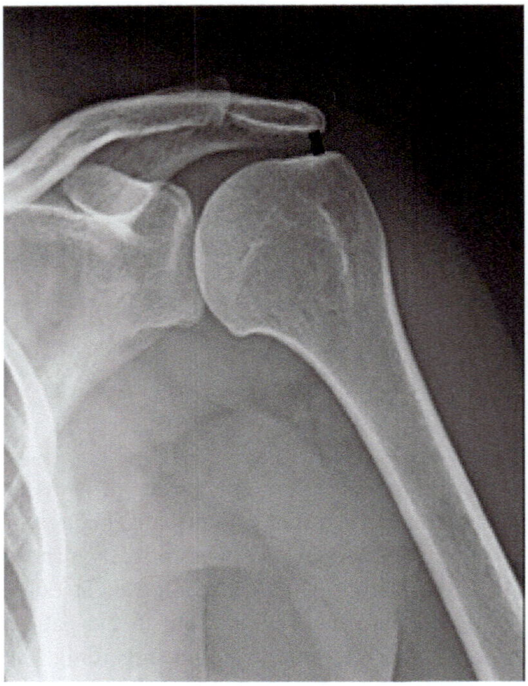

Fig. 16.1 Grashey's view: AP oblique projection. Note the acromion-humeral distance (black line). Between the acromion process and the humeral head

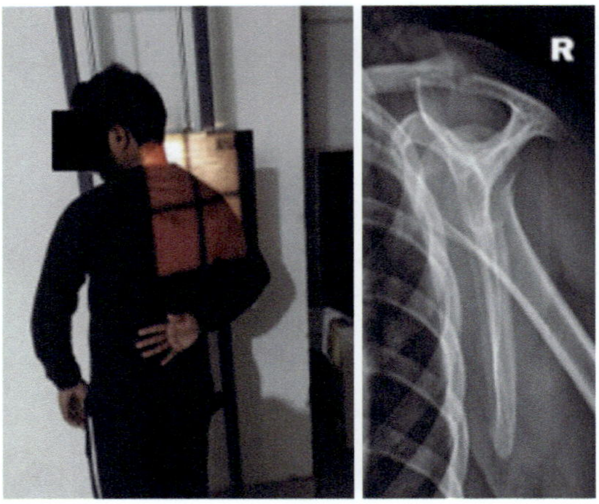

Fig. 16.2 "Y" view: Note the shape of the normal acromion process and the relationship of the humeral head with the glenoid fossa

- **Grashey's View** (Fig. 16.1)

  This view is performed to evaluate the shoulder joint. It is an AP oblique view done in such a way as to project the shoulder joint perpendicular to the image plate. The patient is turned to the side being imaged, unlike in a conventional AP view where the patient lies straight, which results in an end-on projection of the shoulder joint.
- **Zanca View for the Acromioclavicular (AC) Joint**

  The acromioclavicular joint is best evaluated using the Zanca view. In this view, the patient's back is against the imaging plate. The beam is centred at the AC joint and angulated by 10–15° towards the head. In this view, the AC joint is seen clearly without being overlapped by any neighbouring structure.
- **X-ray Assessment for Rotator Cuff Tear**

  There are three views which can be used: an AP view, an axillary view and a "Y" view of the scapula.

The AP view is obtained with the patient supine, the arm by the side, and the thumb pointing outwards. It gives an estimate of the acromion-humeral distance, which is reduced in cases of complete tear/wasting or retraction of the rotator cuff. In these cases, the head of the humerus telescopes towards the acromion process, and may abut it.

The axillary view is a superoinferior view of the shoulder. It gives a good idea about the relationship of the head of the humerus with the glenoid fossa, acromion and coracoid processes.

The scapular Y view (Fig. 16.2) separates the scapula from the posterior ribs. It is a true lateral view of the scapula with a 10–15° caudal angulation. This view is also called the outlet view or Neer's projection (Fig. 16.3). The inferior surface of the acromion process is very clearly seen in this view. It should normally be slightly concave towards the humeral head. If it is flattened, convex or shows a spur (Fig. 16.4), it can impinge on the rotator cuff, restricting its movement.

This view also shows the relationship of the humeral head with the glenoid fossa.

The humeral head should normally be centred on the glenoid fossa. If not, then an anterior or posterior dislocation of the shoulder should be suspected.

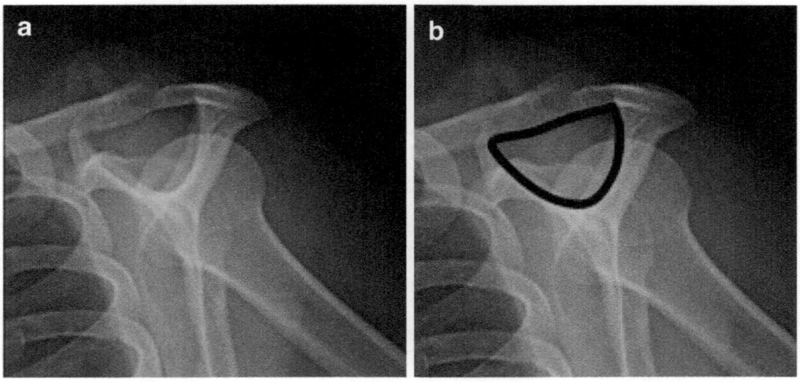

Fig. 16.3 Neer's projection, or Y view of the scapula. This view shows the inferior surface of the acromion process (**a**). The line in (**b**) shows the location of the supraspinatus muscle beneath the acromioclavicular joint

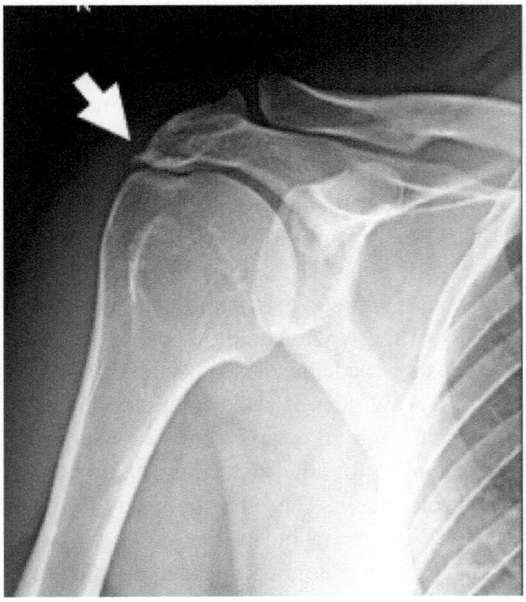

Fig. 16.4 AP view showing an acromion spur impinging on the humeral head (arrow)

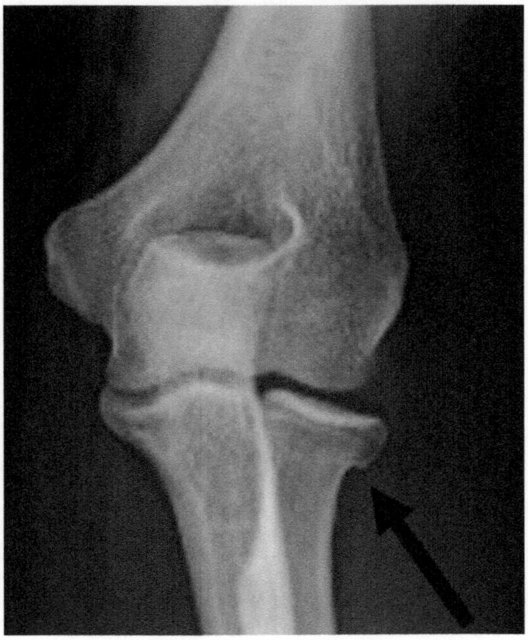

Fig. 16.5 In the AP view, always look out for a tilt of the radial head over the neck and a slight increase in the density of the radial neck. These are signs of a fractured radial neck

- **Views for fracture radial head:**

  Many orthopaedic surgeons ask for standard AP and lateral views of the radius for an elbow injury. In these views, it is very important to look for both direct (Fig. 16.5) and indirect signs (Fig. 16.6) of intracapsular fractures, especially radial neck/head and also intercondylar fracture of the distal end of the humerus.

  Very often, in the conventional lateral view, the radial head fracture is not well made out due to it overlapping with the ulna.

  To clearly visualize the radial head, by throwing it off the ulna, a special view is used (Fig. 16.7). This view is called the **"Coyle's view".** In this view, the elbow is flexed, and the shoulder, elbow, and wrist are positioned in the same horizontal plane. The thumb points towards the ceiling. Centre the X-ray beam on the radial head, angulating it by 45° towards the shoulder [1].

- **Views for Scaphoid Fractures**

  The American College of Radiology [2] has recommended four different views to evaluate the scaphoid (also called navicular) bone. These include a PA view, a lateral view, a semi-prone oblique (45° ulnar oblique) and a PA view with ulnar deviation (Fig. 16.8).

  Additional views include a semi-supinated view (45° radial oblique view) and a "banana view".

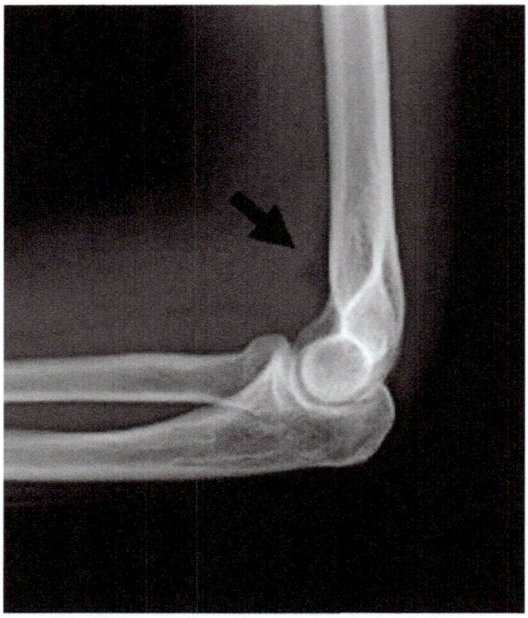

Fig. 16.6 A subtle fracture of the radial neck or head can be missed in this true view. Look out for displacement of the synovial fat pad (arrow). This happens due to the accumulation of synovial fluid/hemarthrosis and is indicative of an intracapsular fracture of the radial head

The "**banana** view" for the scaphoid bone (also called the Ziter's view) [3] is an excellent view to evaluate the scaphoid bone. The wrist is kept in a PA position with slight ulnar deviation. The X-ray beam is focused on the wrist with the tube angled towards the elbow by about 20°. The scaphoid appears stretched out and elongated in this view described by Ziter [4].

Each of these scaphoid views have their own advantage. To understand why these views are useful, one has to take a look at the anatomy of the scaphoid bone. The scaphoid bone has a proximal and distal pole and a waist in between. The blood supply to the scaphoid bone is from branches of the radial artery and flows in a retrograde direction from the distal pole downwards. The different views are taken because fractures are seen better in some views and not in others.

Scaphoid fractures can be missed in up to 20% of cases in X-rays taken within the first week of injury. Therefore, if a strongly suspected fracture is not visible in the X-rays, an MRI of the wrist should be considered. MRI may show oedema caused by trabecular fractures. A CT scan is also sometimes requested even though it is less sensitive than MRI, especially for the detection of trabecular microfractures. The other option is to repeat the X-ray scaphoid series after 2 weeks because it may not be seen in the initial X-rays. The reason why it is important to detect scaphoid fractures is that if left untreated for 4 to 6 weeks, it may lead to non-union of the fractured fragments.

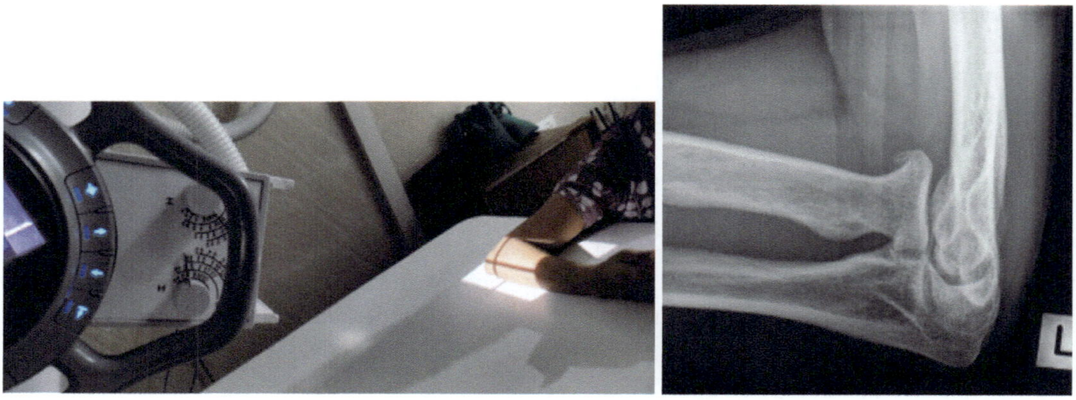

Fig. 16.7 Coyle's view

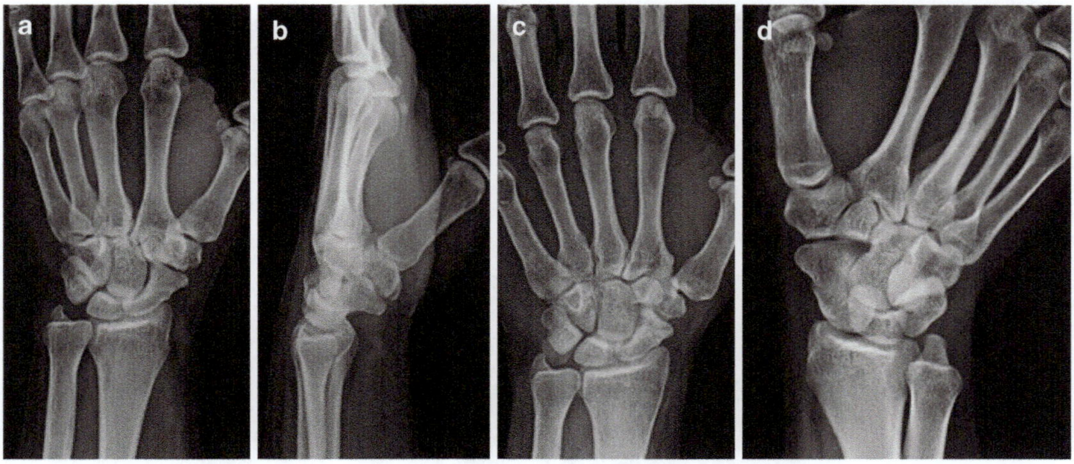

Fig. 16.8 Scaphoid series:- Semiprone (**a**), lateral view (**b**), PA view (**c**) and PA in ulnar deviation (**d**)

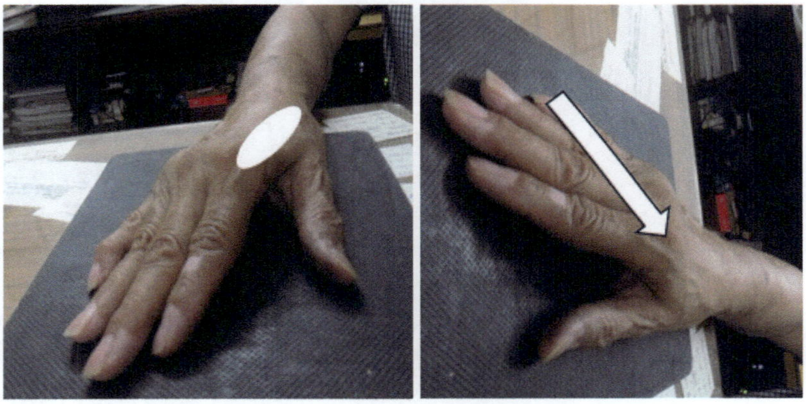

Fig. 16.9 Ziter's (Banana) View for the scaphoid bone

- **The Ball Catcher's View (Norgaard's view)**
  This is a view of both hands often used in suspected cases of RA to detect erosions at the corners of joints (Fig. 16.9). Both hands are cupped by turning them outwards over 40–45°, as if trying to catch a ball. The dorsum of the hands is in touch with the image plate. This view has been replaced by high-resolution ultrasound, which can also demonstrate bone erosions besides other features of rheumatoid arthritis such as synovial thickening, increased synovial vascularity and effusion.
- **Modified Robert's View**
  This is a view used to demonstrate the phalanges of the thumb, the trapeziometacarpal joint and the scaphotrapezial joint [5]. The forearm is internally rotated so that the dorsum of the thumb rests on the image plate. The fingers are kept extended and pulled outwards, away from the thumb, by the other hand so that they do not overlap on the thumb and carpometacarpal joint. The tube is angled 15° towards the wrist.
- **Gaynor Hart's View**
  This is a view used to demonstrate the bony structures forming the carpal tunnel. The forearm and wrist are placed in a prone position. The palm is hyperextended at the wrist joint. The fingers are pulled backwards with the help of a tape or bandage. The X-ray beam is centred at the base of the third metatarsal. The tube is angled 25–30° towards the wrist.

These views are sometimes asked for, hence worth knowing.

- **Cobb's Angle**

  Whenever scoliosis is detected in X-rays of the dorsal spine, a Cobb's angle should be obtained (Fig. 16.10). Cobb's angle is the measurement of spinal curvature obtained by firstly drawing lines along the end plates of the vertebral bodies at the upper and lower limits (extremes) of the spinal curvature (Figs. 16.11 and 16.12).
  This is followed by dropping perpendiculars to these two lines. The perpendiculars cross one another at an angle. This angle is also

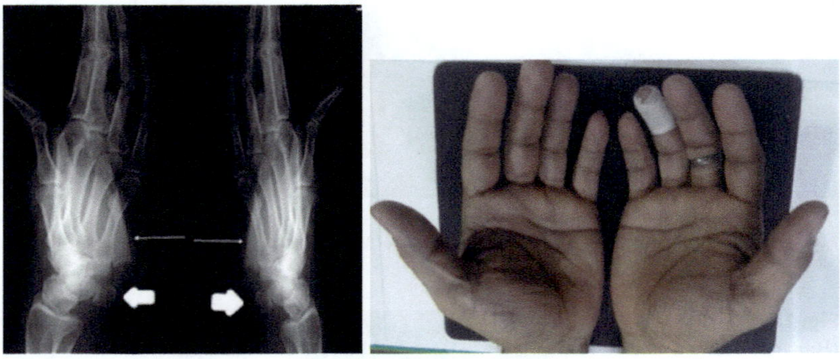

Fig. 16.10 Ball catcher's view (thick arrows)

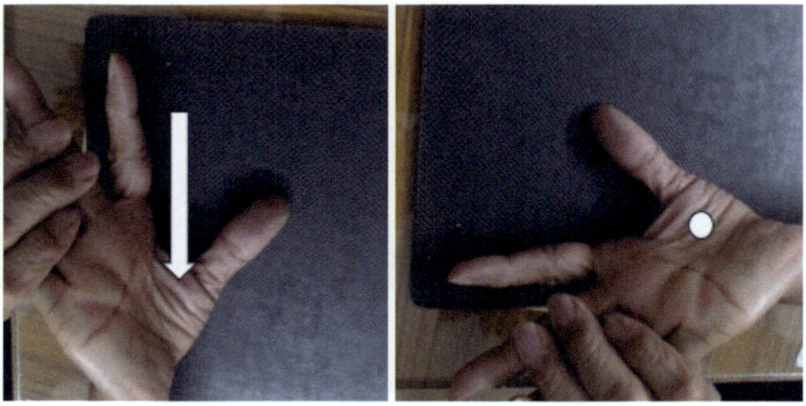

Fig. 16.11 Modified Robert's view

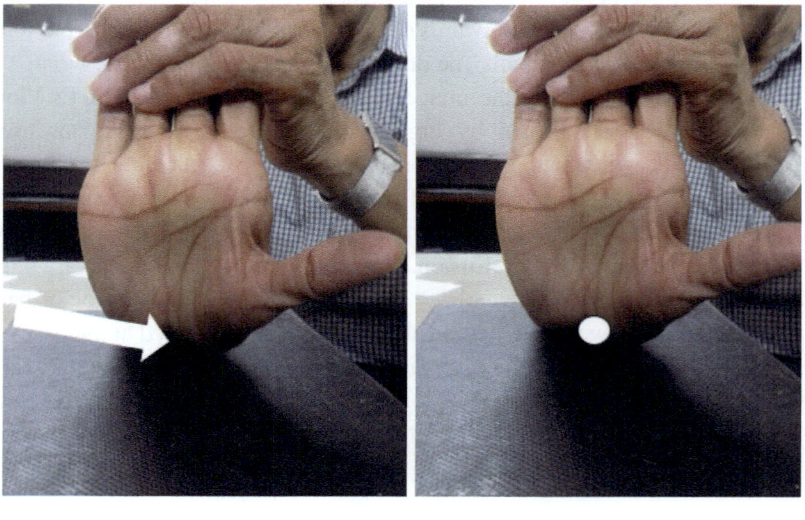

Fig. 16.12 Gaynor Hart's view

known as Cobb's angle. It should not be more than 10°. Between 10° and 20° is mild scoliosis, between 20° and 40° is moderate and over 40° is severe scoliosis [6] (Fig. 16.13).

- **Bohler's Angle**

  A Bohler's angle is meant to detect fractures of the calcaneum. A normal Bohler angle is between 25° and 40° [7] (Fig. 16.14).

  Draw a line joining the uppermost part of the calcaneocuboid articulation and the tip of the posterior articular facet of the talus. Draw another line joining the tip of the posterior articular facet with the calcaneal tuberosity. The angle subtended between these two lines is the Bohler's angle. An angle less than 20° is suggestive of a calcaneal fracture.

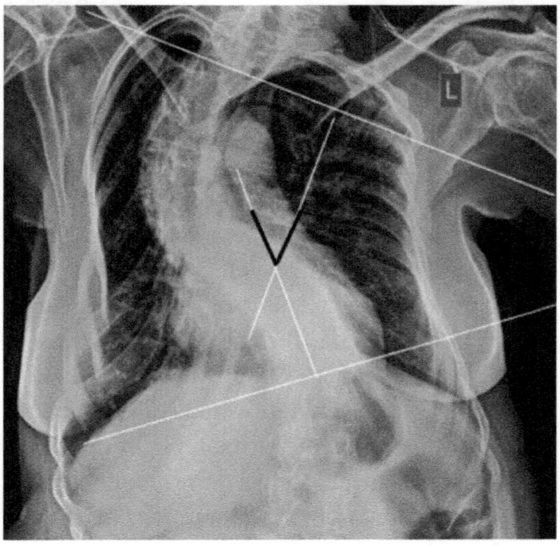

Fig. 16.13 Demonstration of how to obtain the Cobb's angle

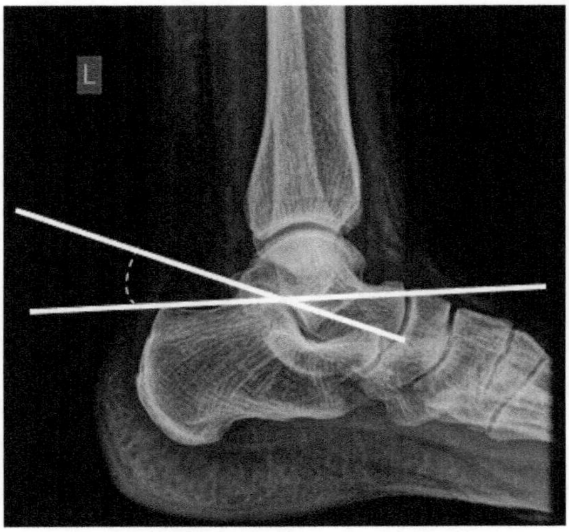

Fig. 16.14 How to calculate the Bohler's angle

16.3 Importance of Obtaining Two Views at Right Angles to One Another

A single view of the skeletal system is often insufficient in demonstrating an abnormality. At least two views taken at right angles to one another must be obtained. Here are two examples (Figs. 16.15 and 16.16)!

16.3.1 Essentials of Skeletal Anatomy

It is important to know a few basic things about the skeletal anatomy, to appreciate normal variations as well as the pathology of bones.

The skeletal system consists of long bones, small bones, flat bones and irregular (vertebral) bones.

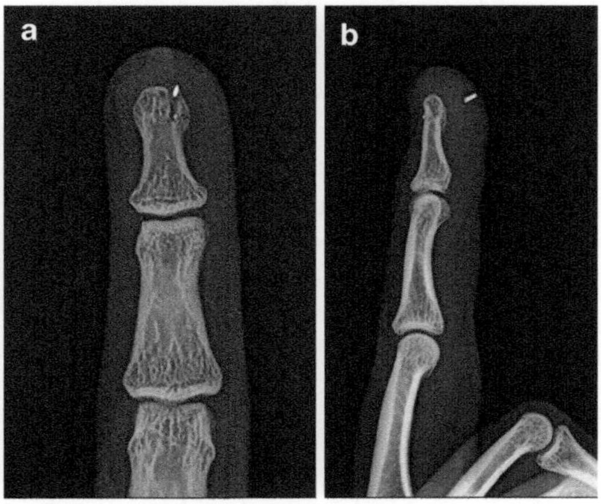

Fig. 16.15 X-ray for the foreign body (FB) (metallic needle tip) localization. In image (**a**), the FB appears to be embedded in the tip of the distal phalanges. The lateral view of the finger (**b**) shows the FB is embedded in the soft tissues and has not penetrated the bone

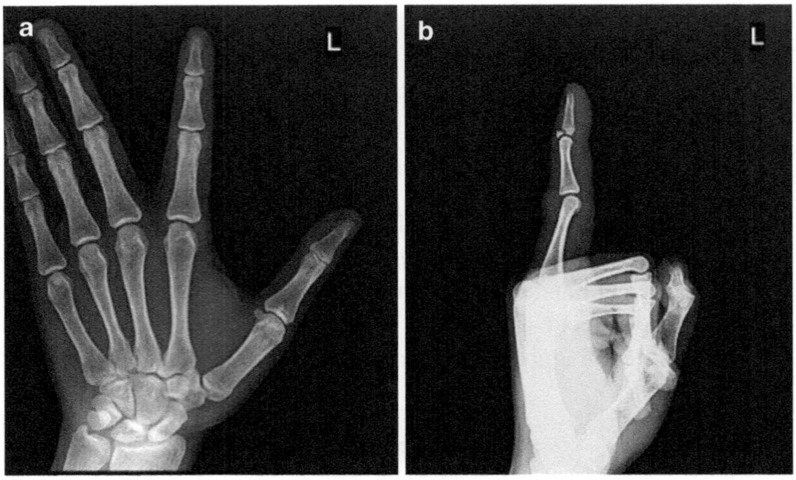

Fig. 16.16 A case of mallet finger. An avulsion fracture of the base of the distal phalanx of the index finger is not seen in the PA view (**a**). The lateral view (**b**) clearly shows it

Each bone has a periosteum and cortex on the outside which cover the inner structure, the medullary cavity, that contains bone marrow.

The cortex of the flat bones of the skull encases what is called the interdiploic space as there is no medulla in flat bones.

The periosteum is a thin fibrous sheath which is not visible on the X-ray unless there is a pathology such as infection, tumour, trauma or a reparative process involving it. It extends from the ends of the long bones, across the diaphysis and does not cover the articular surface.

The cortex is the compact bone which is visible on an X-ray, as a thick, white, dense, solid layer enclosing the medullary cavity or the interdiploic space. On its outer surface, is the periosteal surface and the inner surface is the endosteum.

The medulla, encased by it, consists of trabecular bone and bone marrow.

The long bones are composed of the shaft, also called diaphysis, which is tubular in shape; the metaphysis, which is the flared or broadened distal end; and the epiphysis, the terminal end. The epiphysis is initially separated from the metaphysis by the physis but fuses with it as the skeleton matures.

The terminal ends of two long bones are separated by a joint. A joint is a junction of two bone ends where movement takes place.

Joints are of various types.

They can be ball-and-socket joints, for example, the hip and shoulder joints; hinge joints, such as fingers, wrists, toes and knees; and pivot joints, such as the atlantoaxial joint. Some of the joints are immovable. An example of this is the tooth in a socket. Some are formed by fibrous tissue membranes interconnecting with one another. These joints have slight movement and are called syndesmophytic joints. An example of this is the tibio-fibular and radio-ulnar joint. A membrane, called the interosseous membrane, holds them together, allowing slight movement between the two bones. The articular surfaces of the joints are smooth and take a shape which allows smooth movement against the opposing joint surface. The movement may be large, as in a ball-and-socket joint of the hip. It can also be sliding, where the articular ends, called facets, are almost flat and allow only gliding movement.

Let's look at a typical hinge joint. The ends of the long bones, which form these joints, have a layer of articular cartilage covered by a cushion formed by cartilaginous meniscus. The entire joint is covered by a capsule of fibrous tissue called the joint capsule, which secretes a lubricant—the synovial fluid—to provide smooth, pain-free movement of the joint. These joints are also held together and supported by ligaments and tendons. They have a vascular supply as well as a connection with nerves.

The bony cortex has rough surfaces and irregular outlines. These are meant for either insertion or origin of muscles, tendons, ligaments and fascia. The fascia surrounding the muscles segregates them into different groups.

Bones which are completely embedded in tendons are called sesamoid bones. They are different from accessory bones, which are supernumerary bones, found near the end of short bones. They are present as accessory bones and are well corticated, usually round to ovoid in shape. They should not be mistaken for fractured bone fragments. Fractured bone fragments are geographical in shape with sharp angular borders. Both sesamoid and accessory bones are liable to fracture during a traumatic event; hence, they require careful evaluation.

Sometimes a narrow channel with well-defined walls, called the nutrient canal, is seen entering the bone through an orifice called the nutrient foramen. The vascular supply and nourishment to the bone are through the nutrient artery.

16.4 How Does a Bone Develop?

The bone consists of proteins and minerals such as calcium hydroxyapatite, carbonate, manganese and alkaline phosphatase. The formation of bones is by a complex process called osteoblastic activity performed by osteoblasts. Constant remodelling and reabsorption are by what are called "osteoclasts".

The role of vitamin D in the laying down of minerals in bone matrix is very important. Vitamin D is produced by the skin through exposure to naturally occurring ultraviolet (UV) light. It is initially metabolized by the liver, into the circulating form, 25-hydroxyvitamin D, and further, by the kidneys into 1,25-dihydroxyvitamin D [1,25-$(OH)_2$D]. The 1,25-$(OH)_2$D, by acting on the intestines, stimulates the absorption of calcium and phosphorus from the intestines, thereby maintaining an adequate concentration of these minerals in the bloodstream. This results in the deposition of these minerals on the non-mineralized bone matrix.

16.5 Abnormalities Are Commonly Encountered in X-Rays of the Skeletal System

Note: Only a few cases are being discussed by way of examples. The reader is encouraged to look up more exhaustive books as per requirement during professional life.

- **Metabolic Disease:** These are generalized diseases of nutritional deficiency. Two commonly encountered conditions are discussed here.
  - **Osteoporosis**: This is a condition where, due to a variety of reasons, bone mass reduces and fragility increases. There is a loss of bone from the cortex and medulla. The loss of bone mass is associated with a reduction in the protein and mineral content of the bone. The softened bones are unable to stop the transmission of the X-ray beam through, them resulting in the medulla looking dark on the X-rays, as compared to the denser, more compact cortex. The non-stress-bearing horizontal trabecula disappears first. Hence the number of trabeculae appears less on the X-rays, and the bone appears dark. The vertically orientated trabecula in an osteoporotic bone are still visible, appearing as sieve-like lucencies in the cortex. The causes of osteoporosis include age-related wasting, disuse osteoporosis, steroid-related osteoporosis, vitamin C deficiency or secondary to a malignancy such as myeloma. The tests to determine osteoporosis are to explore bone mineral density by dual-energy X-ray absorptiometry (DEXA) of the hip and spine and quantitative CT

(QCT) of the hip. Scores called the "T score" are then taken out by DEXA equipment, which is then compared with the "T" score values in the normal healthy young population. A "T"-score between +1 and −1 is considered normal. Scores between −1 and −2.5 suggest low bone mass (osteopenia) and a T-score of −2.5 or lower indicates significant bone loss (osteoporosis).

- **Rickets and Osteomalacia** are diseases caused by delayed or insufficient mineralization of the bony matrix due to a deficiency of calcium and vitamin D. It is seen in all age groups, being called rickets in children and osteomalacia in adults. Dietary deficiencies, renal disorders, parathyroid adenomas, lack of absorption from the intestines, and insufficient exposure to sunlight are some of the reasons for developing this mineral deficiency. Patients are brought in with bone and joint deformities, weakness and muscle wasting. On X-rays, unlike in osteoporosis, where the sharpness of the trabecular pattern and bone margins is maintained, the bony outlines of this condition are indistinct and fuzzy. There can be abnormal development of the metaphysis of growing bones, diminished mineralization of the bony matrix, osteoporosis and periosteal reaction. The bones become deformed with resultant bowing, knock knees or varus deformity of the knees. The spine may be deformed with concave vertebral end plates.

- **Lytic and Sclerotic Lesions***:* Destruction of bone can be either due to a benign or an aggressive pathology.

  Lytic lesions result in bone loss at the affected site. Solitary lytic lesions can be benign lesions, malignant primary tumours or secondary deposits from a primary malignant tumour elsewhere in the body. Pathological fractures can happen due to any underlying bony lesion.

  Sclerotic lesions can be primary bone tumours, metastatic deposits or a benign lesion. These lesions can be localized or disseminated.

- **Fractures:** X-rays are most frequently requested for the diagnosis of fractures of various bones. A fracture is the separation of a bone into two or more fragments. It differs from a lytic lesion of the bone by the fact that if the fractured fragments are approximated, they can fit in like pieces of a jigsaw puzzle. A minimum of two views at right angles to one another should be obtained to study fractures. Sometimes multiple views may also be needed, as in cases of scaphoid fracture. The fractured site needs to be evaluated for any malalignment, angulation, number of fractured fragments, distance of fragments from one another, associated dislocation of joints, soft tissue and neurovascular injury. Before doing an X-ray, the request form must be carefully read to avoid unnecessary errors. The injured part must be carefully handled so as not to aggravate the injury. One should always ask the patient, where it hurts most and record that region in the X-ray request form. The radiographed side should be correctly marked using a lead or digital marker. Exposure factors and beam collimation have to be adjusted according to the part being examined. Upon completion of the radiograph, the film should be examined for technical quality and to ensure that the affected area, along with the adjoining joint space, has been fully included in the film (Fig. 16.17).

- **Fractures are of Various Types:**

  A few types will be discussed here.

  In children, before the skeletons mature, the ossific centres are unfused. Do not mistake these unfused epiphyses for fractures. Sometimes, only a soft tissue swelling is seen, as in this X-ray of the elbow (Fig. 16.18). This could be indicative of an intra-articular fracture. In a suspected case of fracture, one should look at the AP view carefully and obtain a lateral view to confirm the presence of the fracture and determine the relationship between the two fractured ends. The lateral view may show displaced synovial fat pads, which is suggestive of an intra-articular fracture (Figs. 16.19, 16.20, and 16.21).

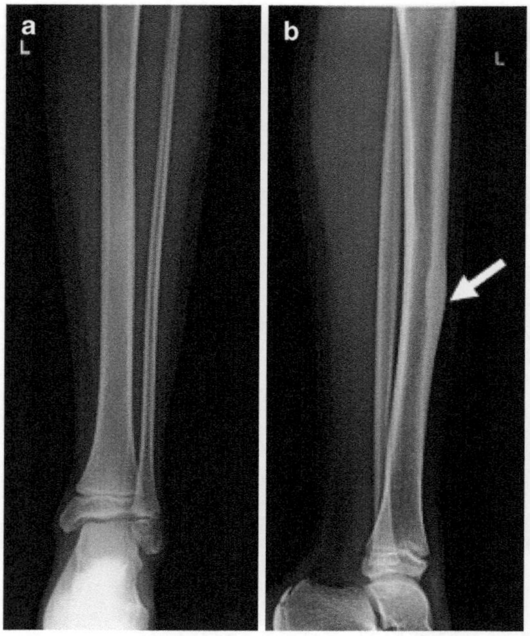

Fig. 16.17 X-ray of the left leg shows a focal area of cortical thickening (arrow in **b**), which is not appreciable in the AP view (**a**). This was a case of osteoid osteoma, which is a benign bony lesion

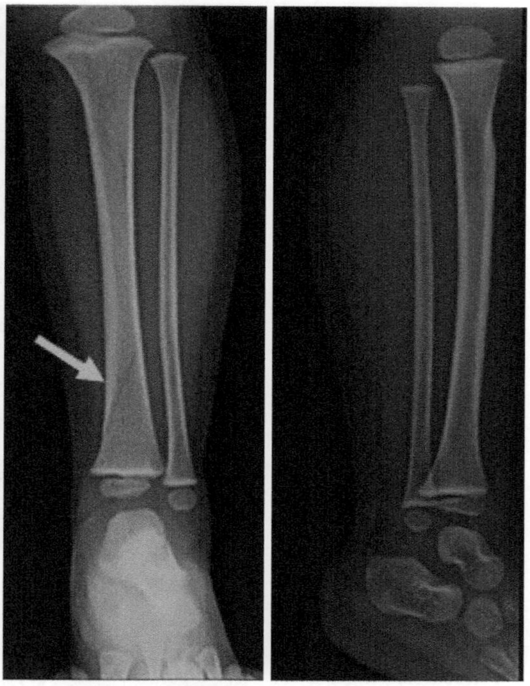

Fig. 16.19 A spiral fracture of the lower end of the left radius, seen well in the AP view but not in the lateral. Thus, exposures have to be a minimum of two, at right angles to one another

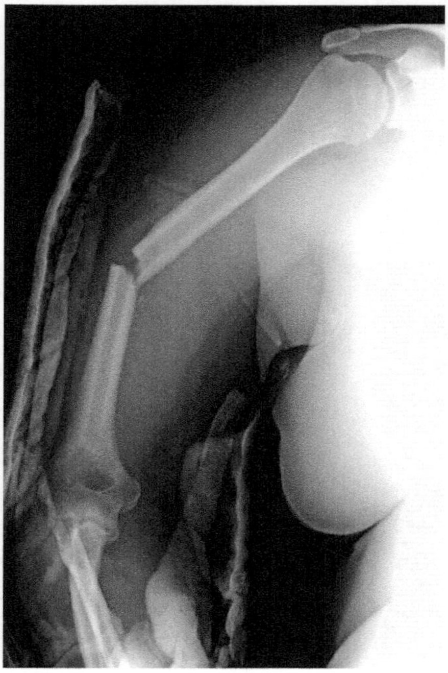

Fig. 16.18 Transverse fracture of the mid-shaft of the humerus. Notice the angulation of the two fractured ends

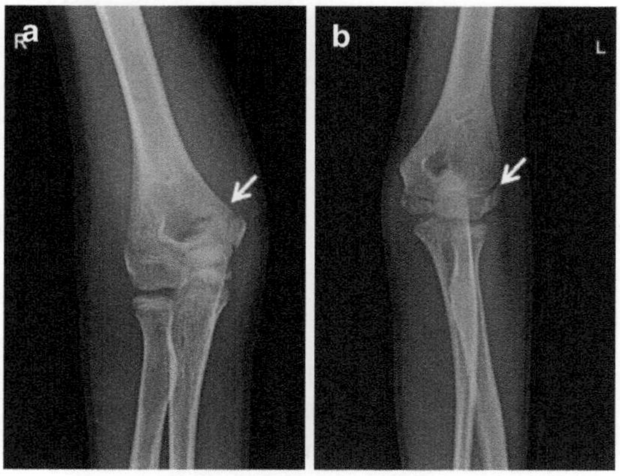

Fig. 16.20 Intraarticular fracture: X-ray of the elbow shows an intraarticular fracture of the humerus (arrow). The view to the left (**a**) is with the forearm in pronation, and on the right (**b**) is with the forearm in supination

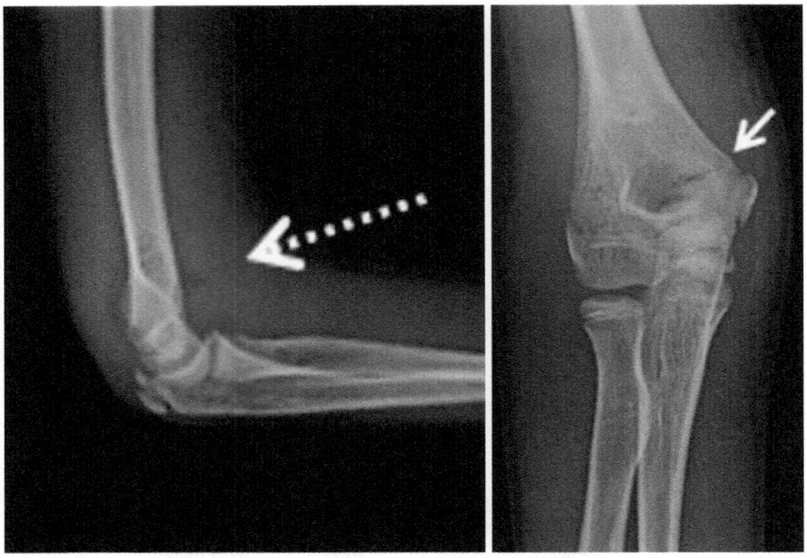

Fig. 16.21 The right elbow shows swelling of the soft tissues with displaced synovial fat pads (dotted arrows). This is indicative of an intra-articular fracture which can now be appreciated in the AP film also (white arrow)

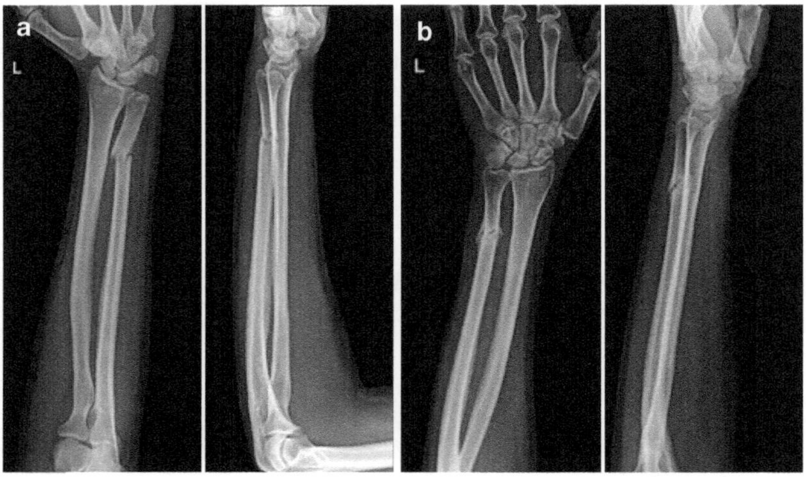

Fig. 16.22 X-ray of the left forearm. Figure (**a**) is before treatment, and (**b**) is after a few weeks of treatment. The x-rays show adequate reduction and formation of the callus

When the fracture is treated either by a cast or by internal fixation using plates and screws, the process of healing starts. A new bone, called callus, is formed around the fracture site. Check x-rays are obtained after treatment to determine the adequacy of correction, formation of callus and healing of the fracture.

A callus is better seen in fractured long bones which are treated with a cast, rather than with implants (Figs. 16.22 and 16.23)

- **Dislocation**

  During an accident, not only can a bone break, but the joint can also get dislocated. In such cases, the movement of the limb may be extremely painful and restricted. X-rays

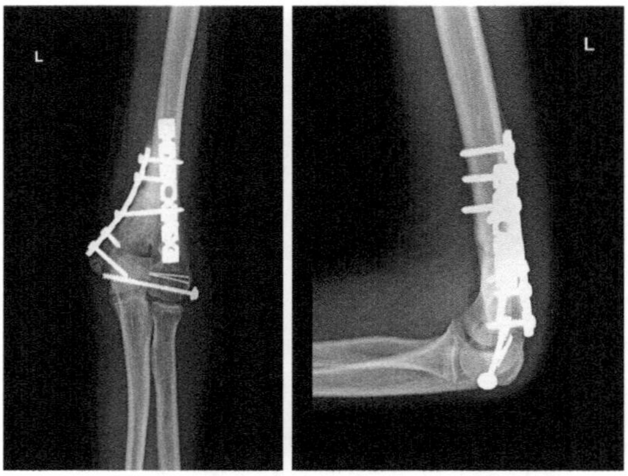

Fig. 16.23 X-rays of the distal humeral fracture, showing internal fixation using plates and screws. Callus formation and healing are difficult to demonstrate whenever internal fixation using metallic implants, is performed

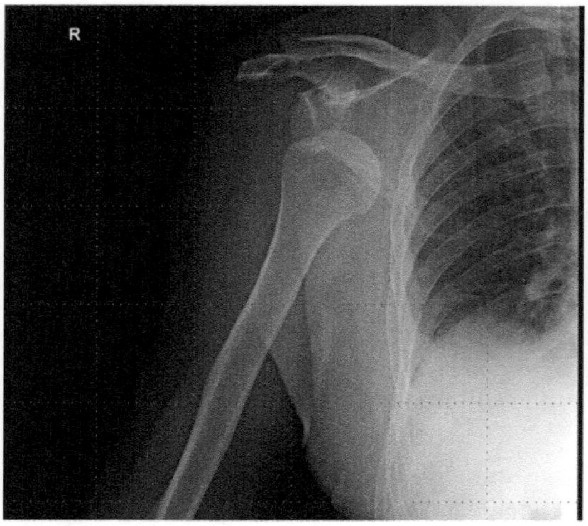

Fig. 16.24 X-ray of the right shoulder, showing anterior dislocation of the humeral head. Note the malalignment of the humeral head with the glenoid fossa. Also note the position of the dislocated humeral head, which is seen below the anteriorly located coracoid process. This is a case of "subcoracoid anterior dislocation" of the shoulder

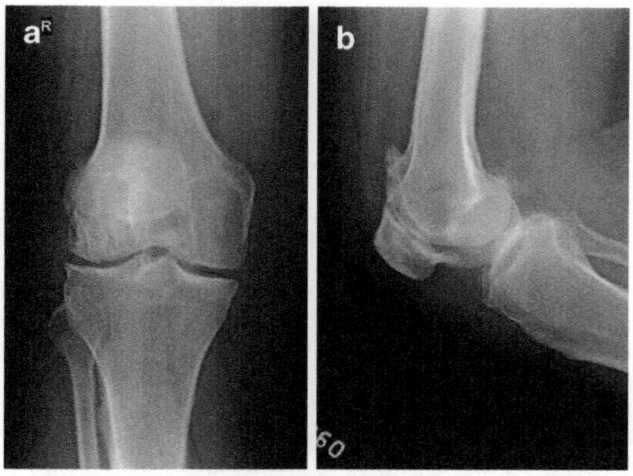

Fig. 16.25 Osteoarthritic changes in the knee. Note the presence of a lucency indicates degeneration in the medial aspect of the knee joint space (**a**). The lateral view shows degenerative changes in the patellofemoral joint (**b**)

should be performed without causing additional pain to the patient. They should be done in the position, most comfortable for the patient and the best possible view or views, under the circumstances, should be obtained. The X-ray should be immediately reviewed by the treating physician and radiologist so that the problem is identified, and a decision regarding additional X-rays can be taken on the spot (Fig. 16.24).

- **Joint Disorders Such as Osteoarthritis and Rheumatoid Arthritis.**
- **Osteoarthritis (OA):** Osteoarthritis is a disorder of joints; when age-related, it is called primary osteoarthritis. When caused by old trauma, underlying avascular necrosis of the bone, connective tissue disorders or previous infection, it is called secondary osteoarthritis. Weight-bearing joints, especially the knee joints, are more prone to developing osteoarthritis. However, even small joints of the hands, toes and wrists can be affected by OA. In this disorder, the articular surfaces of the joints lose their normal smooth fit and become irregular and deformed, resulting in tears and degeneration of the cartilage covering them. The joint space narrows with the subarticular surface showing evidence of necrosis. The bony surfaces rub against each other, resulting in painful movement accompanying the wear and tear. Occasionally a vacuum phenomenon can also be seen in a degenerated joint space. The knees, shoulders, cervical spine, and distal interphalangeal joints are most frequently involved. In the cervical spine, changes can be seen both in the lower and especially in the upper cervical region. The lumbosacral and the temporomandibular (TM) joints also show degenerative changes in the form of asymmetric sclerosis, localized curvature, asymmetric or symmetric disc space reduction and development of anterior and lateral osteophytes. The latter probably provides support to the relatively unstable spine (Figs. 16.25, 16.26, and 16.27).
- **Rheumatoid Arthritis**: This is a connective tissue-related pathology which can be seen at both early and late ages, especially in females. It usually affects small joints of the hands and feet, single large joints, the upper cervical spine and TM joints. The pathology is essentially in the synovial membranes, which are inflamed and hypertrophied. They cause erosions at the site of attachment to the joint margins. At a later stage, the hypertrophied synovium burrows into the joint cartilage and bony surfaces. The affected joints swell and show periarticular (around joints) rarefaction,

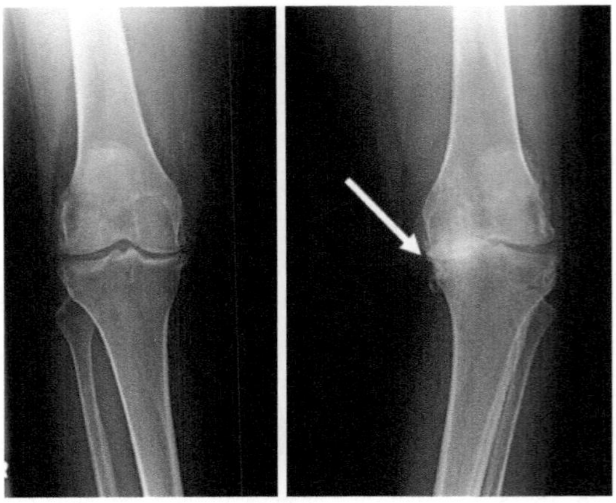

Fig. 16.26 A case of bilateral osteoarthritis. Note sclerosis, deformity and joint space reduction in the left knee (arrow)

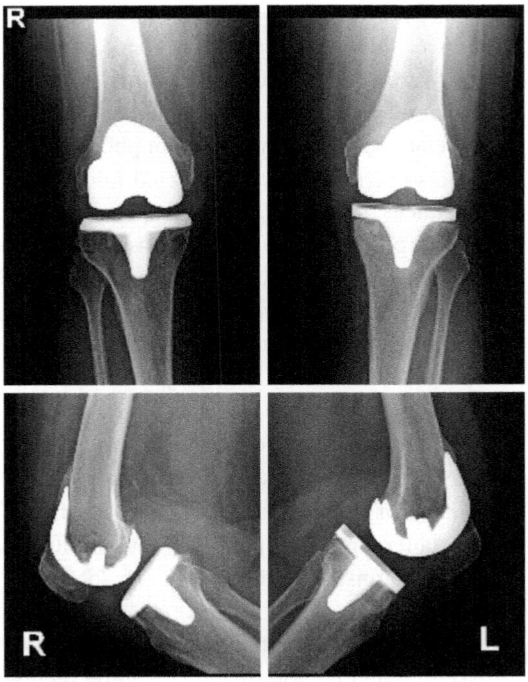

Fig. 16.27 A case of severe osteoarthritis in both knees, treated by total knee replacement (TKR)

joint space reduction followed by bony destruction close to the joint margins. There is usually no osteophytosis or sclerosis, which enables distinction from osteoarthritis. In untreated cases, the hands and wrist show various types of deformities.

Although RA involves the feet as frequently as the hands, it is the hands which are most often x-rayed. The views include PA of the hands and wrist as well as the ball catcher's view (NorGaard's view). Both hands should be radiographed for comparison. The PA view helps evaluate the alignment of the bones to each other, determine the presence of juxta-articular rarefaction, if any, evaluate joint margins for any erosions and examine the soft tissues for any swelling.

The "ball catchers" view can be performed as an additional view to further evaluate the edges and corners of the joints for any erosions, which may not be apparent in the PA view.

Evaluating the cervical spine for any changes due to RA entails obtaining a lateral view in flexion, extension and neutral positions. Usually, the C1-C2 vertebra shows erosions with synovial soft tissue swelling. Later on, there may be subluxation with progressive bone destruction.

The soft tissues are best evaluated by high-resolution musculoskeletal ultrasound. The swollen tendon sheaths, inflammatory changes in colour/power Doppler and even bony erosions can be appreciated on high-resolution ultrasound. Bone changes, such as erosions, subchondral cysts, osteolysis and fusion, occur much later and are infrequently seen nowadays.

- **Other common joint lesions for which x-rays are frequently requested**: These include gout, other crystal deposit diseases, tuberculosis as well as non-tubercular infections of joints. The bony erosion in gout is likened to a rat bite. There is usually associated soft tissue swelling which may show faint calcification. A dual-energy CT can help in demonstrating gouty deposits. One may be asked to take an X-ray of the hands of patients with psoriasis and shoulders, wrists, knees and symphysis pubis in crystal deposition diseases.
- **Chondrocalcinosis:** Calcification in the articular cartilage, particularly of the knee, wrist, and spine, can occur due to a variety of lesions.

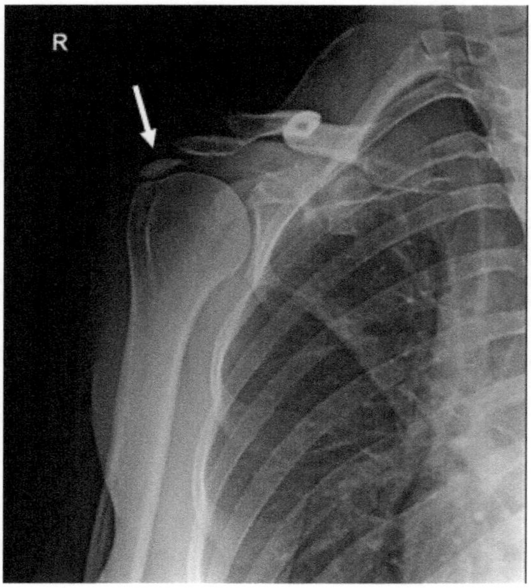

Fig. 16.28 Crystal deposition in the rotator cuff region of the right shoulder

These include **W**ilson's disease, **H**yperparathyroidism, **H**emochromatosis, **I**diopathic, **P**seudogout (CPDD), **A**cromegaly, **D**iabetes Mellitus, **O**chronosis and **G**out (WHIP A DOG). A knowledge of the clinical profile helps in arriving at the correct diagnosis (Fig. 16.28).

The skeletal system, as seen above, occupies a large chunk of the radiologic technologists and radiologists time. In trauma patients, positioning may not be easy. The technologist must learn to work around the situation so that the radiological findings may be appropriately demonstrated. Also, the technologist is in a good position to examine and talk to the patient. The role of the technologist is of paramount importance in the field of skeletal radiology.

References

1. Coyle GF. Unit 7. Special angled views of joints—elbow, knee, ankle. In: Radiographing immobile trauma patients. Denver: Multi-Media Publishing; 1980.
2. Torabi M, Lenchik L, Beaman FD, Wessell DE, Bussell JK, Cassidy RC, Czuczman GJ, Demertzis JL, Khurana B, Klitzke A, Motamedi K, Pierce JL, Sharma A, Walker EA, Kransdorf MJ. ACR Appropriateness Criteria® acute hand and wrist trauma. J Am Coll Radiol. 2019;16(5, Supplement):S7–S17. https://doi.org/10.1016/j.jacr.2019.02.029.
3. Stirling PHC, Strelzow JA, Doornberg JN, White TO, McQueen MM, Duckworth A. Diagnosis of suspected scaphoid fractures. J Bone Joint Surg. 2021;9(12):e20.00247. https://doi.org/10.2106/JBJS.RVW.20.00247.
4. Ziter FMH. A modified view of the carpal navicular. Radiology. 1973;108(3):706–7.
5. Ladd AL. Guest editorial: the Robert's view: a historical and clinical perspective. Clin Orthop Relat Res. 2014;472(4):1097–100. https://doi.org/10.1007/s11999-013-3428-2.
6. Horng MH, Kuok CP, Fu MJ, Lin CJ, Sun YN. Cobb angle measurement of spine from X-ray images using convolutional neural network. Comput Math Methods Med. 2019;19(2019):6357171. https://doi.org/10.1155/2019/6357171.
7. Amini B, Worsley C, Weerakkody Y, et al. Böhler angle. Radiopaedia.org. https://doi.org/10.53347/rID-1002.

17 The Peritoneal Spaces

Abstract

A thin serous membrane, called the peritoneal membrane outlines the abdominal cavity. It wraps the solid and hollow organs and anchors them loosely to the abdominal wall. It divides the abdominal cavity into spaces called the intra- and extraperitoneal spaces. These spaces hold the abdominal organs and help localize the spread of diseases.

The peritoneal membrane itself can be the site of a primary disease. It can also be secondarily affected by diseases spreading from neighbouring and remotely located organs. Hence the need to know something about the peritoneum!

Keywords

Abdominal cavity · Peritoneum · Peritoneal spaces

The abdominal cavity is outlined by a thin translucent serous membrane called the peritoneal membrane. This membrane divides the cavity into intra- and extraperitoneal spaces. The intraperitoneal space contains most of the solid and hollow organs which are anchored to the posterior abdominal wall by the peritoneal folds. The extraperitoneal space, which is outside the peritoneal cavity, contains some hollow organs and blood vessels. It is divided into three spaces: the retroperitoneal space, which is posterior to the peritoneal cavity; the subperitoneal space, which is below the peritoneal cavity; and the preperitoneal space, which is between the anterior abdominal wall muscles and the peritoneal cavity. The peritoneal membrane enclosing the abdominal viscera is called the "visceral peritoneum", and the membrane outlining the parietal wall is the "parietal peritoneum".

The parietal peritoneum anchors the abdominal viscera to the abdominal wall by forming suspensory ligaments and mesenteric folds [1], through which vessels, nerves, and lymphatics traverse to reach the organs they supply. It also forms a protective covering over the viscera, called the greater and lesser omentum.

The peritoneum also forms several pouches as it wraps over the viscera. These pouches are normally not visible because, under normal circumstances, they are opposed to each other. Whenever there is fluid or air in the abdominal cavity, these pouches fill up and become visible. Examples are "Morison's pouch" between the liver and right kidney, "Pouch of Douglas", between the uterus and rectum, rectovesical space, and right and left subphrenic spaces.

R. Gothi, *Radiographic and Imaging Techniques for Radiology Residents and Technologists*,
https://doi.org/10.1007/978-981-96-4816-0_17

The normal peritoneal reflections and spaces are easily seen in patients with a large amount of intra-abdominal fat deposition in cross-sectional imaging studies such as CT scans and MRI.

We will now examine the peritoneum through images of the abdomen obtained through different imaging modalities. We shall start with plain films first because they are the most basic views for recognizing the peritoneal spaces.

17.1 Plain X-Rays of the Abdomen

The peritoneal folds are not seen in a normal X-ray of the abdomen. However, in the presence of air and fat (Fig. 17.1), some of the spaces can be recognized (Figs. 17.2, 17.3, 17.4, and 17.5).

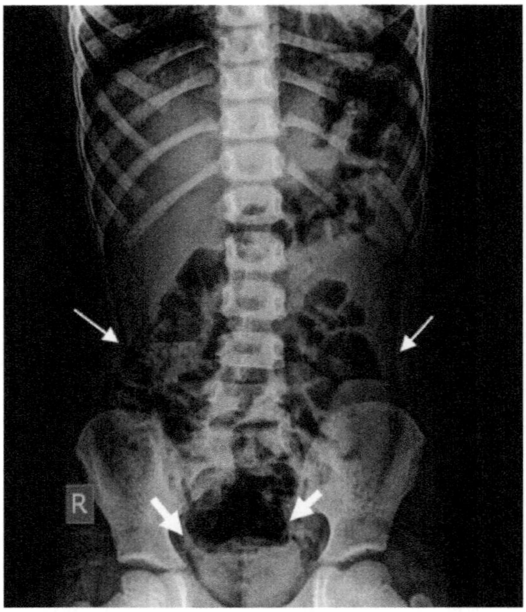

Fig. 17.2 Thin arrows showing extraperitoneal fat. The extraperitoneal fat plane can also obliterated by local inflammatory processes and lateral bending, as in scoliosis. Thick arrow showing perivesical fat. The perivesical fat planes are obliterated by subperitoneal fluid collection. Fluid in the peritoneal cavity also obscures it

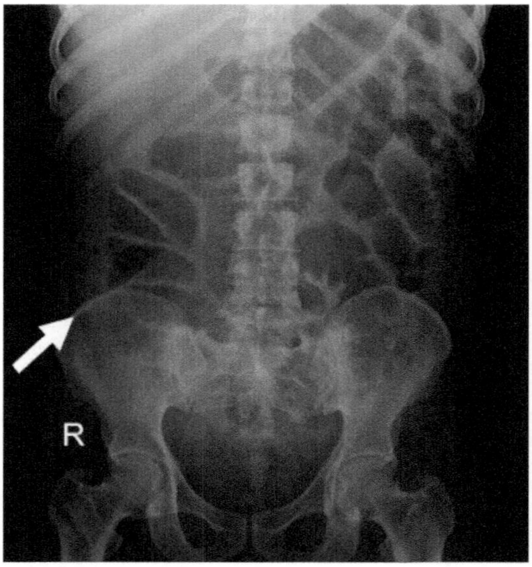

Fig. 17.1 The extraperitoneal space can be recognized by the presence of fat within it (arrow). This space gets compressed and obliterated whenever there is distension of the abdominal cavity due to bowel gas shadows or massive ascites

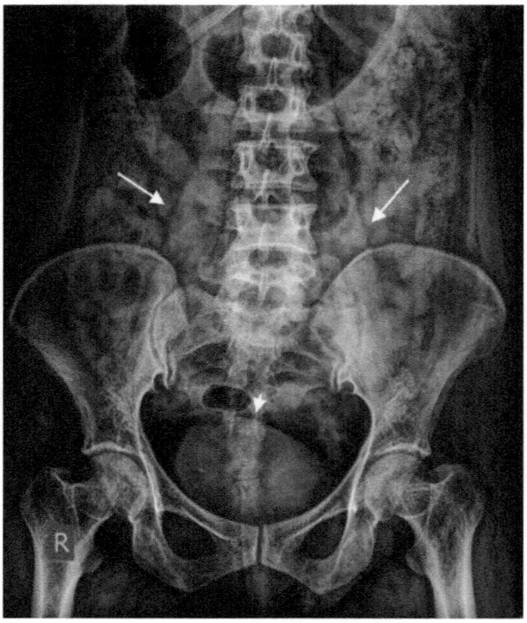

Fig. 17.3 Arrows showing extraperitoneal (retroperitoneal) fat outlining the normal psoas muscles. This retroperitoneal fat stripe is obliterated by a scoliotic deformity as well as by paraspinal abscesses. If the retroperitoneal fat is replaced by air, consider the perforation of a retroperitoneally located bowel loop, especially the duodenum

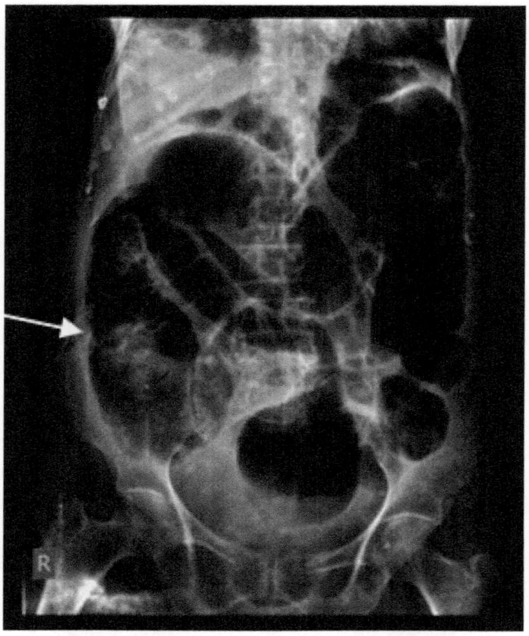

Fig. 17.4 Extraperitoneal fat planes obliterated by distended gas-filled bowel loops (arrow)

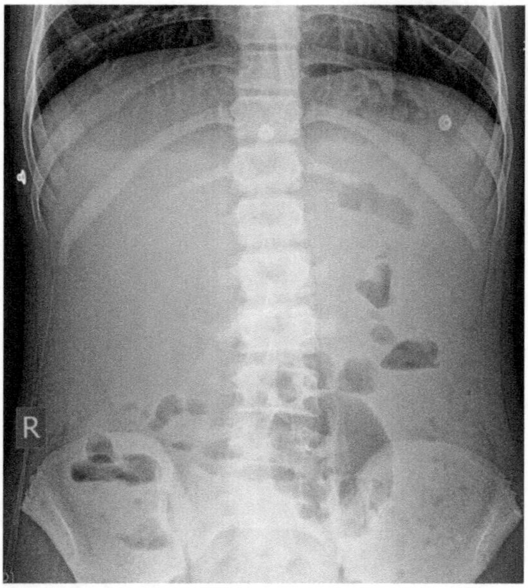

Fig. 17.5 Loss of extraperitoneal fat stripe due to the compressive effect of fluid in the abdominal cavity

17.2 Peritoneal Anatomy as Seen in CT and MRI

The peritoneal reflections as well as spaces are easily seen in most patients, provided they have some fat in the peritoneal and extraperitoneal spaces. A pictorial study using both CT and MRI images will be used to drive home the point that these cross-sectional imaging studies are excellent for examining the peritoneal spaces. (Figs. 17.6, 17.7, 17.8, 17.9, 17.10, 17.11, 17.12, 17.13, and 17.14).

These are some of the examples of how the peritoneal layers and the peritoneal spaces look in various imaging modalities. The peritoneal layers form large spaces, and knowledge of anatomy helps localize the disease process and better treatment planning.

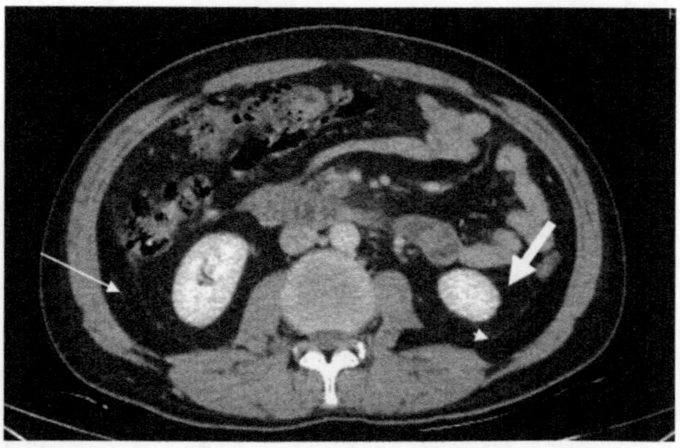

Fig. 17.6 CT scan of the abdomen showing extraperitoneal fat (thin arrow), peritoneal membrane (arrowhead) and peritoneal cavity (thick arrow)

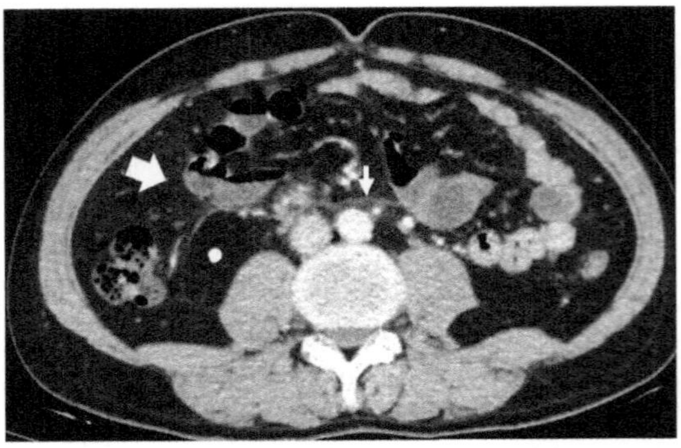

Fig. 17.7 CT scan of the abdomen showing the peritoneal cavity (thick arrow), containing bowel loops, thick peritoneum overlying the aorta and IVC, which are retroperitoneal structures, and retroperitoneal fat (white dot), surrounding the psoas muscle

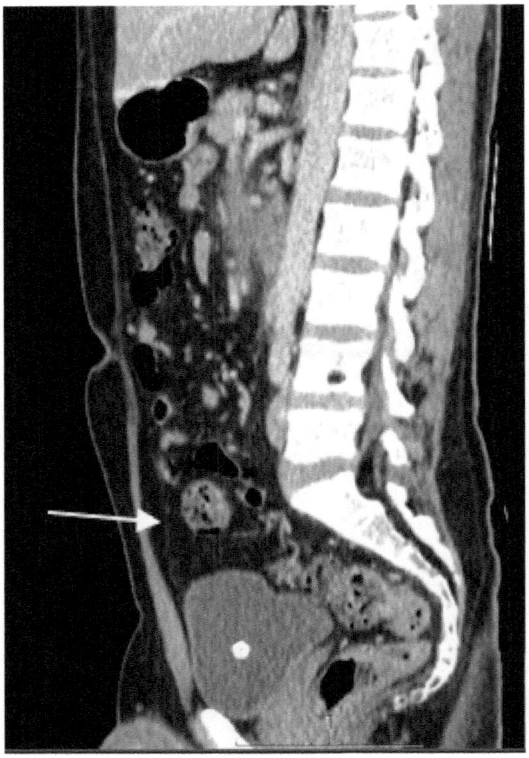

Fig. 17.8 Sagittal reformation, showing preperitoneal space (arrow). The urinary bladder (white dot) is located in the subperitoneal space

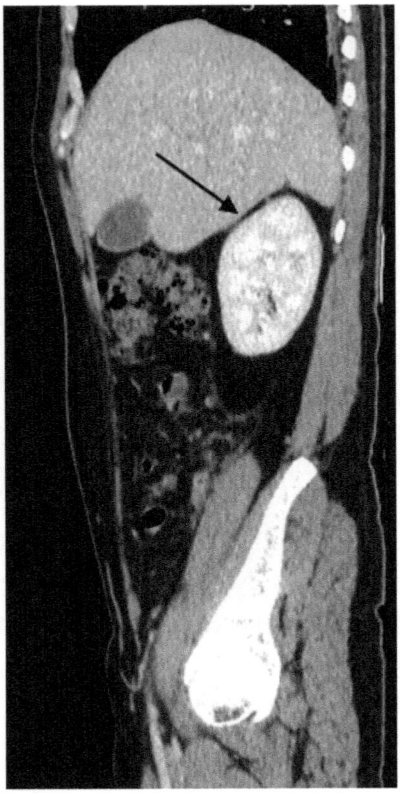

Fig. 17.9 Morison's pouch (arrow), between the liver and right kidney

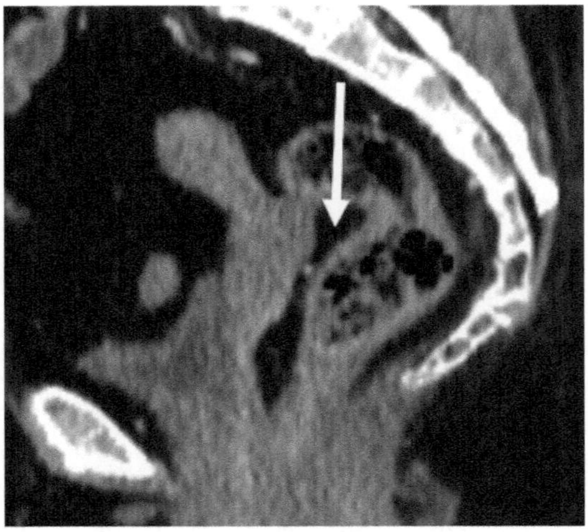

Fig. 17.10 CT scan showing the location of the Pouch of Douglas between the uterus and rectum. In males, this space is simply called the rectovesical pouch

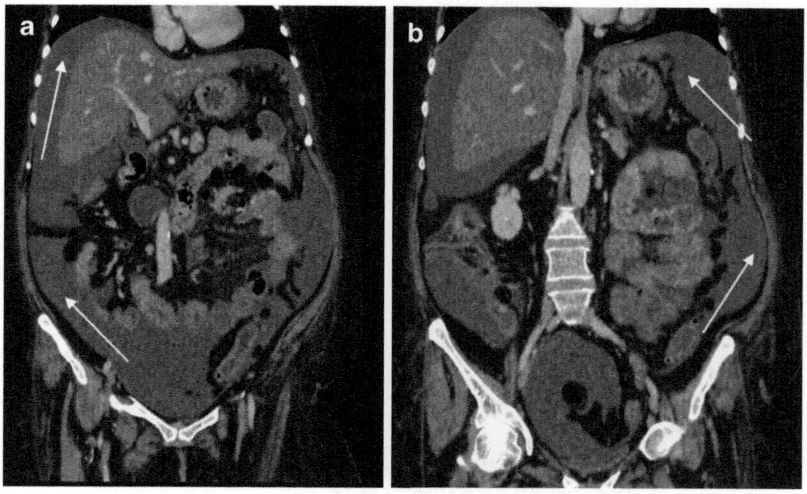

Fig. 17.11 Demonstration of fluid-filled peritoneal cavity. Note how the fluid fills the right (**a**) and left flanks (**b**) and extends upwards to the bare area of the liver

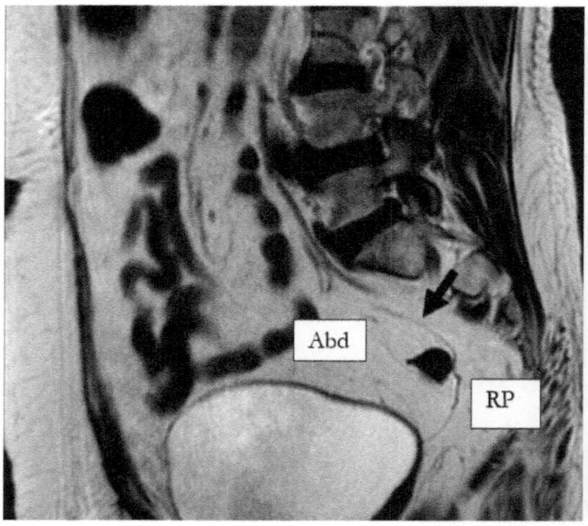

Fig. 17.12 MRI of the abdomen, showing the peritoneal membrane (black arrow) separating the intra-abdominal fat (Abd) from the retroperitoneal fat (RP)

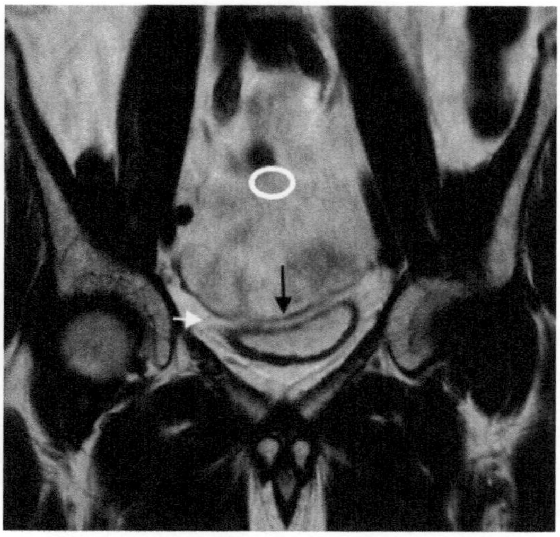

Fig. 17.13 MRI image of the pelvis. The peritoneal layer (black arrow) is seen separating the abdominal cavity (circle) from the subperitoneal fat (small white arrow), which surrounds the urinary bladder

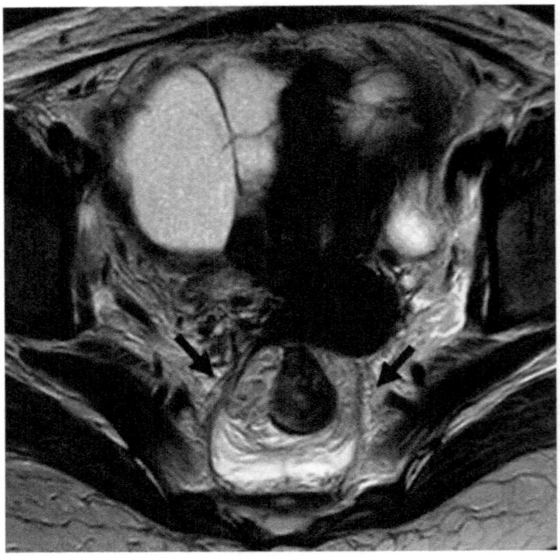

Fig. 17.14 MRI of the pelvis, showing mesorectal fascia (black arrows) surrounding the rectum, which is an extraperitoneal structure. The mesorectal fascia is a continuity of the posterior layer of the peritoneum [2] which separates the presacral fat plane from the abdominal cavity

References

1. Marques DT, de Brito Siqueira LT, Bezerra ROF, Menezes MR, de Souza Rocha M, Cerri GG. Resident and fellow education feature: imaging evaluation of peritoneal disease: overview of anatomy and differential diagnosis. Radiographics. 2014;34(4):962–3.
2. Santiago I, Figueiredo N, Parés O, et al. MRI of rectal cancer—relevant anatomy and staging key points. Insights Imaging. 2020;11:100. https://doi.org/10.1186/s13244-020-00890-7.

18 X-Rays of the Skull

Abstract

With the advent of CT scans, the utility of X-rays of the skull has reduced significantly. Nevertheless, x-rays are still requested for medico-legal purposes, evaluation of paranasal sinuses, teeth, post-cochlear implant surgery, as a part of the skeletal survey for metabolic bone disease, congenital anomalies, and skeletal metastasis. Hence, it is important to know at least some of the positions still in use in skull radiography.

Keywords

Skull · Cochlear implants · Paranasal sinuses Skeletal survey · Skull · Waters view · Lateral view · TM joints · OPG · Cadwell's view

The commonly requested skull x-rays in the present time are the PA and lateral views, the Waters view for paranasal sinuses, the open and closed mouth of the TM joints, the orthopantomographic view (OPG) of the teeth, and Stenver's view for evaluating the position of the electrode array in cochlear implants. A coned-down view of the Sella is rarely asked for these days. These views will be discussed in this chapter. The reader is encouraged to look up books specializing in radiography for descriptions of various other views of the skull, which were commonly used previously but are rarely asked for these days.

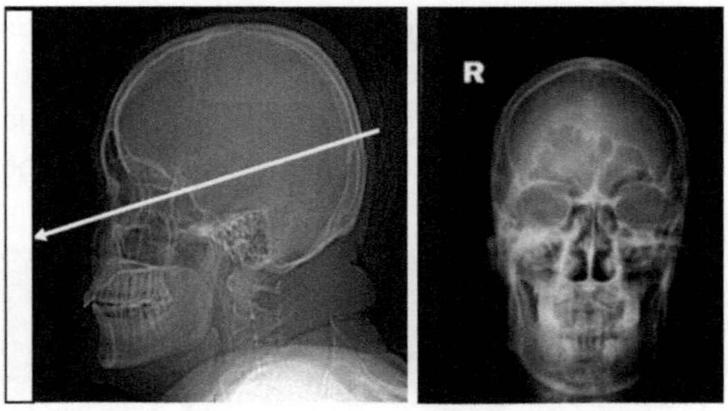

Fig. 18.1 Cadwell view

- **Cadwell's view**: This is an x-ray skull PA view (Fig. 18.1), also called "the Cadwell's view". Note the position of the petrous bones in the x-ray. They are projected just below the orbital margin. This view allows easy assessment of the orbital margins. The frontal sinuses are also projected better in this view, as they are parallel to the imaging plate, unlike in a Water's view, where they are projected at an angle to the image plate. Unlike in a trans-orbital view where no angulation is given and the petrous bones are projected within the orbital margins, this view is obtained by about 15% caudal angulation.
- **Water's view (also called occipitomental view) for paranasal sinuses** (Fig. 18.2): This is a PA view of the skull performed for evaluating the paranasal sinuses. The chin should touch the image plate while the tip of the nose should be just away from it. The mouth should

R. Gothi, *Radiographic and Imaging Techniques for Radiology Residents and Technologists*,
https://doi.org/10.1007/978-981-96-4816-0_18

be kept open. The orbitomeatal (OM) line makes an angle of 45° with the horizontal plane. The X-ray beam is centred above the upper lip, just below the nasal septum without any need for angulation. Note the clear visualization of the maxillary sinuses. However, this view does not provide an adequate assessment of the frontal and ethmoid sinuses. The sphenoid sinus is seen through the open mouth. If the neck is extended further, it is possible to get good images of the odontoid process.

- **Orthopantomographic view:** This is a panoramic view (Fig. 18.3) of the upper and lower sets of teeth, obtained by using a special type of X-ray machine called the orthopantomograph (OPG). This view not only shows the entire rows of teeth but can also be used in the evaluation of the mandible, including the temporomandibular joints (Figs. 18.4 and 18.5) and maxillary sinuses.

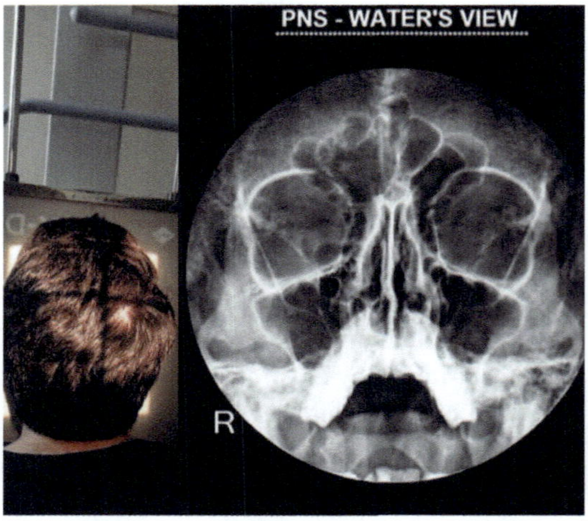

Fig. 18.2 Water's view

These days, radiographs are rarely requested, for evaluation of temporal bone pathologies. They have been replaced by high-resolution CT scans and MRIs of the temporal bones. However, we still come across requests for Stenver's view, especially following a cochlear implant to assess the position of the electrode array. The Stenver's and modified Stenver's views require some understanding of the anatomy to get it right in the X-rays.

Stenver's view demonstrates the triangular-shaped petrous bone as a longitudinal structure. The superior surface is the tegmen tympani. The middle ear cavity with the ossicular chain and the snail-like cochlear turns are also well demonstrated, making it easy to evaluate the electrode of the cochlear implant.

The principle of this view is to align the petrous temporal bone, parallel to the image

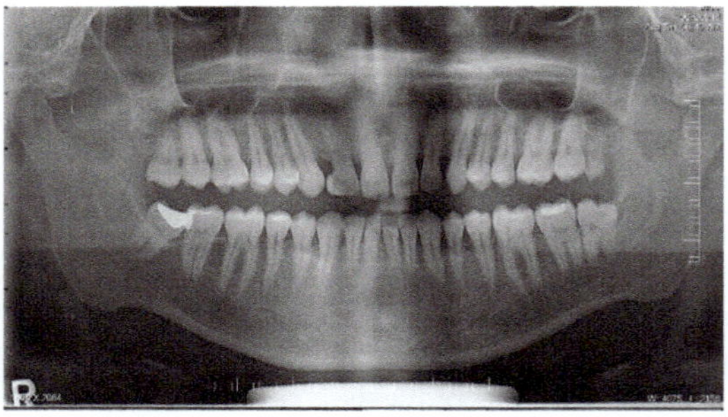

Fig. 18.3 Orthopantomograph (OPG)

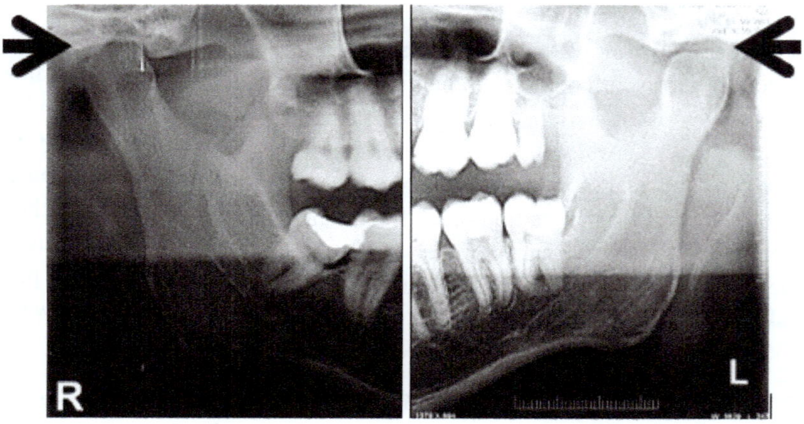

Fig. 18.4 OPG for TM joints. The OPG images can be put to good use in the evaluation of the TM joints (arrows). Both open and closed-mouth views can be performed to evaluate TM joint mobility

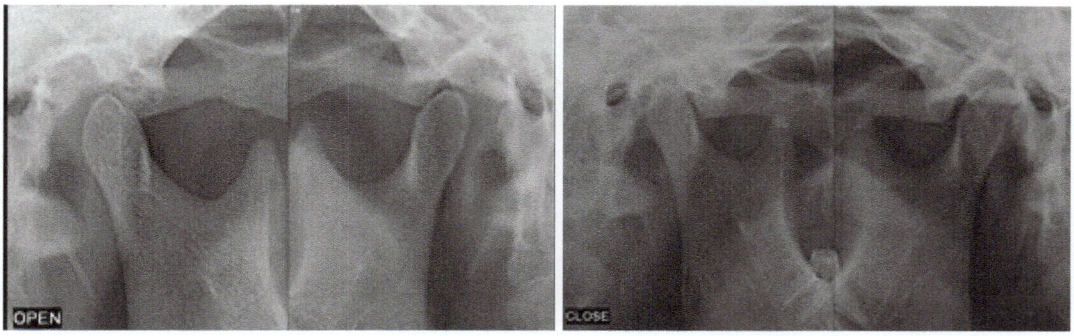

Fig. 18.5 OPG for open and close mouth views: These views are requested to evaluate the mobility of the mandibular condyles relative to the mandibular fossa. Although this is not how a TM joint X-ray should be obtained, the OPG works well because of the additional capabilities of the OPG machine

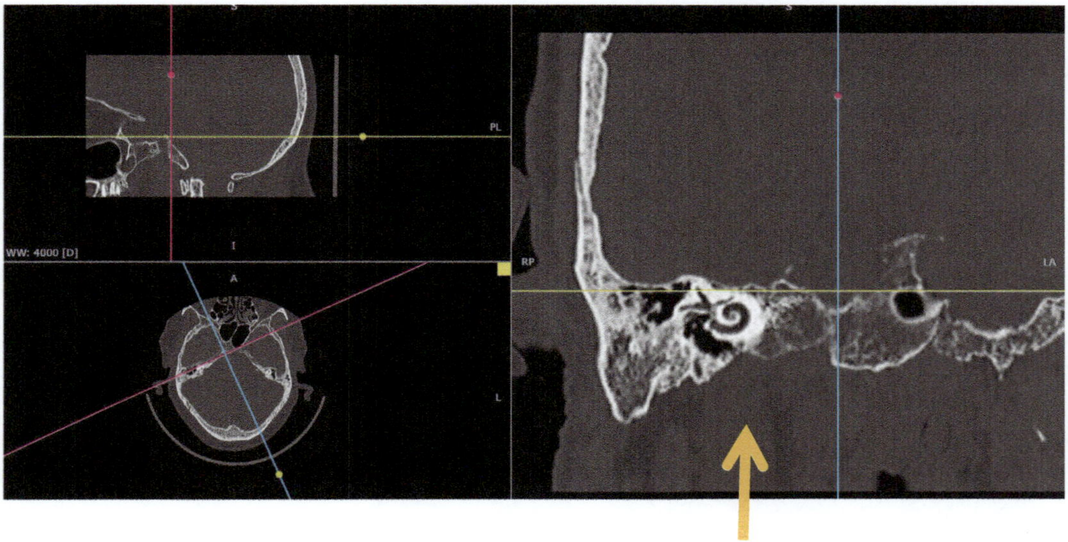

Fig. 18.6 Note how a Stenver's view can be created using CT images of the temporal bone

plate. The triangular appearance of the petrous temporal bone allows adequate visualization of the cochlear turns. The ENT surgeon can then see the electrode properly curled into the cochlear canal and can count the number of electrodes within the canal. The higher the number of electrode counts, the better the positioning, hence the better the hearing.

So if we look at the HRCT of the temporal bone and obtain a section along the length of the petrous bone in axial view as shown in Fig. 18.6, we can obtain Stenver's view (arrow).

If a Stenver view x-ray is requested, then position the patient is positioned (either sitting or lying prone) with the side to be x-rayed kept at 45° to the image plate, the chin extended and the head tilted backward. This positions the petrous bone parallel to the image plate. The X-ray beam should pass 2–3 fingers above and 2–3 fingers behind the opposite external auditory canal.

In a modified Stenver's view, which provides a better view of the cochlear turns and implant, the angulation of the head is by approximately 30°. The chin is not extended as in Stenver's view, and the head is also not tilted backwards.

With the availability of high-resolution CT scans, requests for most skull X-rays other than these views are infrequent. The reader can refer to standard textbooks or authoritative websites for further information and techniques.

Further Reading

1. du Boulay GH. Principles of X-ray diagnosis of the skull. 2nd ed. Butterworths; 1980.
2. Sloan C, Holmes K, Anderson C. Clark's pocket handbook for radiographers. CRC Press; 2014.
3. Moller TB, Reif E, Stark P. Pocket atlas for radiograph anatomy. Thieme; 1993.
4. Swallow RA, Naylor E. Clark's positioning in radiography. 11th ed. CBS Publisher; 1990.

Part II

CT Scans

19 CT Scans: Basics of CT Scanning

Abstract

Computed tomography, also known as CT scan, is a significant advancement over conventional radiology. The term "computed" stands for calculation and "tomography" stands for sectioning a part of the anatomy, using X-rays, and displaying the image of that section (Jung, Prog Med Phys 32:117, 2021). The CT scan consists of a gantry with a wide bore, which houses an X-ray tube. The tube faces the couch on which the patient lies. Behind this couch and within the CT gantry (housing), are an array of photoelectric detectors which are on the opposite side of the X-ray tube, facing it. A finely collimated X-ray beam passes through the part of the body being examined. This X-ray beam is attenuated to varying degrees by the structures in the body part,it traverses through on its way to the photoelectric detectors. The photoelectric detectors light up to different degrees, producing light energy which is converted into electrical energy. This electrical energy carries data of the structure traversed by the X-ray beam. The data which is in the form of attenuation differences between various tissues encountered in the scanned field (and measured in Hounsfield units—HU), is converted into an image through a complicated process using mathematical principles.

Keywords

X-ray · CT · Detectors · HU · Hounsfield units · Gantry · Filter · Table CT numbers · Slip rings

19.1 Basics of Scanning

In conventional radiology, an X-ray beam passes through a patient and leaves an impression of the tissues it has encountered on the image plate placed behind the patient. The image plate provides a summated image of all the structures, the X-ray beam has traversed. From this image, it is not easy to distinguish all the soft tissue components present in the path of the X-ray beam. To see more than mere bones, air and some shadows of soft tissues, studies using barium, iodinated contrast, and air contrast are required. These studies allow visualization of hollow viscus and blood vessels but not the other soft tissues so abundantly present in the body.

To examine other soft tissue structures, conventional X-ray tomography was introduced. The rotation of the conventional tomographic unit was usually 45° on either side of the median. This resulted in blurring of all structures located infront and behind the layer of soft tissues under evaluation. However, many of the soft tissues such as the liver, cardiac chambers, renal paren-

R. Gothi, *Radiographic and Imaging Techniques for Radiology Residents and Technologists*,
https://doi.org/10.1007/978-981-96-4816-0_19

chyma, pituitary gland, and brain were still not clearly delineated by this method.

This limitation of conventional X-ray tomography has since been removed by a cross-sectional tomographic technique called the CT scan, in which the X-ray tube rotates 360° about the patient, emitting radiation. The beam of radiation gets attenuated as it passes through the section of the body under investigation. This attenuated beam is captured by detectors which are arranged in an array, opposite the incoming X-ray beam and finally converted into an image which is then displayed on a viewing monitor.

The CT scan consists of an X-ray tube and an array of detectors. The detectors could be scintillation detectors (more commonly used) or solid-state detectors. When the X-ray beam passes through the patient, the radiation is absorbed to varying extents by tissues having different densities. Those with low density allow most of the radiation to pass through, while others with higher density, restrict the passage of the X-ray beam. Hence the X-ray beam is variably attenuated.

When this attenuated X-ray beam reaches the scintillation detectors (composed of a scintillator made of rare earth elements and a photomultiplier tube), it emits light of varying intensity, which is converted by the photomultiplier tube into electrical signals. The output of the electrical signals depends upon the brightness of the light emitted by the scintillation detectors. This leads to differences in the electrical signal strength, which enables the assignment of values to the tissues through which the X-ray beam has passed. The values are then converted from an analogue to a digital form which is displayed as an image.

The CT image consists of pixels that are assigned numbers according to the difference in attenuation of the X-ray beam as it traverses through the different density structure present in the anatomical section. The ultimate image production is thus a complex process involving radiation, light, electrical signals, and mathematical processing of the data generated. The images are displayed in two-dimensional and even three-dimensional formats, called cinematic rendering.

If the detector happens to be a solid-state detector, the stage of light emission is excluded. The X-ray data is directly converted into electric signals.

19.2 A Word About Pixels and Voxels

Pixels, also known as picture elements, are small squares that add up to form an image matrix. A typical CT image matrix consists of 512 by 512 pixels or even more. The greater the number of pixels, the sharper an image will look. Since CT scan images have a certain thickness also, each pixel represents a small volume of tissue—called a voxel (which is pixel area multiplied by slice thickness). The size of the voxel depends upon several factors, including the matrix used, slice thickness, and the selected field of view [1].

Each pixel represents a minute focus of light, the intensity of which varies from position to position in the image matrix. This results in the variable density of the pixels. Actually, the pixel represents a replica of the inside of the body traversed by the X-ray beam, which is displayed by the image matrix [2].

Since the image matrix is composed of pixels, if the number of pixels is large, the pixels will blend imperceptibly into one another, and the image will be of high quality (sharper, smoother) and not grainy.

The density of the pixel is represented by a number called the CT number or HU (Hounsfield unit) value. The CT number/HU value represents the attenuation value of the imaged tissue, normalized with water. It varies with individual organs and fluid collections inside the selected slice.

19.3 Composition of a CT Scanner

The CT scanner is composed of numerous components, which enable it to provide a 2D image of 3D structures [3]. It is a rotate-fixed type of scanner, in which the X-ray tube rotates around a fixed detector ring.

The scanner is composed of a couch, a gantry, and a workstation. The couch and gantry are in the scanner room. The workstation is in an adjacent room. It is a computer-based system where the technologist sets the examination protocols and processes the acquired images.

Scanning Table/Couch The scanner table is made of materials that do not produce artefacts in the images. The material could be acrylic or carbon fibre. The table is elevated or lowered using hydraulics and is motorized, which enables it to slide in and out of the gantry. The table should be able to withstand the weight of at least a 200 kg patient.

Scanning Unit (Gantry) The gantry housing is a hollow square-shaped or cylindrical box-like structure with a central bore through which the table can slide in or out during exposure. The gantry, or the scanning unit located within it, consists of an X-ray generator, X-ray tube/tubes, collimators, and filters on one side and a row of detectors on the opposite side. It is capable of tilting 25–30° in either direction. The cooling unit of the X-ray tube is also within the gantry. The gantry aperture needs to be at least 70 cm to take in a large patient. There is an infrared laser cross-hair beam for accurately positioning the patient. The gantry has a display unit in the front, showing parameters such as the height of the table and positioning (head or feet first) being applied.

Generator The generator used in the spiral CT scan, resides in the gantry. It provides a high-voltage supply between 20 and 150 kV to the X-ray tube, which determines the strength of the generated X-ray beam. There is another smaller 10 kV supply provided to the cathode, which results in continuous emissions of X-ray photons [3]. The mA range of a helical CT scanner varies from 10 to 500 mA. The range applied depends on the patient size as well as the area being scanned. Low kVp and low mA are used when imaging children. Low kVp in the range of 80–100 is also preferred in low-dose CTs and when performing vascular studies, where it helps highlight the difference between the high atomic number of iodine and the surrounding low-density soft tissues. Low mA also results in lowering the radiation dose because a lesser number of X-ray photons are produced. But this happens at the cost of increased noise and reduced image quality. Low mA is used in paediatric patients, in low-dose CT scanning for the detection of lung cancers, and in CT scans of the paranasal sinuses and bones.

X-Ray Tubes The X-ray tubes used in CT scans differ from the conventional X-ray tubes. The tubes used in CT scans are motorized so that they can rotate at fast speeds within the gantry. They are, therefore, capable of taking images from every angle, which enables 3D reconstructions of the organs being studied. The tubes in a conventional X-ray machine are static and can produce only 2D images. The radiation dose given by a CT tube is much higher than that given by a conventional X-ray tube. The maximum energy of the X-ray beam emitted by the cathode is up to 140 keV. The anode of the CT scan tube is larger, and cooling is either by air, water, or some other form of liquid coolant. The focal spot size of the CT scan tube ranges from 0.5 to 2.0 mm. The shape of the X-ray beam emitted is controlled by dynamic collimators, which not only reduce scatter but also adjust the slice thickness as per requirement of the anatomical area being studied. The emitted X-ray beam can be fan- or cone-shaped. A parallel or pencil-shaped beam emission is possible but needs flat panel detectors, while the detectors used in the current scanners are curvilinear shaped.

There are different types of X-ray tubes that different manufacturers use. GE uses a variable rotational tube (VRT), Siemens uses" Straton" tubes, and Philips uses MRC tubes, which stands for "mega rotational capacity" tubes.

Filters Filters are made of aluminium or tin [4]. These are juxtaposed between the X-ray tube and collimators. Their purpose is to cut off low-intensity X-ray photons, thus enabling a uniform monochromatic exposure, which results in improved image quality and reduction in noise and radiation dose. Filters are bowtie-shaped, wedge-shaped, removable, and also post-collimator positioned, which improves their performance [5]. Bow-tie filters are used for body imaging. The head, having a smaller area, needs a smaller-sized filter as compared to the body. The thickness of the aluminium filters can range from 0.1 to 2.0 mm.

Gantry The gantry of a helical CT scanner can rotate continuously at the speed of 3 or 5 times a second and even faster for cardiac applications. In the past, its movement and speed were restricted by the power and data cables attached to the X-ray tube. Now, the fast continuous rotation has been made possible by replacing the cables with "slip-ring" technology. The slip-ring consists of an outer stationary ring and an inner rotating ring. This allows unrestricted circular motion at a very high speed. By means of brushes on the rotating ring which contact the stationary ring, a power supply is provided to the equipment. In the same way, data signals are also collected from the stationary part of the slip ring and provided to the detectors for generating an image.

Collimators Collimators used in CT are dynamic collimators. There are two types of collimators: a diaphragm (source) type, which collimates the beam, and a grid type (also called detector collimator), which absorbs the radiation scattered from the patient's body [3]. Two sets of collimators are therefore present in CT scanners, one below the X-ray tube aperture and the other just in front of the detector array. The collimators help in cutting off the scattered radiation as well as in adjusting the slice thickness.

Detectors There are a large number of detector rows within the rotating ring of the gantry, arranged in parallel, in the current helical scanner. Their numbers can range from 4 to 256 depending on the equipment. Each row consists of 1000–2000 detectors and acquires data independently, thus enabling imaging of a large area of the patient. The detector array in the current CT is arranged in a curvilinear/circular manner, opposite the rotating X-ray tube. Each row consists of two layers, an inner scintillator layer (earlier detectors were ionizing chambers having either krypton or xenon gas) which converts the incoming X-ray photons into light photons. The outer layer is called the photodiode layer, which converts the emitted light photons into electrical signals.

Temperature and Humidity Control in the Scanner Room The CT scanner generates a lot of heat. Hence, a low temperature is required in the scanner room to cool the X-ray tube. The temperature should range between 64 and 75 °F (approximately 17–24 °C). The humidity should be between 30% and 70%. Both overheating and excess temperature can damage the equipment, including the boards and cables.

Console Room Outside the scanner room is another room which has the operating and viewing consoles. The technologist uses the operating console to plan a study and record and print the generated images. The slice thickness which can be chosen, ranges from under 1 to 10 mm. The interface has to be DICOM and PACs compatible.

The viewing console is used to study the images by both the radiologist and the technologist. Some of the complex reconstructions are also carried out using the software loaded in the viewing console (Figs. 19.1, 19.2, 19.3, 19.4, 19.5, 19.6, and 19.7).

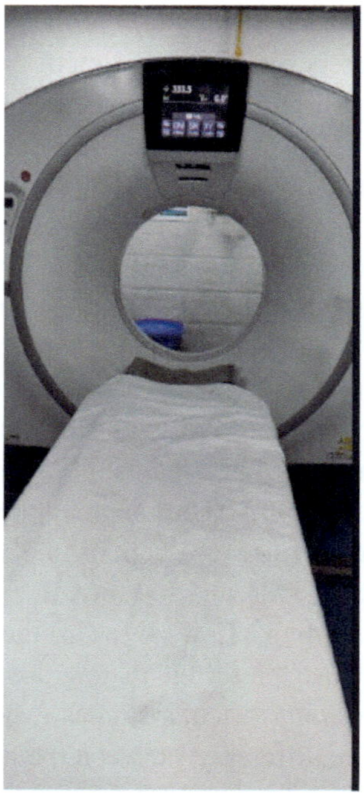

Fig. 19.1 CT scanner showing motorized table/couch in the line of the gantry aperture

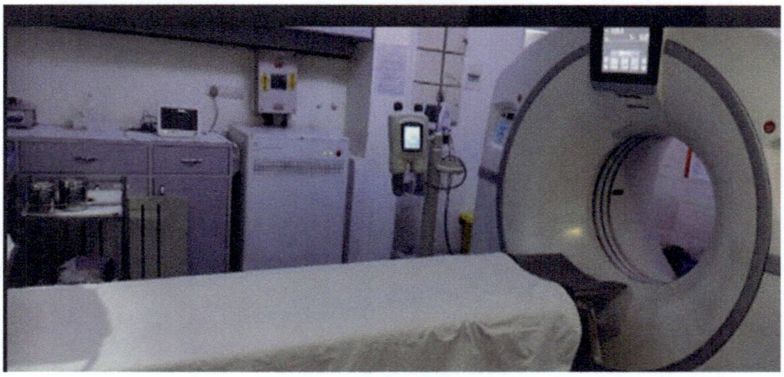

Fig. 19.2 The table moves continuously through the aperture during helical scanning, while during axial scanning, it stops at the time an exposure to the body section is being given. It then moves on to the next spot for the next exposure

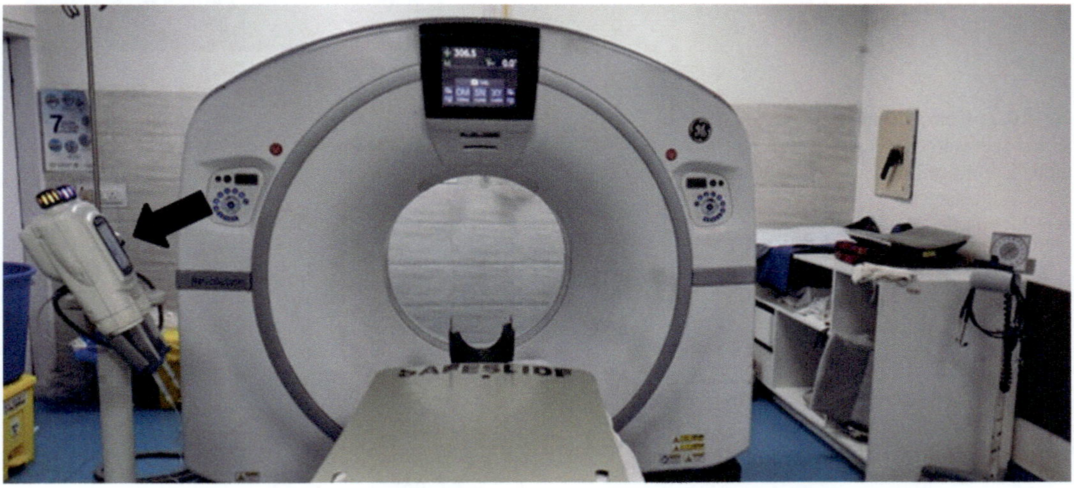

Fig. 19.3 CT scanner with pressure injector (arrow)

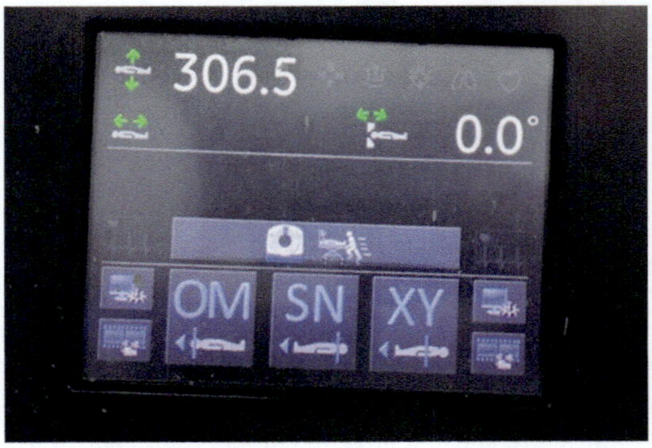

Fig. 19.4 Display on the gantry showing table position. The abbreviations stand for OM-orbitomeatal line, SN-sternal notch, XY-xiphisternum

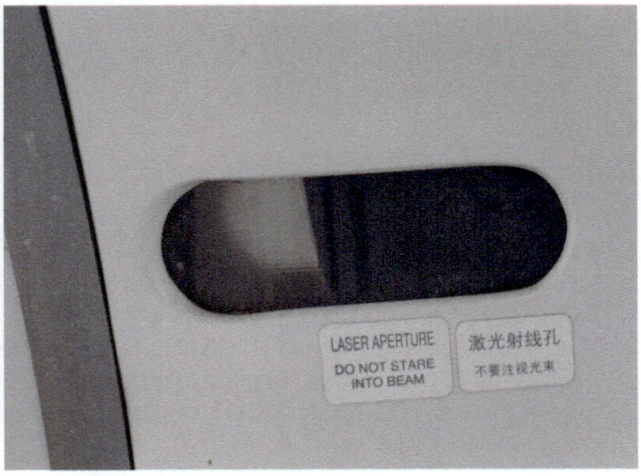

Fig. 19.5 Laser light aperture in the gantry for accurately positioning the patient

Fig. 19.6 CT gantry

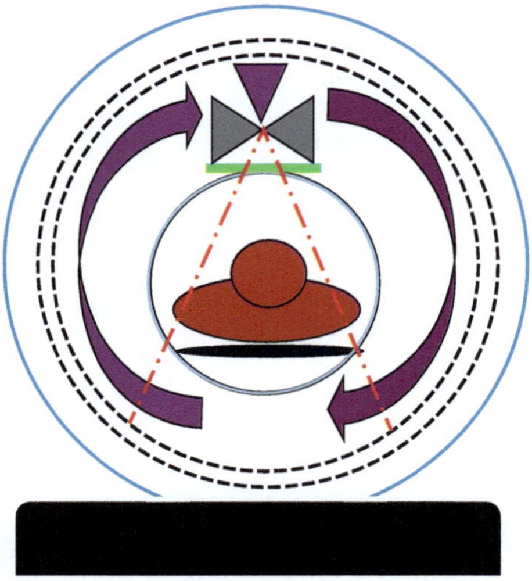

Fig. 19.7 Components within the gantry: X-ray tube, bow tie collimator, filter, solid state, or scintillation detector and photodiode

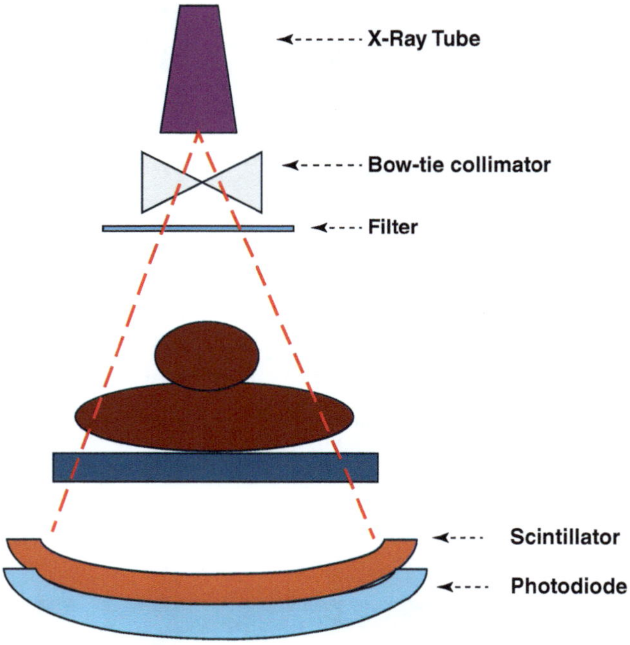

References

1. Jung H. Basic physical principles and clinical applications of computed tomography. Prog Med Phys. 2021;32:117. https://doi.org/10.14316/pmp.2021.32.1.1.
2. Hata A, Yanagawa M, Honda O, Kikuchi N, Miyata T, Tsukagoshi S, et al. Effect of matrix size on the image quality of ultra-high-resolution CT of the lung: comparison of 512 × 512, 1024 × 1024, and 2048 × 2048. Acad Radiol. 2018;25:869–76.
3. Hermena S, Young M. CT-scan image production procedures. [Updated 2023 Aug 8]. In: StatPearls. Treasure Island, FL: StatPearls Publishing; 2024. https://www.ncbi.nlm.nih.gov/books/NBK574548/.
4. https://www.siemens-healthineers.com/en-eg/computed-tomography/technologies-and-innovations/tin-filter?trk=article-ssr-frontend-pulse_little-text-block.
5. https://www.diagnosticimaging.com/view/filters-spectral-shaping-quality-computed-tomography.

Types of CT Scanners

20

Abstract

A brief history of the evolution of CT scanners from the time X-ray tomography was conceived till the present-day computed tomography (CT) scanners, makes interesting reading.

This chapter includes some of the main events leading to the evolution of the current generation of CT scanners. Additionally, the chapter also introduces the readers to the various types of CT scanners available and the way they work. Readers may want to know more about scanners. A few references are provided for those with a historical and technical bend of mind.

Keywords

History of CT scanners · Tomography · Computed tomography

It's a given that all radiographs can show bones and soft tissues. The delineation of the various parts of the bones, such as the cortex and medulla, their shape, thickness, length, and density, are also easily made out in the X-ray film. However, conventional X-rays produce 2D images; hence, they do not provide a clear picture of the composition of the soft tissues projected in the image. This is because soft tissues, with the exception of calcium, air, and fat, have similar densities. Only the known anatomical arrangement of the organs in the body, as well as their outlines and patterns, helps in distinguishing one soft tissue structure from the other. An X-ray film also does not possess the latitude to distinguish an abnormality lying within a soft tissue from the adjoining normal tissue [1]. Unlike a CT scan, which can produce multiplanar and 3D images, X-ray films also do not give a quantitative assessment of the density of various soft tissue components present in the image [2]. Many researchers using conventional radiology have explored ways of improving soft tissue resolution. Allesandra Vallebona [3], in 1930, constructed a tomographic equipment that could provide sectional images of the body. The equipment produced linear tomographic images, and not cross-sectional images, as we see today. The question of being able to differentiate tissues of differing density was a far cry in the early days of radiography.

The limitations of conventional X-rays were addressed with the development of other imaging modalities such as CT scans, ultrasound, MRI, and nuclear scans.

In 1963, Allan M. Cormack provided the mathematical model for calculating the absorption of ionizing radiation as it passed through tissue. In 1971, Godfrey Hounsfield, using this mathematical model and combining it with the available technology, developed the first CT scanner. This scanner could only produce images of the brain. With improvements in technology, the whole body is now examined, leading to the

R. Gothi, *Radiographic and Imaging Techniques for Radiology Residents and Technologists*,
https://doi.org/10.1007/978-981-96-4816-0_20

development of innumerable applications available to meet the growing needs of the medical profession. **Let us now see how CT technology has evolved over the years.**

20.1 CT Scanners Have a Pedigree

- The first-generation CT scanners (Fig. 20.1) had a single tube and a single detector. This scanner was used to obtain images in a step-by-step manner. The tube and detector combination first moved around the patient (which is called "translate") and then "rotated" to the next spot. This process of "translate-rotate" continued around the patient in a circular motion till the area of interest was completely scanned. The attached power and data cables needed to wind, unwind, and rewind during the scanning process, which slowed the speed of rotation.
- The second-generation scanner (Fig. 20.2) was also a translate-rotate type, but unlike the first-generation scanner, it had up to 30 detectors.
- The third generation was called the "rotate-rotate" scanner (Fig. 20.3). This scanner first rotates around one cross-section of the patient, producing its image before moving to the next cross-section. This is called "axial scanning". The 360° rotation was also slow, being restricted by the length of cables of the X-ray tube, located within the gantry housing. With this technique, only axial imaging was possible, not spiral! (Axial images are still obtained for immobile structures such as the brain. They can also be obtained at predesignated

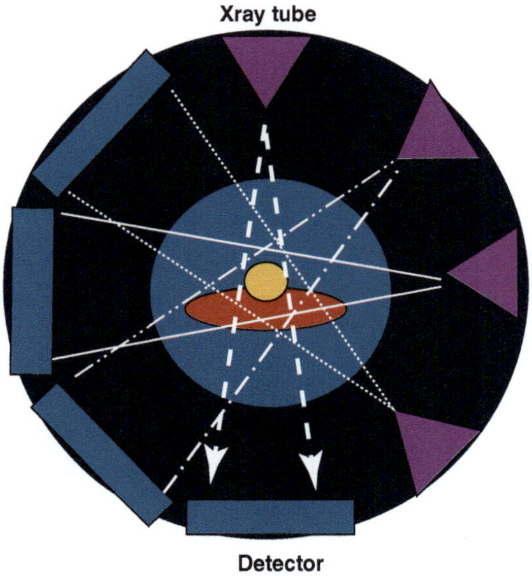

Fig. 20.2 Second generation scanner. This is also a translate-rotate scanner with an array of up to 30 detectors

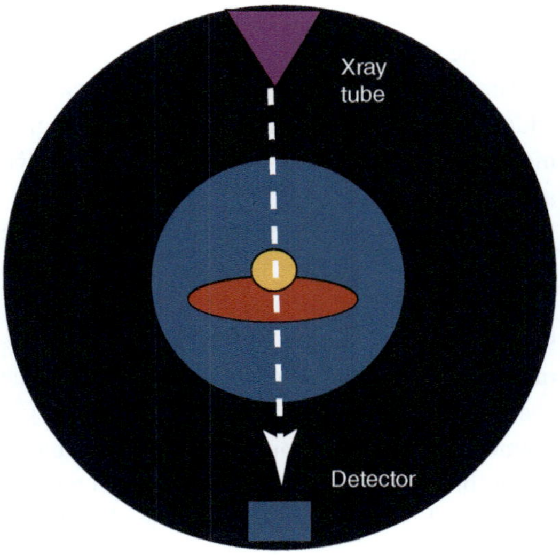

Fig. 20.1 First generation scanner. This is a "translate-rotate" scanner with a single tube and a single detector

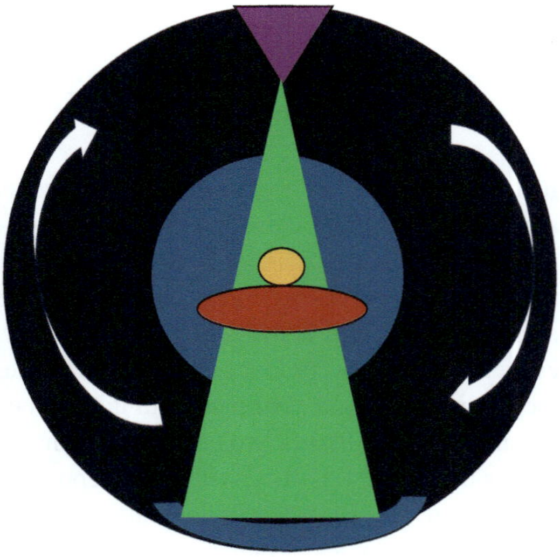

Fig. 20.3 Third generation scanner: This is a "rotate rotate" scanner which makes a continuous 360° movement around the patient

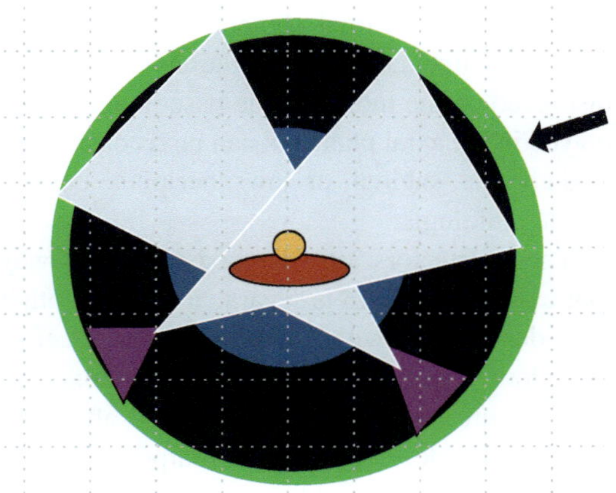

Fig. 20.4 The fourth generation scanner, which is a "rotate-fixed" type of scanner. Here, only the tube rotates. The detector array (arrow) is fixed

spots in helical scans of the lungs, used for producing high-resolution CT images (HRCT).

- The fourth-generation scanner improved further (Fig. 20.4). It was a "rotate-fixed" scanner having a stationary ring of detectors encircling the patient, while the X-ray tube rotated around the patient. The entire gantry, with the tube rotating within it, could move continuously from one level to another in a spiral mode, hence called a spiral CT scanner. With this equipment,however, axial scanning is also possible.
- The fifth-generation scanner was the "**electron beam scanner**" scanner (Fig. 20.5). These are ultrafast CT scanners that use an electron beam produced by an electron emitter. The electron beam is deflected towards a curved 210° tungsten target, located below the patient. The beam sweeps through the target which releases X-ray photons. These photons pass through the patient and are detected by a fixed detector ring located in front of the supine patient. There is no moving part; hence, the scanning is ultrafast, taking 50 to 250 ms. The main use of this scanner is for cardiac evaluation [4].

The "non-volumetric or axial CT scanners" (Fig. 20.6) have now been replaced by helical or spiral CT scanners which use the third-generation technology with upgraded hardware and software.

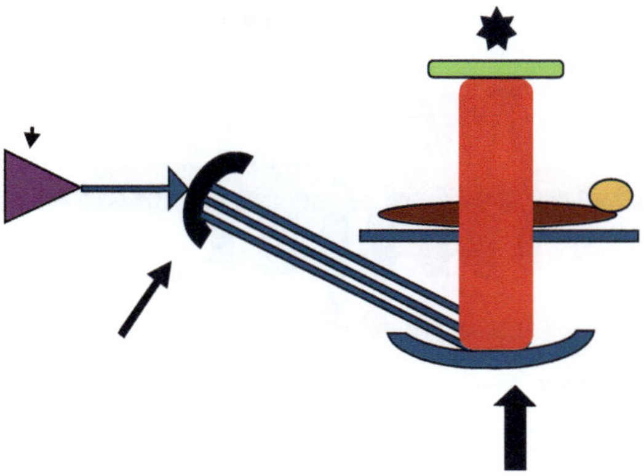

Fig. 20.5 Electron Beam CT: The electron gun (arrowhead) produces an electron beam, which is deflected by a coil (long arrow) towards a curved x-ray anode. As this beam sweeps across the curved anode, the target ring, (block arrow), X-ray photons are generated, which pass through the patient, reaching the detector array (asterisk)

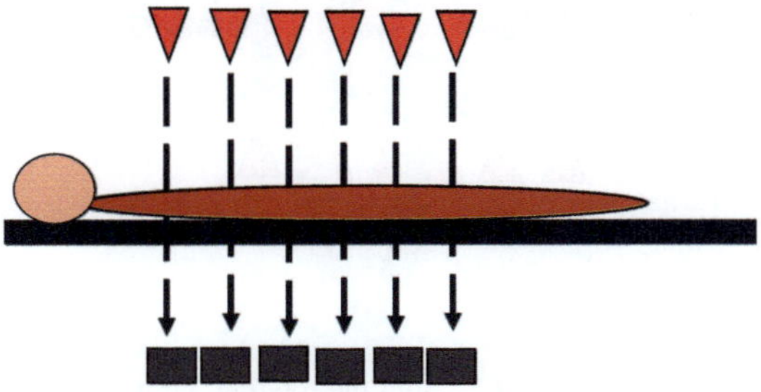

Fig. 20.6 Axial scanning: The patient moves from one slice to the next. The tube is switched on only during the exposure and switched off during patient movement to the next slice

20.2 Spiral CT (Also Called "Helical/Volume CT) Scanners"

Spiral/helical/volume CTs have a single tube on one side and an array of "energy-integrating scintillation detectors (EID)", made of ceramic, on the opposite side. During exposure, the motorized scanning table moves at a controlled speed through the gantry aperture in the "z" axis direction. The X-ray tube continuously rotates around the patient during the table movement (Fig. 20.7). The X-ray beam traverses through the patient and reaches the detector array (Fig. 20.8), resulting in a spiral scanning of the area of interest.

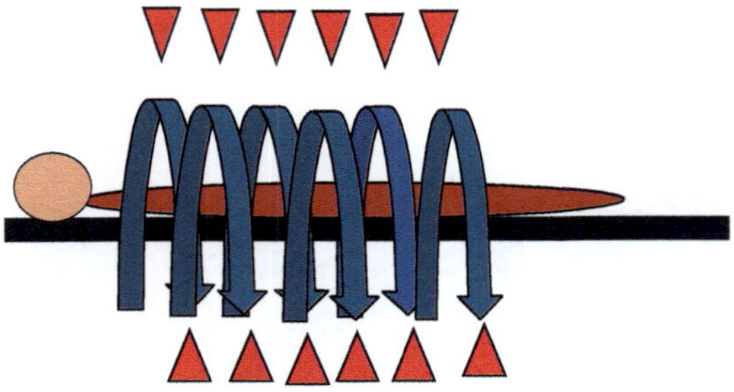

Fig. 20.7 Spiral motion of the single tube (triangle)

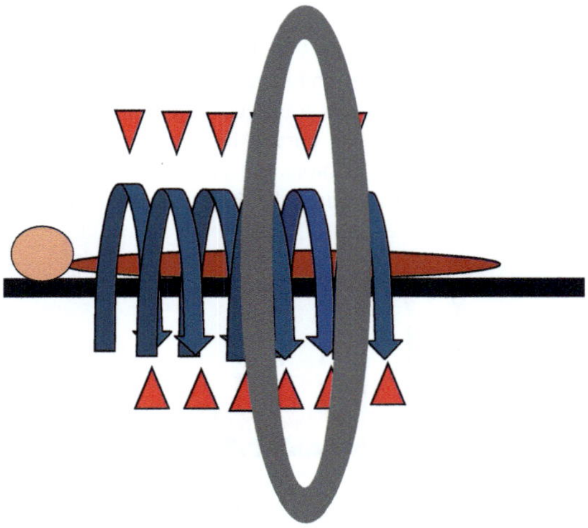

Fig. 20.8 Helical CT: Both the rotating X-ray tube and detector array are within the gantry (gray ring) and rotate about the patient. The tube rotates continuously during the study. The motorized table slides through the gantry during the scanning, resulting in a spiral scanning of the region under investigation

The detectors are arranged in rows which can number from 4 to 16 to 64 to 128 or even 320. The rows are arranged to form a matrix of 800–1000 detectors, composed of a scintillator and a photodiode. The volume of data provided by the incoming X-ray beam and passing through the selected area of the patient's body is continuously acquired at a much faster rate than can be acquired by a non-helical CT scanner. The photon energy of this outgoing attenuated X-ray beam is converted by the individual scintillation detectors into visible light. The emitted visible light signals are added up as a sum of all light generated by the incident X-ray beam falling on the detectors. This emitted light is converted into electrical signals by the photodiode, which also amplifies the electrical signal. Then, through a series of mathematical computations, an image is displayed on the monitor. The base image is displayed in the axial plane but can be reconstructed into coronal, sagittal, or any other plane desired by the radiologist.

These detectors are designed in such a way that each one of them is separated from the other by a dead space, which minimizes the effect of afterglow from the scintillation detectors [5]. This feature of eliminating unwanted afterglow results in the development of a sharper image.

The high-tension cables, present in the earlier scanners to join the static and rotating components of the CT gantry, have been done away with in these modern scanners. They have been replaced by "slip-ring" technology. This technology, using brushes, allows continuous transference of electric current and data between the rings, which enables fast and continuous gantry rotation. The physical restrictions imposed by the electricity cables are eliminated. A single rotation time is now under 50 ms. Slip-ring technology provides multiple varieties of acquisition modes, including helical CT, cine CT, cardiac CT, CT perfusion, gated lung imaging (i.e., 4D CT), and CT Fluoroscopy.

Spiral CTs are much faster than the previous generation scanners and can complete an examination within 15–20 s. They can also perform the traditional non-spiral (axial) scanning of relatively immobile parts such as limbs, head, and paranasal sinuses. They can also provide single-shot breath-hold HRCT images of the chest. Because of their speed and capability of covering a large area in seconds, they are used for vascular studies, including cardiac angiography and angiography of the brain and extremities.

20.3 Dual Source and Dual-Energy CT

In a conventional CT scan, soft tissues with different densities merge and produce a single contrast image. The pixel-sized unit of the detector is unable to distinguish the various constituents of the tissues because a single kV is applied in a typical spiral CT scanner to produce the image. To distinguish the different components of a tissue, dual-energy CT (DECT) scanners are now available. These scanners can vary the kVp from low to high to mixed [6] and produce both conventional and colour-coded images, based on the chemical composition of the soft tissues present within the sections imaged.

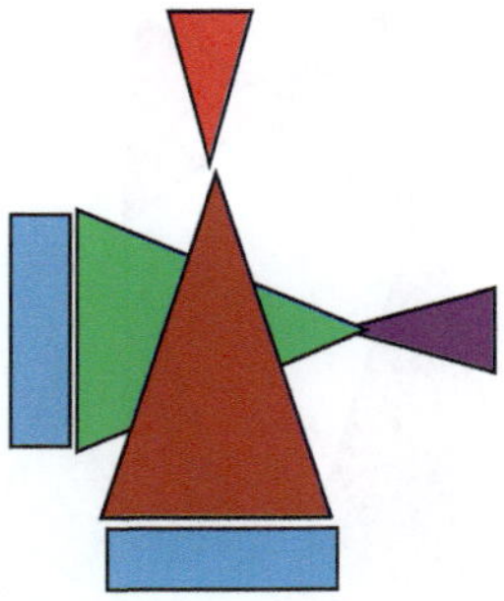

Fig. 20.9 Dual Source scanners DECT. The two X-ray sources (triangles) are at a right angle to one another, each facing their own detector arrays (rectangle shaped boxes). The kVp of each source is different

20.4 Dual-Energy CT Scanners

In a dual-energy CT scanner (also called "spectral CT scanner"), by using two different energy spectrums, (typically 80 and 140 kV), two different data sets can be obtained. Using this method, it is possible to distinguish many constituents of the body section under investigation. Dual energy CT not only provides the usual anatomic information but also information about the metabolic status of the constituents of the sections scanned.

Dual-energy CT images can be acquired by using a single X-ray source or two sources of X-ray energy production (Figs. 20.9, 20.10, 20.11, 20.12, and 20.13).

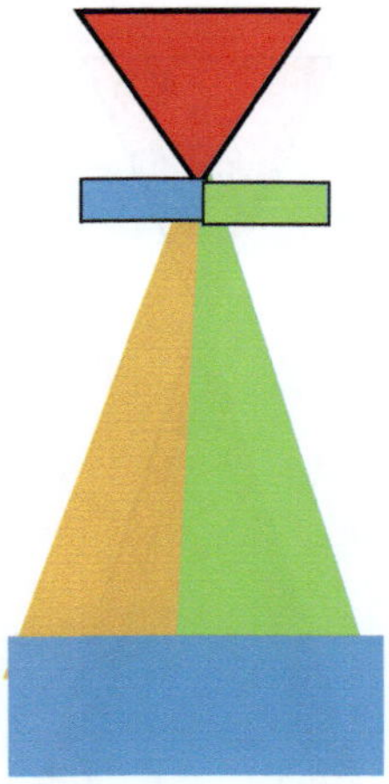

Fig. 20.10 Single source DECT with two filters (yellow and green) which are used to split the voltages into low and high voltages

The single-source scanner has a single tube. The dual energy images (using two different kVps) can be produced by **(a) continuous fast switching of the kVp** from low to high in a single acquisition, **(b) rescanning the same section at low and high kVps**, that is, scanning the same area twice, **(c) using two filters placed side by side**, outside the X-ray source for separating high and low energy, and **(d) using two arrays of detectors** (sandwich detectors based spectral CT) which can detect two different sets of kV [7].

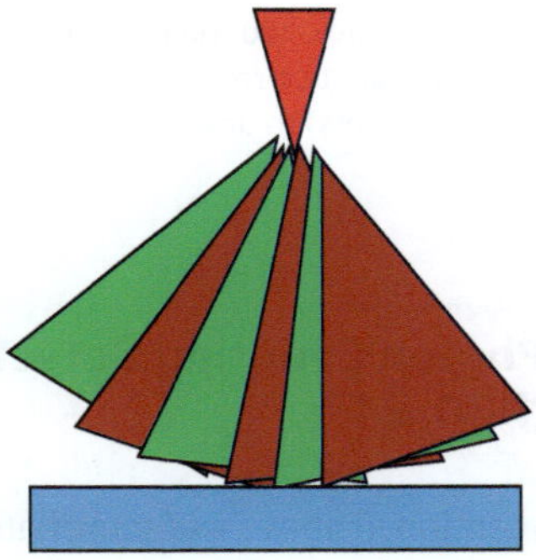

Fig. 20.11 Single source DECT with fast kV switching. The X-ray beam (red triangle) switches between high and low kVp (green and brown shaded) during the same rotation

CT images acquired from a dual-energy are sharper and reconstructed faster than by the conventional Helical CT scan. The acquired datasets can be single, as in conventional CT, or multiple, which include iodine maps, virtual unenhanced images (like non-contrast CT), monoenergetic images (like CECT), or atomic number maps. The X-ray tube life is the same as that of a conventional CT. Further advancement beyond dual energy is towards multi-energy CT and photon counting CT [8]. Besides dual energy scanning, a single source of X-ray can also perform "multi-energy scanning" [9].

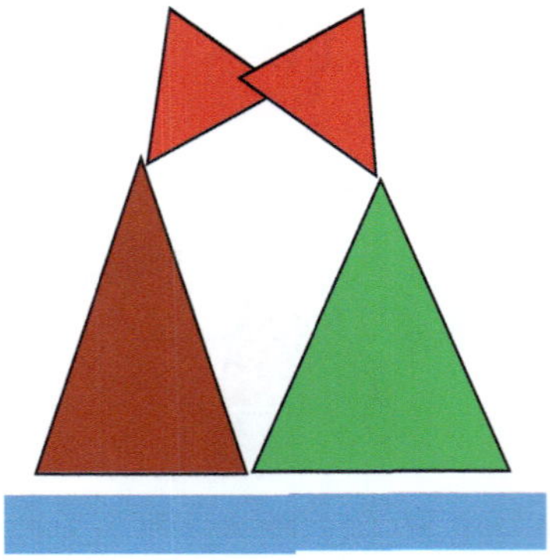

Fig. 20.12 Single source DECT (red triangle) detectors scanning the area of interest twice (brown and green triangles). The scanning is done at low and high kVp

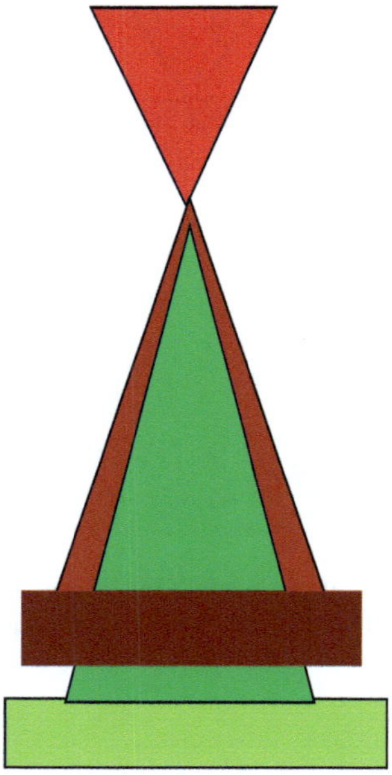

Fig. 20.13 Single source (red triangle) DECT with sandwich detector: There are two rows of detectors (brown and green sandwich detectors) to absorb x-rays having different kVps

20.5 Photon Counting Detector (PCD) CT

The CTs mentioned above use scintillation detectors, which work based on the production of light photons upon being exposed to an X-ray beam. The light generated upon exposure to the incoming

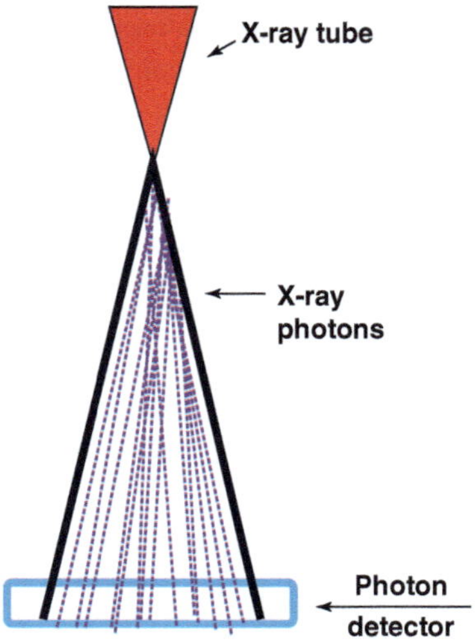

Fig. 20.14 Photon counting CT: The emitted x-ray photons are directly counted by the detector. There is no scintillation detector

X-ray beam is measured by photodiodes locate behind these detectors and is converted into electrical energy. These detectors are called "energy-integrated detectors". In the photon-counting CT scanner, the process of conversion of the incoming X-ray photons to light photons first, is eliminated (Fig. 20.14).

In a photon-counting CT, the photon energy of the incident X-ray beam is counted by the pixels within the detectors and converted directly into an electronic signal. The semiconductor detectors used in PCD CT are different from the conventional CT scan detectors and are made of silicon (Si)/cadmium telluride or cadmium zinc telluride. (The detectors in a conventional scanner are made of calcium tungstate, bismuth, or some other rare earth ceramics). The pixel size is also much smaller than in the energy-integrating detectors.

This process of skipping the "light photon stage", results in much sharper images being produced rather than having a slightly blurred edge to the image, produced by the afterglow, which is expected if light photons are to be used to produce images. There is also improvement in contrast-to-noise ratio (especially for higher z materials), improved spatial resolution, reduction in the radiation dose as well as the dose of IV contrast required for a contrast-enhanced studies.

Photon counting CTs can be used for all clinical situations and can migrate images from greyscale to colour [10, 11].

This brief overview is meant to provide the reader with basic information about CT scanners. Interested readers may look at the references and explore many resources available on this subject.

References

1. Praestholm J. Fremstilling af det flade röntgenbilledes tredie dimension analog tomografi—computer Tomografi [producing the third dimension of flat radiographic images: analogue tomography—computer tomography]. Dan Medicinhist Arbog. 1995:122–44. Danish.
2. Hounsfield GN. Computed medical imaging. Nobel lecture, December 8, 1979. J Comput Assist Tomogr. 1980;4(5):665–74.
3. Schulz RA, Stein JA, Pelc NJ. How CT happened: the early development of medical computed tomography. J Med Imaging (Bellingham). 2021;8(5):052110. https://doi.org/10.1117/1.JMI.8.5.052110.
4. Kulkarni S, Rumberger JA, Jha S. Electron beam CT: a historical review. Am J Roentgenol. 2021;216(5):1222–8.
5. Heiken JP, Brink JA, Vannier MW. Spiral (helical) CT. Radiology. 1993;189(3):647–56.
6. Fletcher JG, Takahashi N, Hartman R, Guimaraes L, Huprich JE, Hough DM, Yu L, McCollough CH. Dual-energy and dual-source CT: is there a role in the abdomen and pelvis? Radiol Clin North Am. 2009;47(1):41–57. https://doi.org/10.1016/j.rcl.2008.10.003.
7. Goo HW, Goo JM. Dual-energy CT: new horizon in medical imaging. Korean J Radiol. 2017;18(4):555–69. https://doi.org/10.3348/kjr.2017.18.4.555.
8. Mileto A. Ten frequently asked questions about dual energy CT. AJR Am J Roentgenol. 2017;208 https://doi.org/10.2214/AJR.16.16462.
9. Alavandar E, Venkatesh KA, Narappulan N, Gowtham SM, Kashyap R, Mehta P, Cherian M. Principles and available hardware in DECT. J Gastrointestinal Abdominal Radiol. 2022;5:76–84. https://doi.org/10.1055/s-0042-1742772.
10. Esquivel A, Ferrero A, Mileto A, Baffour F, Horst K, Rajiah PS, Inoue A, Leng S, McCollough C, Fletcher JG. Photon-counting detector CT: key points radiologists should know. Korean J Radiol. 2022;23(9):854–65. https://doi.org/10.3348/kjr.2022.0377.
11. Kreisler B. Photon counting detectors: concept, technical challenges, and clinical outlook. Eur J Radiol. 2022;149:110229.

21 Meaning of Commonly Used Acronyms and Words in CT: A Beginner's Guide

Abstract

During the course of posting in the CT department, residents and trainees will keep hearing some commonly used words, acronyms and abbreviations (Silverman PM et al., Am J Roentgenol 176, 1135–1136, 2001). In this chapter, the meaning of some of these terms will be explained. (The meaning of many of the terms is already explained in the previous chapters, also). After reading this chapter, hopefully, the student will not feel out of place in their initial days of CT training.

Keywords

CT acronyms · Abbreviations used in CT · CT terminology

21.1 Axial CT

This is a sequentially performed cross-sectional scanning of the area of interest, in the "Z" axis. The patient lies on the motorized scanning table. The table slides through the gantry aperture and stops at the upper edge of the scanning field. Radiation exposure of the first slice takes place. Then the table moves to the next slice, stops again for the exposure and moves on to the next stop. In this way, the table stops and starts till all sections are acquired. The images obtained are sequential and not helical.

Beam Collimation: Radiation exposure needs to be restricted to the slice being investigated with none or minimal scattering of the X-ray beam beyond the perimeters of that slice. This process of restricting the X-ray beam is called collimation. Collimation is achieved by using collimators.

Collimators in CT: Collimators are made of high-density materials such as lead, molybdenum, tungsten or copper which absorb the extra radiation, thus eliminating undesirable radiation. Beam collimation can also be performed by increasing or reducing the slice thickness.

21.2 CT Gantry Housing

This is a box-like or circular hollow structure at the head of the CT table. It houses the gantry, which has X-ray tube/tubes, detectors, and electronic components of the CT scanner, as well as the collimators. The housing has a wide aperture in its centre, leading into a tunnel, which is surrounded by the gantry. The tunnel is the central hollow area through which the CT table, carrying the patient, slides in and out. A slit-like window is present on the inner surface of the gantry housing through which the X-ray beam emerges. It traverses the patients, gets attenuated by absorption and reaches the detector array on the opposite side (Figs. 21.1 and 21.2).

R. Gothi, *Radiographic and Imaging Techniques for Radiology Residents and Technologists*,
https://doi.org/10.1007/978-981-96-4816-0_21

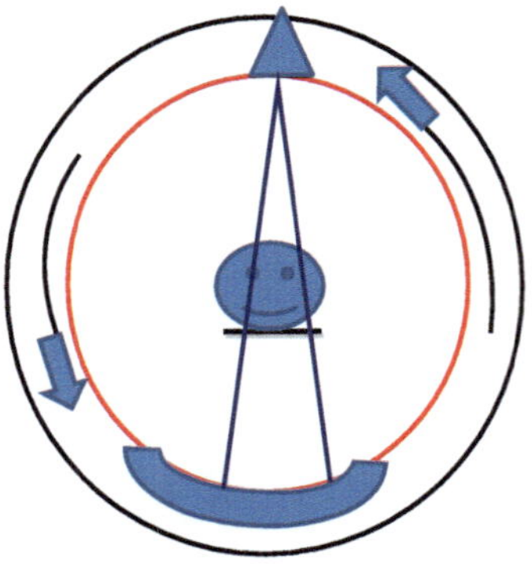

Fig. 21.1 Cross-section of the CT gantry showing, the X-ray source (blue triangle), the emerging beam passing through the patient and falling on the detector array located opposite the X-ray source

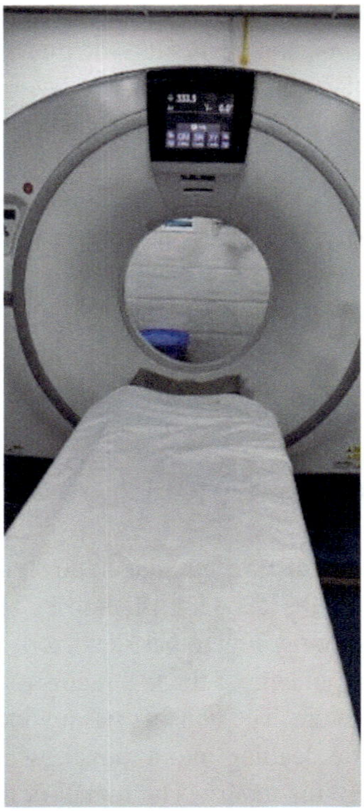

Fig. 21.2 CT table with gantry housing showing the circular aperture on either end of the tunnel through which the table slides in and out

Within the gantry, there is a source of laser beams, which form a crosshair. The anatomy under investigation must be positioned at the point of crossing of these beams. This enables the appropriate distribution of radiation through

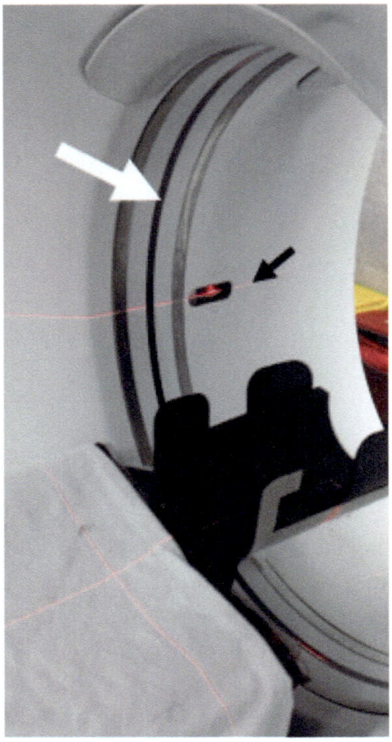

Fig. 21.3 Figure showing inside the gantry housing. There is a slit-like aperture (thick arrow) for the X-ray beam to emerge. Note the source for laser light (small arrow)

that part. The patient's position should be adjusted, prior to the commencement of scanning, by moving the motorized table up or down (Fig. 21.3).

21.2.1 CT Table/Couch

The CT table has a foot and a head end. The table is motorized. It can be made to move up or down and slide in or out of the gantry. At its head end, one can attach a headrest which is used to position the head during imaging.

21.2.2 Contrast Medium

Many CT studies require the use of intravenous, oral, rectal and intrathecal contrast administration. Contrast administration is also needed to study fistulas, urethra and urinary bladder. The IV contrast used is non-ionic, which has a much lesser risk of reaction as compared to ionic contrast agents, used previously. Oral contrasts can be positive, that is, of high density, such as diluted barium or iodine; can be neutral (water, mannitol); or even have a negative density (air). Positive, neutral and air contrast can also be introduced rectally. Intrathecal contrast, used to study the intracranial CSF spaces, is non-ionic iodinated contrast.

21.3 CT Dose Index (CTDI)

It is a measure, in mGy, of the radiation dose given to a phantom (which simulates a patient), placed in the "Z" axis, by a primary X-ray beam emerging from a single rotation of the CT gantry. The beam width used to measure CTDI is kept at 10 mm [2–5]. CTDI is a measure of the actual absorbed dose (in mGy) given to a patient during scanning. It is not the skin entrance dose and does not give the measurement of radiation dose given to the internal organs because of the variable size of the patient and the scanning protocol used. CTDI can be CTDIw, CTDI vol and CTDI 100.

21.3.1 CTDI Weight

The periphery of the human body is thinner than the central area. To compensate for this variation, CTDI*w* (in mGy) is used. This takes into account the higher dose received by the relatively thinner peripheral portion of the slice. The dose is calculated by adding a two-third peripheral region dose to the one-third dose given to the central region. This gives a weighted average across the selected slice (that is, in the X-Y axis) and gives the CTDI*w*. In order to make the CTDI*w* measurement more accurate, data acquired from 12, 3, 6 and 9° clockwise rotation of the scanner is averaged [5].

21.3.2 CTDI Vol

In the helical scanning mode, a volume of tissue is being examined and not a single slice. CTDI*vol* is, therefore, radiation exposure to a volume of tissue examined. The volume of tissue scanned and the tissue left out depend upon the pitch, which is the table movement in the "Z" axis per slice thickness. If the table movement (pitch) is more than the slice thickness, some areas will be left out and not be exposed. Hence the total radiation dose given will be reduced. CTDI*vol*, therefore, is CTDI*w*/pitch. Its measurement unit is mGy.

CTDI $_{100}$: This is a measure of radiation dose given over a length of 100 mm ionization chamber (phantom). It is calculated by dividing the dose given over 100 mm by the beam width. Since it does not take into consideration the variation of the thickness of the body at different sections, it is used in a single-slice CT scanner and not in helical CT scanning.

21.3.3 Dose Length Product

This is the total radiation dose given to a patient or a phantom during the "Z" axis movement (i.e. distance covered during scanning) through the gantry. It is calculated by multiplying CTDI*vol* with the scan length (distance travelled) in the Z axis (mGy × cm).

21.3.4 Effective Dose

The effective dose stands for the radiation dose each organ receives during scanning. It is not the same as the total dose. Each organ has varying levels of sensitivity and is therefore affected differently. The effective dose is measured by the unit, millisievert (mSv), and can be calculated by adding an age- and sex-specific conversion factor to DLP [6].

21.3.5 Filtered Back Projection

This is one of the initial methods of image reconstruction. The incoming X-ray beam is attenuated by the subject through which it has passed. The attenuated beam reaches the detectors, which project back the acquired attenuated data along the path it came—a mathematical process called back projection—after filtering it to remove the blurring and make the final image sharp. This is called filtered back projection.

21.3.6 Hounsfield Units (CT Numbers)

The density of various bony and soft tissue structures is measured in units called Hounsfied units named after Godfrey Hounsfield, the inventor of the CT scan [2]. Low-density structures like air and fat are dark while water and other soft tissues are intermediate-density structures, presenting in various shades of gray. Blood, calcium, bones and metals are of high density, and show different densities of whiteness (Figs. 21.4 and 21.5).

The approximate HU values (densities) of various structures are as under:

Free Air	−800 to −1000 or even lower units
Air in the lung parenchyma	−500 to −700
Fat	−30 to −80 or lower, but higher than air
Water (transudate)	0–10
Fluid (exudate)	0–30
Blood	70–90 (over 90 almost certain)
Muscles	30–45
Soft tissues including solid organs	25–45
Brain—Gray matter	35–45
Brain—White matter	25–35
Calcium	50–500
Intravenous or oral positive contrast	100–600
Bones	800 or more

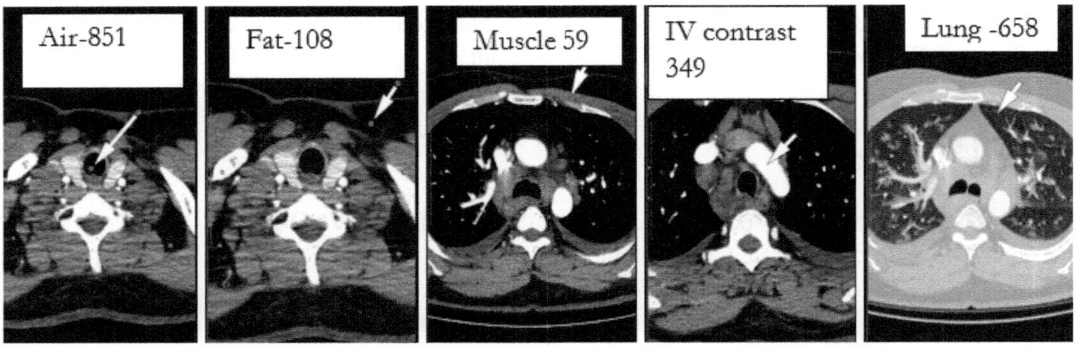

Fig. 21.4 Examples of HU values of air (-851 HU), fat (-108HU), muscle (59HU), IV contrast (349HU) and lung parenchyma (-658 HU), in these images

Fig. 21.5 Examples of HU values in these NCCT sections of the abdomen. Liver 54, spleen 46, fluid in stomach 2, kidney 23, bony cortex 756

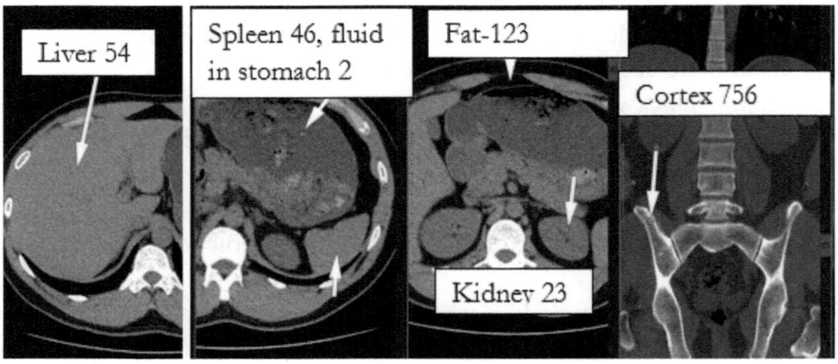

21.4 Multiple Scan Average Dose (MSAD)

It represents the average dose in mGy, received the skin entrance dose.

21.4.1 Pitch

The term "pitch" is used in spiral CT scanners. It implies the distance a table moves in the Z axis (table feed) during a single rotation. This distance is correlated with the slice thickness, which is determined by the total thickness of the detector array utilized during scanning of a particular slice. The relationship between the distance moved and the slice thickness, in one rotation, gives the pitch factor (table movement (pitch) / slice thickness). For example, if the pitch is 10 mm and the slice (total thickness of the detector arrays used) thickness is also 10 mm thick, then the table movement and the slice thickness are the same and the pitch factor is 1. If the pitch is 8 mm (a smaller distance covered by the table movement as compared to the slice thickness of 10 mm,) then the pitch factor is 8/10, i.e. 0.8. If the pitch is 12 mm and the slice thickness is 10 mm, it implies that the table has covered a larger distance as compared to the slice thickness. The pitch factor will, therefore, be 12/10, that is, 1.2.

Short table movements with a broader slice thickness mean a shorter gap between the images, resulting in overlapping of images. The image quality improves at the cost of increased radiation dose and time. A short pitch is used while examining the internal auditory canal.

When the table movement is greater than the slice thickness, the pitch factor is larger, and a gap is present between the two adjoining images. While this leads to faster scanning and reduced radiation dose, it affects the quality of sagittal and coronal reconstructions. A higher pitch is used when performing a low-dose CT or when large areas have to be covered, as in angiography of the lower limbs (Figs. 21.6, 21.7, and 21.8).

21.4.2 Pressure Injector

A pressure injector is an equipment capable of rapidly injecting a large volume of intravenous contrast. It is managed by the technologist at the operator console. The technologist regulates its function and activates it to coincide contrast injection with the x-ray exposure.

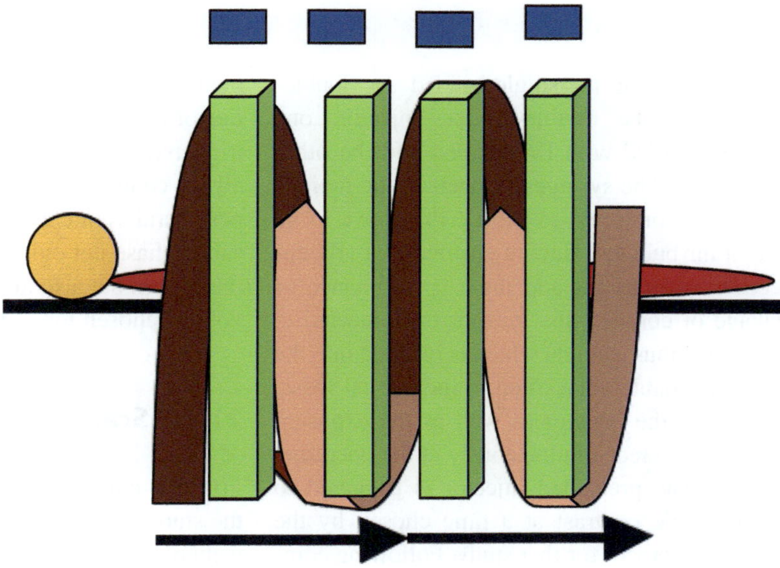

Fig. 21.6 Pitch (spiral turns in this image) and slice thickness (bars). The movement of the table is more than the slice thickness. The pitch ratio will therefore be more than 1

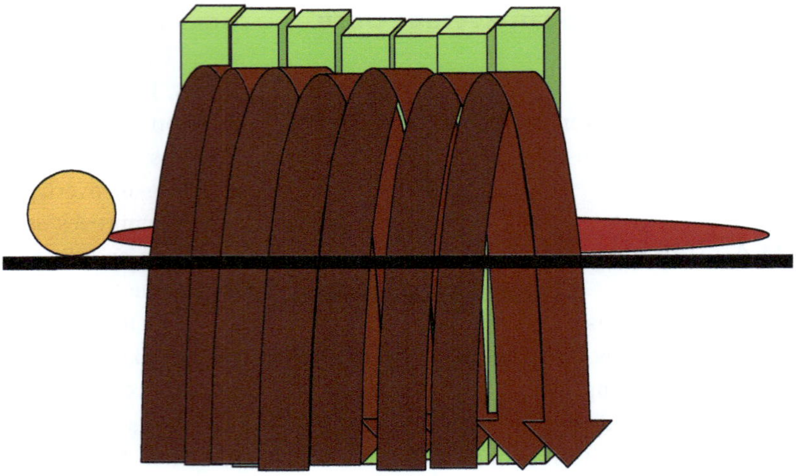

Fig. 21.7 The slice thickness and the pitch are the same. The pitch ratio is 1

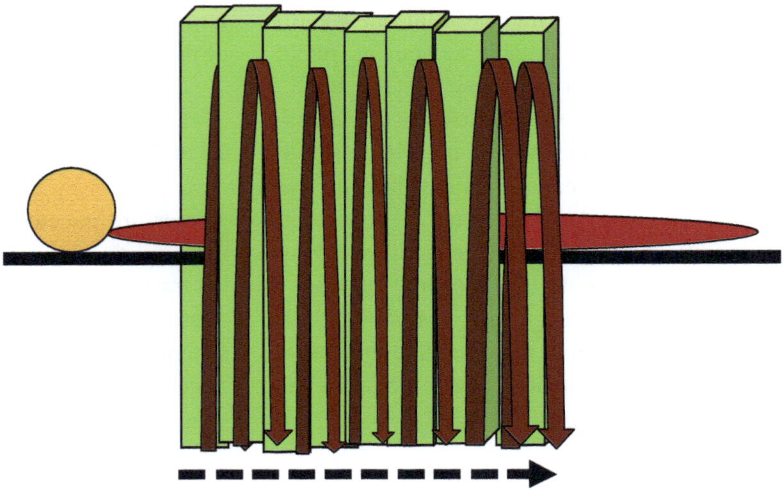

Fig. 21.8 In this diagram the pitch (spiral turns) is smaller than the slice thickness (bars), resulting in a pitch ratio being less than 1.0. The slices overlap at the end of each spiral turn, thereby improving image details in all planes. This happens at the cost of increased scan time and radiation dose

Injectors can be single-headed or double-headed. In the double-headed injector, one syringe is filled with IV contrast and the other with saline. The syringes, as well as the tubings which are connected to the IV line, have to be free of air bubbles. Having ensured that all connections are airtight and there is no chance of leakage of contrast, the injector is connected to the intravenous cannula which is inserted into the largest available vein, often in the cubital fossa. Thereafter, the injector as well as the exposure button is pressed simultaneously at the operating console. The preloaded injector is triggered to inject the IV contrast at a time chosen by the scanning protocol for that study. Following completion of IV contrast injection, automatic injection of saline (called saline chase) is automatically triggered. The saline chase is meant to push out all the contrast from the tubing, cannula and the peripheral vein chosen as the injection site. The saline chase not only pushes all the contrast into the system but also makes full use of the contrast volume chosen for a given protocol.

21.5 Scanogram

Prior to commencing cross-sectional imaging, the study needs to be planned. This is done by a technologist at the CT console. The protocol chosen for the study has an inbuilt capability of acquiring AP and lateral x-ray-like views of the area of interest. This is called a "scanogram", also known as a "topogram". The studies are mapped out on the scanogram.

21.6 Single Shot High-Resolution CT (High-Resolution CT-HRCT)

These are axial snapshot images obtained at predetermined levels. The table slides from one spot to the next, where the scanner stops and takes an image at that slice. This stop, shoot and shift method of scanning is slower than helical scanning but is used while performing HRCT of the chest, in temporal bone imaging and in brain imaging. It can also be used wherever there is minimal chance of movement. Multiplanar reconstructions by this method are suboptimal because no data is available from the sections skipped during scanning. The HRCT quality is affected by movement artefacts such as breathing movements.

Axial scanning is built into a helical CT scanner, which can therefore perform both axial and helical (spiral) scanning (Fig. 21.9).

21.6.1 Spiral CT/Helical CT

In a spiral CT scan, the X-ray tube is continuously on, rotating all the while, during table movement through the gantry (in the Z direction). The table also moves continuously ("translates") during exposure, along the "Z' axis, through the gantry tunnel. Because the scanning is continuous, the examination time is reduced; hence, examination of moving objects such as vascular and cardiac structures is possible. The X-ray beam is fan-shaped and activates many detectors. The data acquired from the scanned area is volumetric; hence, any number of sections of any thickness can be recreated (Fig. 21.10).

21.6.2 Slice Thickness

The thickness of a slice imaged is the slice thickness. Since the data acquired is in the form of a volume, ranging from 1 to 10 mm, several thinner sections can be sliced off from this data set. For example, in HRCT of the chest or the temporal bone scanning, the slice thickness can be reduced to as low as 0.625 mm. If the slice thickness is reduced further, the number of photons used to make the image is reduced, resulting in a grainy

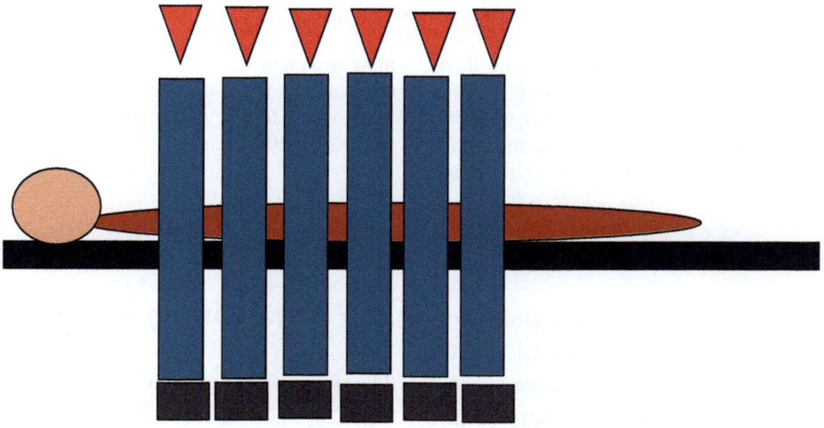

Fig. 21.9 Axial CT. Sections are obtained by stopping, shooting and then sliding down to the next slice

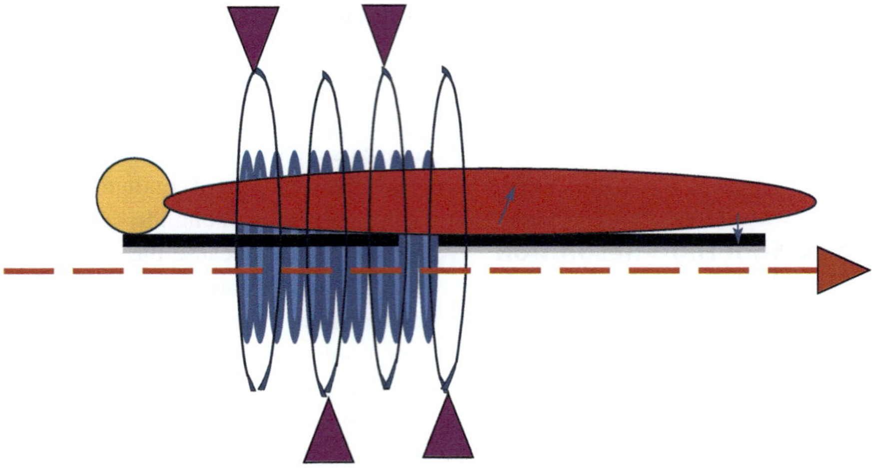

Fig. 21.10 Spiral or Helical CT. The continuous rotation of the X-ray tube and the table sliding through the gantry create a spiral-shaped exposure pattern. Volumetric data is acquired in a few seconds. The scan length can be increased to cover large parts of the body, such as extremities and the both abdomen and pelvis, in one contrast injection

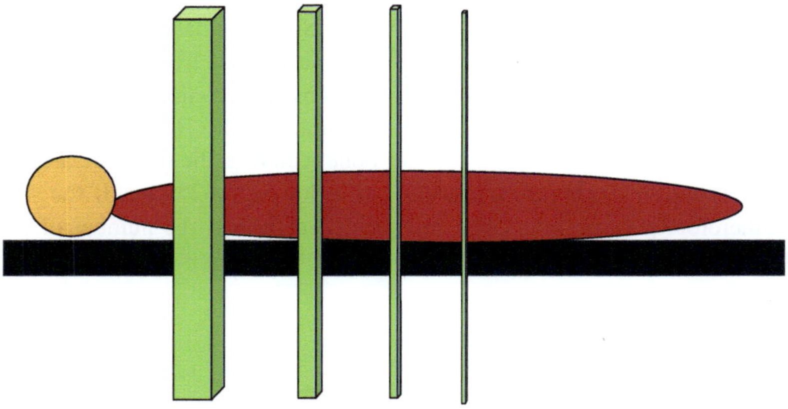

Fig. 21.11 Image showing sections of differing thickness which can be acquired while performing a helical CT. This is done by stimulating a few or a larger number of detectors during scanning. When large objects, such as the liver, kidneys or urinary bladder need to be evaluated, more detectors are stimulated to get a thicker slice or slab of the image. When high-detail structures are being examined, only a few detectors are stimulated to increase the sharpness of the images

image. Therefore, by using an optimal slice thickness the noise in the image is reduced and the image quality improves. The multiplanar reconstructions also look adequate for interpretation (Fig. 21.11).

21.7 Windowing in CT Scan

There are two terms most frequently used when looking at CT scan images. These are "window width (WW) and window level (WL)".

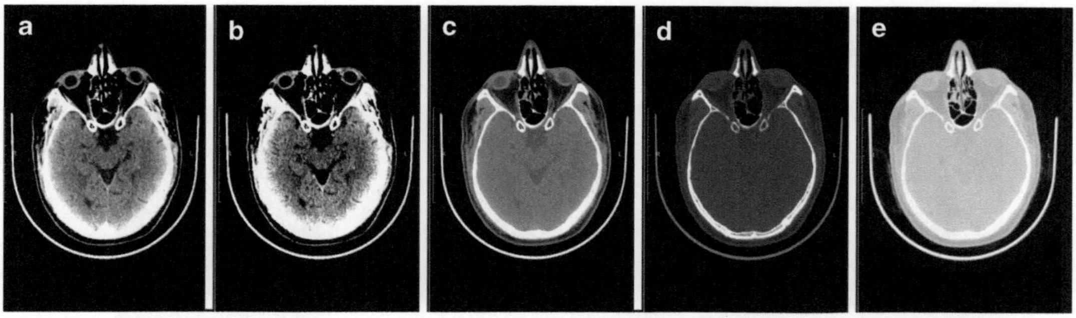

Fig. 21.12 Images of the head showing from left to right (**a**) normal brain parenchyma, (**b**) increased gray-white differentiation in the brain (called stroke window), (**c**) soft tissue window, (**d**) bone window and (**e**) window to show air in the sinuses

By adjusting the WW and WL, various shades of gray from dark to bright can be included or excluded in a CT image (Fig. 21.12).

21.7.1 Window Width

CT scan images are made of pixels which have different shades of gray. The varying densities of the pixels are dependent on the attenuation of the X-ray beam as it traverses a body section. The detector detects the residual photons which have reached it, leading to the differing density of the pixels in the final image. Each density of the gray shade is assigned a number called "Hounsfield Unit or CT number (HU)".

Window width (WW) allows viewing of a range of densities, having HU values ranging from extremely low (indicated by a minus sign) to extremely high values (indicated by a plus sign). The window width is adjustable. It can be widened or narrowed, to include only the relevant pixels needed to form the image. The window width for soft tissues, bones and air-containing structures is different. WW is set by the vendor but can be manually adjusted during the viewing or printing of the images.

21.7.2 Window Level

While window width is the range of densities selected for viewing in a CT scan image, window level (WL) is the centre point of this range. By shifting this centre point up or down and keeping the window width unchanged, it is possible to shift the scale of densities being viewed anywhere from the positive side of the zero baseline to the negative side. WL is essentially the centre point of the range of densities, chosen for viewing an anatomical area under investigation. For example, if the non-contrast CT of the abdomen is being performed, the WL of the liver would be between 30 and 50. As compared to the window width, which can be up to 400 HU.

21.8 Some Examples (Figs. 21.13 and 21.14)

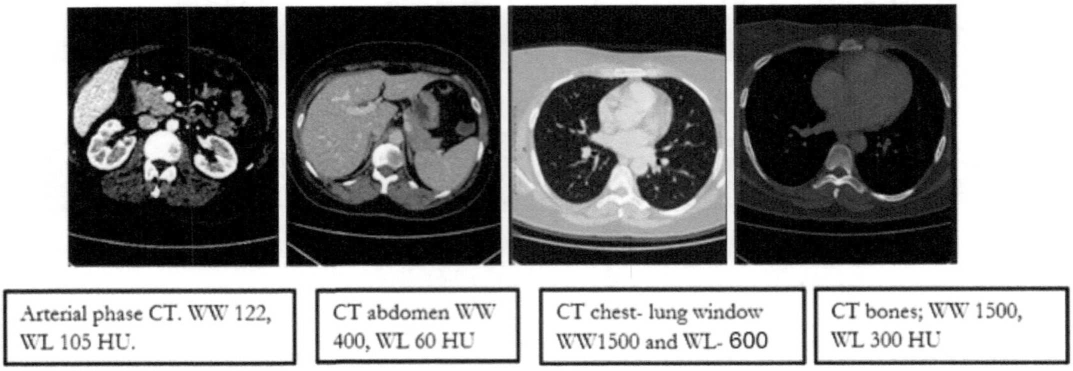

Fig. 21.13 Some examples of HU values based on organ-to-organ differences

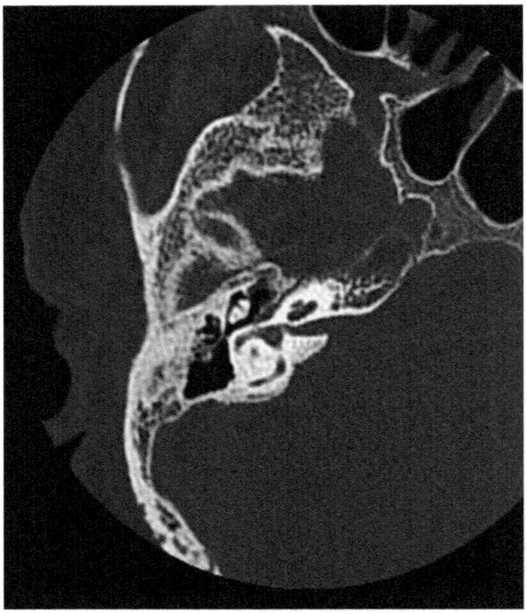

Fig. 21.14 CT scan of the temporal bone: WW 4000, WL 700. This window width setting is used because a wide range of densities are present in the temporal bone. Densities ranging from air to bone can be seen in the temporal bone. The central point (WL) is kept high as the structures are mainly of bone density

References

1. Silverman PM, Kalender WA, Hazle JD. Common terminology for single and multislice helical CT. Am J Roentgenol. 2001;176(5):1135–6.
2. Raman SP, Mahesh M. CT scan parameters and radiation dose: practical advice for radiologists. J Am Coll Radiol. 2013;10(11):840–6. https://doi.org/10.1016/j.jacr.2013.05.032.
3. Farr's physics for medical imaging, 2nd ed. Saunders. 2008. p. 116.
4. https://www.sciencedirect.com/topics/medicine-and-dentistry/computed-tomography-doseindex#:~:-text=The%20CT%20dose%20index%20(CTDI,scan%20width%20or%20beam%20collimation.
5. Treb K, Li K. Accuracy of weighted CTDI in estimating average dose delivered to CTDI phantoms: an experimental study. Med Phys. 2020;47(12):6484–99. https://doi.org/10.1002/mp.14528. Epub 2020 Nov 6. PMID: 33034041.
6. Smith-Bindman R, Miglioretti DL. CTDIvol, DLP, and effective dose are excellent measures for use in CT quality improvement. Radiology. 2011;261(3):999; author reply 999–1000. PMID: 22096003; PMCID: PMC6940005. https://doi.org/10.1148/radiol.11111055.

22 Artefacts in CT and How to Deal with Them

Abstract

There are often many shadows in the CT images which are unrelated to the part of the body being examined. These shadows may degrade image quality, and produce spurious additions in the image which can be mistaken for a pathology. These shadows may even mask a pathological finding. They are called artefacts and are produced due to various causes. Recognizing and eliminating or minimizing them, wherever possible, is important. Both the radiologist and the technologist must be able to recognize artifactual shadows and take measures to discard them or minimize their effect.

Keywords

Artefacts · Patient-related · Physics-related · Machine-related · Beam hardening · Streak · Cupping · Truncation artefacts · Partial volume averaging · Stair-step artefacts · MARS

Artefacts are fallacious shadows seen in images, which are not due to a disease or normal anatomy. They can affect the image quality negatively, mimic diseases and obscure findings. They can be related to patients, physics-related or hardware-related.

Let us look at some of the artefacts we encounter in daily practice.

Patient-Related Artefacts: These could be caused by respiratory or cardiac motion during scanning or by the presence of any metal or high-density object within or in the area of the body being imaged.

- **Breathing-Related Artefacts**:
  For chest CTs, patients are expected to breathe in deeply and hold their breath while the scanning is on. This results in outward bulging of the trachealis muscle and ligament, giving the trachea a round shape. A good inspiration results in the expansion of the lungs and the homogenous lucency of the normal lung parenchyma. The intrapulmonary vessels can be traced to nearly a few millimetres from the lung periphery. During the expiratory phase, the trachealis muscle assumes a concave shape, thereby compromising the tracheal lumen. The bronchial lumen may also be compromised and appear narrow and concave. The lung volume is reduced. There may be a ground-glass haze of the lung parenchyma. A few (not more than 3–5) areas of air trapping may also be seen. Because the diaphragms also move up, the orientation of the cardiac shadow is more horizontal, and it may appear prominent. The outlines of the diaphragms may show mirroring artefacts if the respiratory rate is high. The pulmonary parenchymal vessels may appear tortuous and kinked in the expiratory scan. Uncontrolled breathing

R. Gothi, *Radiographic and Imaging Techniques for Radiology Residents and Technologists*, https://doi.org/10.1007/978-981-96-4816-0_22

motion-related artefacts result in indistinct outlines of the vascular markings, giving them a comma-shaped or "bird flying with their wings spread" like appearance (Fig. 22.1).

Solution: Patients should be instructed about how to breathe during scanning and given a demonstration before the scanning is commenced. For chest CT, the patient should be instructed to take in a deep breath, simultaneously distend the abdomen (which brings the diaphragms down) and remain still till the scanning is over. Some patients are unable to hold their breath for more than a few seconds. In these cases, chest scanning can be done caudocranially to get adequate images of the lower lobes where breathing-related artefacts are mostly seen. The pitch can be increased to speed up the scanning. Scanning in quiet breathing, in which no breathing instructions are given, can also be tried. Scanning in a prone position also helps because it restricts motion of the anterior chest wall, which results in limiting diaphragmatic excursions and allows the lower lobes to expand maximally. Breathless and ICU patients will not be able to hold their breath, so one has to learn to recognize and accept breathing-related artefacts. In these cases, if a pulmonary angiogram has to be performed, then a quiet breathing technique, short scanning time and no scan delay once a high threshold (100 HU) bolus trigger is achieved produce satisfactory results [1]. The advantage of quiet breathing over breath-hold after deep inspiration is that the abrupt inflow of unopacified blood does not happen and the vessels are adequately filled with contrast.

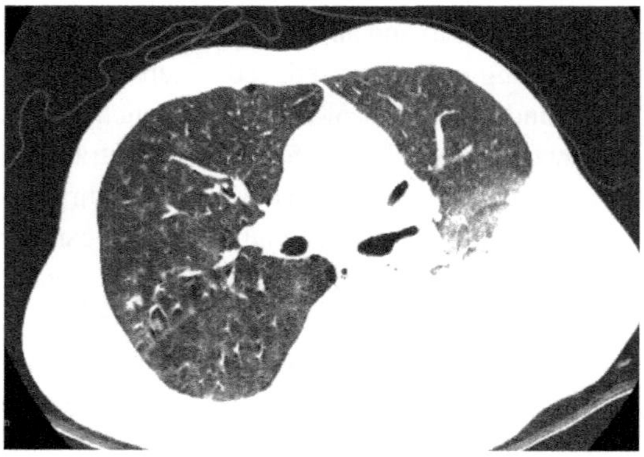

Fig. 22.1 Breathing motion artefacts are seen as "birds flying with their wings spread" in the right upper and lower lobes

- **Movement-Related Artefacts**

  Motion artefacts are seen in restless patients and in children. Scans can be delayed for a few moments to allow patients to settle down. Some patients can follow instructions and abide by them, staying still while the scanning is in progress. Others may need restraints or sedation.

Physics-Related Artefacts: These artefacts can be beam hardening artefacts, partial volume effect-related artefacts, aliasing artefacts or artefacts related to the photon starving effect.

- **Beam Hardening Artefacts** [2, 3]. Three types of beam hardening artefacts are generated, namely streak artefacts, metal artefacts and cupping artefacts.
  1. **Streak Artefacts** [4].

     The X-ray beam consists of photons having varying energy levels (that is, it has polychromatic energies). Upon passing through a dense object, the low-energy photons are absorbed, resulting in the detectors being deprived of these photons. This leads to lower HU values (hypodense attenuation) being assigned to the photon-deprived area, resulting in the production of dark streaks in those areas. The high-energy protons can pass through, producing bright streaks, and reach the detectors, thereby being assigned higher HU values. Streak artefacts are seen in the posterior fossa due to the difference in density between the thick petrous temporal bones and the adjoining CSF spaces and soft tissues residing in the posterior fossa. In these images, there will be the appearance of dark and bright streaks till the hard bone of the posterior fossa is crossed. Similar streak artefacts are also seen at places where high-density intravenously administered contrast is seen mixing with relatively low-density contrast (unopacified blood or fluid), such as at the level of the superior vena cava (SVC) and right atrial (RA) junction, especially during CT pulmonary angiography.

Solution: Streak artefacts can be resolved to a certain extent by increasing the kVp and mAs, by using a high pass filter (bow-tie filters), smoothening filters during post-processing or by using dual-energy CT scans. The high-pass filters absorb the low-energy photons and allow only high-energy photons to reach the object, thus reducing the beam hardening artefacts. Streak artefacts in the posterior fossa can also be reduced by changing the direction of the X-ray beam. This is done by tilting the gantry so that the beam is focused over the posterior aspect of the neck rather than on the petrous temporal bones. In situations where the gantry cannot be tilted, tilt the chin down as close as possible to the neck.

2. **Metal Artefacts**: These are commonly seen wherever metals such as dental implants and metallic prostheses are present.
   Solution: Artefacts resulting from metals can be reduced by using the metal artefacts reduction sequence (MARS) (Figs. 22.2 and 22.3).
3. **Cupping Artefacts**: These are also beam hardening effects in which there is absorption of the low- energy photons in the thicker centre of the object, while the high- energy protons can pass through. The reduced number of photons which pass through the central area makes it appear darker as compared to the periphery. The periphery of the object being comparatively thinner allows all the photons to pass through to the detectors, thereby producing a stronger, brighter peripheral signal. Cupping artefacts are mostly seen in the skull, where a cup-shaped low density is seen in the centre of the image. The image, looks darker in the centre as compared to the periphery.
   Solution: The patient should be correctly centred. Scatter must be reduced, as it provides more photons to the detectors in the periphery of the image and less protons to the centre. A bow-tie filter and applying iterative reconstruction also helps.

- **Aliasing** [4]: The quality of a CT scan image depends upon how much data is collected by the detectors to produce an image. Collecting a sufficient amount of data from an object being imaged leads to better image quality and undistorted reconstructions. When only a small amount of data (which is also known as undersampling of data) is collected, as it happens in lung cancer screening CT, it leads to aliasing artefacts. The homogeneity of the image is compromised. Artefacts resembling distortions, serrations and streak artefacts close to the hardware, such as around aneurysm clips in the brain, are seen in the image.

  Solution: Some of the solutions include increasing the number of slices taken through the region which is causing aliasing. Reducing the gantry rotation speed leading to more pho-

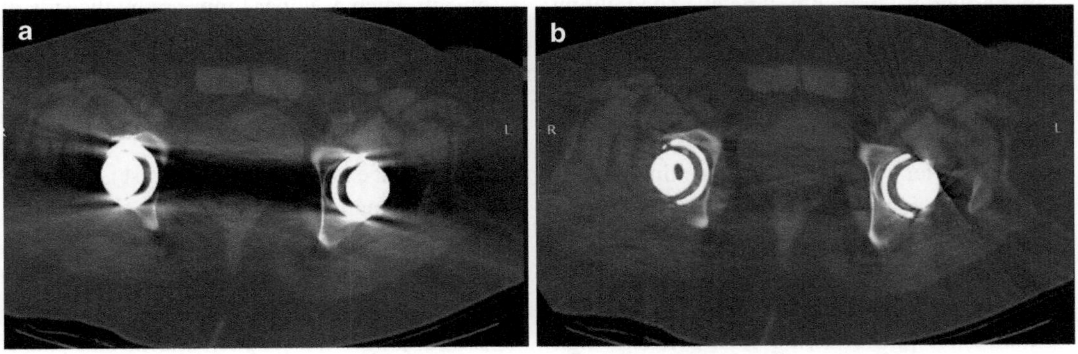

Fig. 22.2 (A) Metal artefacts. Before (**a**) and (**b**) after applying metal artefact reduction software (MARS)

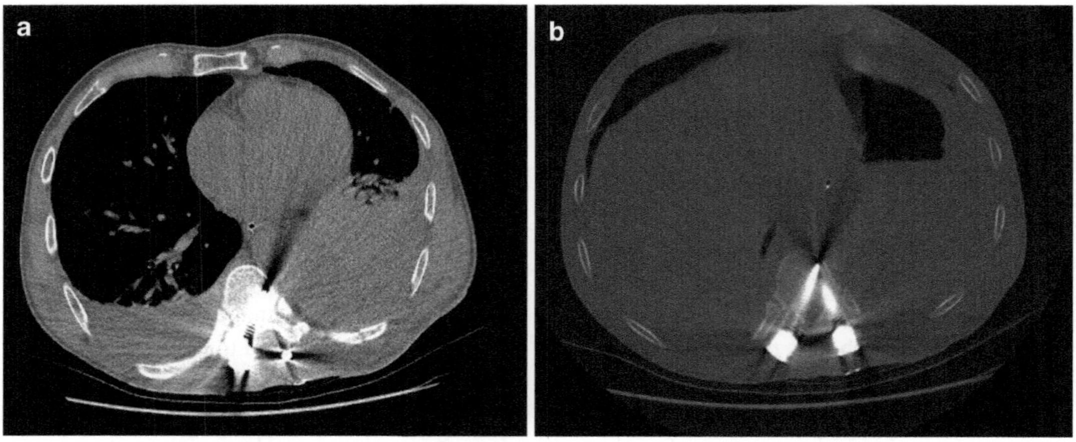

Fig. 22.3 Metal artefacts. No metal artefact reduction software was used (**a**). Note the dark shadow at the tip of the screws (**a**) caused by photon starvation. Scanning the following usage of metal artefact-reducing software (**b**)

tons reaching the detectors and the use of iterative reconstruction also reduces the aliasing artefact. However, these solutions are not foolproof.

- **Partial Volume Averaging**:

  When tissues of different densities are included within a slice, the HU value of the imaged tissue, present within that section, is averaged. For example, if in a slice, an IV contrast containing a blood vessel and the adjoining soft tissue is included, the HU value of that slice will be the average of the two densities. It will be lower than that of the IV contrast density but higher than the soft tissue density. This can also happen if a thick section which includes the perivascular interstitium is used to image a pulmonary artery branch. In a suspected case of pulmonary thromboembolism, the HU value of the contrast-containing pulmonary artery branch will be averaged out by the soft tissue present in that slice. The attenuation value will therefore be lower than that of the IV contrast, thereby giving a false impression of the presence of a thrombus in that pulmonary artery branch. If the slice thickness is reduced to include just the pulmonary artery branch, the HU value will be high if no thrombus is present and low if a thrombus is present. This artefact, which results when a large number of pixels having both soft and high densities are present within a slice, is called a "partial volume averaging" artefact.

  Solution: Use thinner slices for reconstructing images, especially of those regions needing high definition, such as in temporal bone imaging and HRCT chest for studying interstitial lung diseases.

  Another important cause of the partial volume effect is that if there is a high-density object at the outer perimeter of an X-ray beam, the detectors will be able to see this object and include its density in the main image. For example, if the upper limb is included in a CT scan of the abdomen, a partial volume effect will be seen as streak artefacts in the sections which include the limb and adjoining abdominal soft tissues. This also leads to an increase in radiation dose in this region.

  Solution: Ensure that no high-density objects, such as upper limbs are by the side of the body during the scanning of the chest or abdomen. Also ensure that there is no metallic object including wires or tubes, in the area under investigation.

  A different example! If IV contrast is administered to a patient having a small simple renal cyst and a slice includes it in the nephrographic phase of the study, owing to the presence of high-density contrast in the surrounding renal parenchyma in that phase, the HU values of the cyst may also appear fallaciously high (pseudo enhancement).

Solution: Use a thinner section or compare the study with non-contrast CT images, ultrasound or MRI.

- **Photon Starving Effect**. When, during rotational movement, the X-ray beam is travelling horizontally through two high attenuation areas, such as across the shoulders or both hips with metallic implants, the attenuation of the X-ray beam is significant. This results in the intervening area being starved of photons, hence appearing dark (low HU value) and riddled with noise. In the case of shoulders, the thoracic inlet is affected, while in patients with bilateral total hip replacement, the intervening pelvic area shows low attenuation with noise-related artefacts. The artefacts are streak-like and are seen between the shoulders and hip joints.

  Solution: Increase the radiation dose by automatic exposure control mode. Increase the tube current, use thicker slices or reduce the pitch. In those areas, where there is an abrupt change in thickness, as happens at the root of the neck, longitudinal tube current modulation can be turned on [5] (Fig. 22.4).
- **Noise**:

  This is an electronic phenomenon caused by either by variation of photon flux at the level of the source of x-rays or by electronic disturbance around the detectors, which can overlap on an image. This casts a shadow on the image, making the image sometimes uninterpretable. Noise can also produce streak artefacts due to electromagnetic interference.

  Solution: Noise reduction can be done by increasing mAs [7]. Try changing the scan parameters, because improper scan parameters can also add noise to the image.

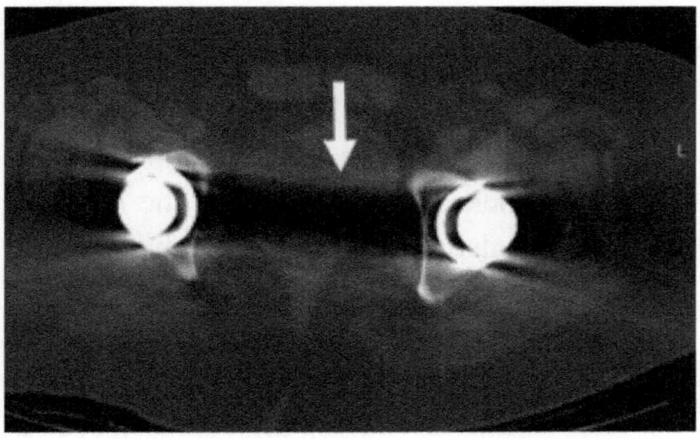

Fig. 22.4 The photon starving streak is seen as a dark area between the two total hip implants

- **Truncation Artefact**:

  If a part of the body, is outside the imaging field of view, especially in a large patient or with the arms resting by the side, in a CT chest or CT abdomen, it will produce an arc-like shadow having increased HU values at the periphery of the image. This artefact does not affect the inner area of the image.

  Solution: To eliminate this artifactual shadow, the field of view will have to be increased to include the entire area in the scanning field. In the case of arms by the side, reposition them above the head.

22.1 Hardware-Based Artefacts

These include ring artefacts, noise, cone beam artefacts and spiral scanner-related artefacts.

- **Ring Artefacts**: These artefacts are produced as a result of the malfunctioning of one of the detectors. They can also be due to reduced radiation dose falling on some detectors or contrast droplets overlying the polyester film covering the detector array. Depending upon the signal intensity that those detectors give out to the photoelectrode diode, the rings can be light or dark. These ring-shaped circular artefacts and their number depend upon the number of detectors which are malfunctioning or giving incorrect readings while revolving around the patient. Ring-shaped artefacts can be easily appreciated in a CT image, as they are generally in the centre of the image and may not cause much disturbance to the reader of that image. However, if excessive, they may seriously degrade the image.

  Solution: The machine may require preventive maintenance, recalibration, cleaning of the polyester covering over the detector window or increasing the radiation dose.

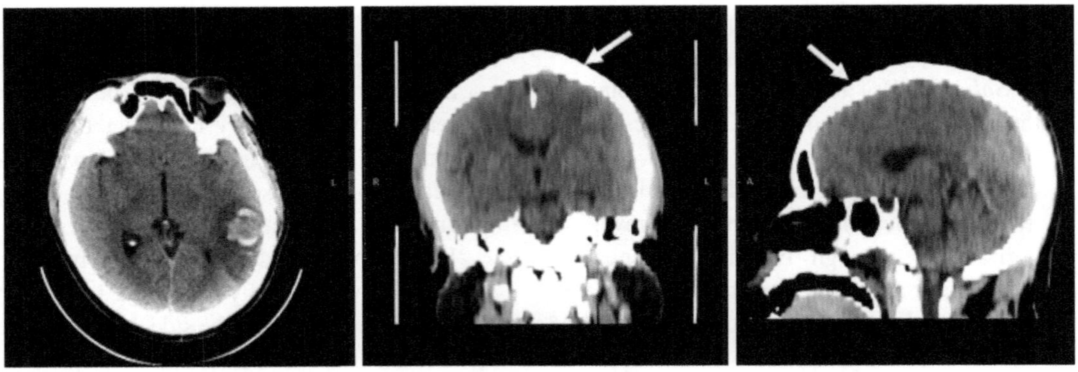

Fig. 22.5 CT scan of the brain using 5 mm contiguous, non-overlapping slices shows stair-step artefacts in the coronal and sagittal reformatted images (arrow)

- **Stair Step Artefacts**:

  When non-overlapping and large sections are obtained, for example, 5 mm non-overlapping sections in cranial CT, a stair-step-like artefact is generated in the coronal and sagittal reformatted images (Fig. 22.5).

  Solution: This artefact can be eliminated by obtaining overlapping images. For example, if the original image in the CT head was 5 mm thick, reduce the thickness to 1.2 mm for soft tissue evaluation and 0.6 mm for evaluating bones (Fig. 22.6).

- **Tube Arcing Artefact**:

  If for some reason, there is a short circuit within an X-ray tube, there will be a sudden stoppage of X-ray generation, and artefacts will be seen. These artefacts can be linear, parallel streaks, or horizontal hypodense bands [6]. Voltage fluctuations and ageing of the tube can also cause the development of these types of artefacts.

  Solution: Use the equipment at a lower power setting. If the tube is ageing, it may emit ions. The glass covering may need degassing. The equipment may need a call to the service engineer. Try changing the algorithm.

- **Spiral Scanner Related Artefacts**:

  These are cone beam artefacts, helical motion-related artefacts and windmill artefacts.

  (a) **Cone Beam Artefacts**:

  When a spiral scanner tries to include a large number of rows of the detector array, the flat beam emitted by the scanner (slice-selecting beam which selects a few slices only) becomes more like a large volume-seeking "cone-shaped beam". The apex of the cone is the X-ray machine and the base is formed by the row of detectors at the other end. The cone beam scanner results in a variety of artefacts, such as noise, streak and stair-step artefacts. The artefacts are more in the region of the peripherally mounted detectors. These artefacts are also seen with dental implants and metal hardware (Fig. 22.7).

  Solution: There are several ways to reduce these artefacts. These include reducing the field of view, using metal artefact-reducing software, increasing the kV, and increasing the scanning speed to minimize motion-related artefacts. In the case of dental implants, try placing a gauze roll or cotton between the upper and lower rows of teeth.

  (b) **Helical Motion-Related Artefacts**:

  If during the helical motion of the scanner, any object within the scanning field also moves, its image and size may be distorted.

  Solution: Reduce the pitch.

  (c) **Blooming Related Artefact**:

  Materials having high density, such as calcium, radio-opaque calculus, and high-density foreign bodies, appear

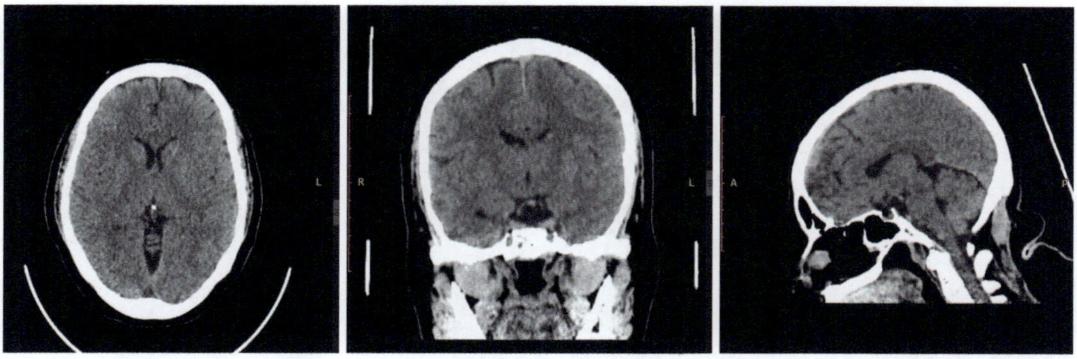

Fig. 22.6 Scans obtained with 1.2 mm thickness sections. Note that the stair-step artefacts have disappeared from the coronal and sagittal reformatted soft tissue images. In order to remove it from bone window images, the slice thickness was reduced to 0.6 mm

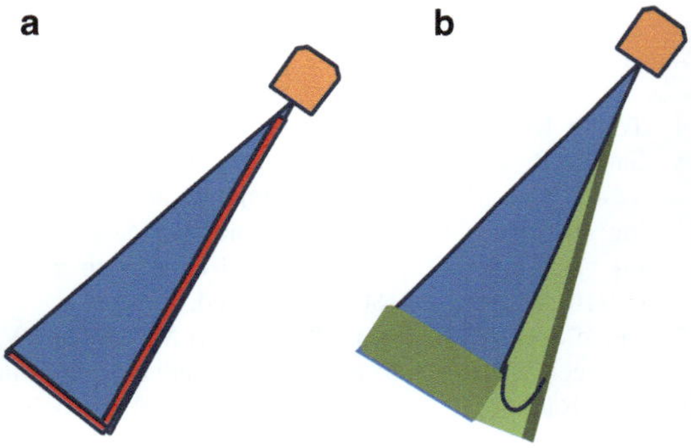

Fig. 22.7 (**a**, **b**) Images showing slice selecting beam (**a**) and cone beam (**b**)

larger than they are. The blooming effect changes with changes in WW and WL (Fig. 22.8).

Solution: Use a sharp bone algorithm filter, thin section and reduce the field of view.

(d) **Windmill Artefact**:

A windmill artefact [7] is seen in a helical CT, wherein streak artefacts arise from a high-density material and are seen rotating like propeller blades during the back-and-forth scrolling movement of the images. These artefacts are actually aliasing artefacts. They are caused either by inadequate data sampling or increasing the pitch.

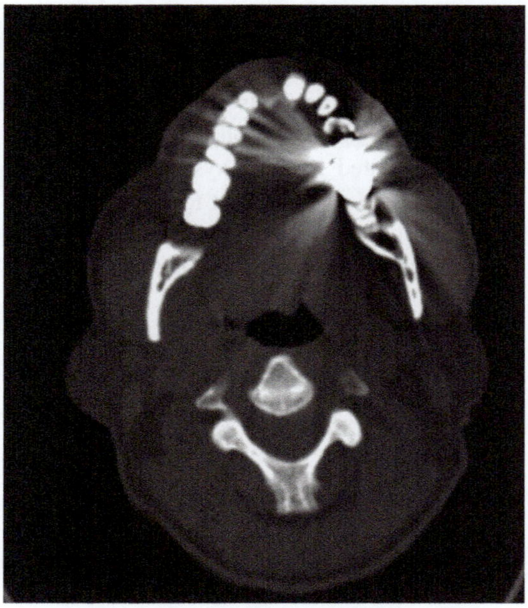

Fig. 22.8 Blooming artefacts caused by dental implants

Solution: Reduce the pitch and increase data sampling in the Z axis (axial plane) by altering the focal spot [8] (Fig. 22.9).

(e) **Multiplanar Reconstruction-Related Artefacts**:

There are two types of artefacts which can be related to multiplanar reconstructions. These include stair-step artefacts as described above, and “zebra artefacts”, which are seen in MRI images.

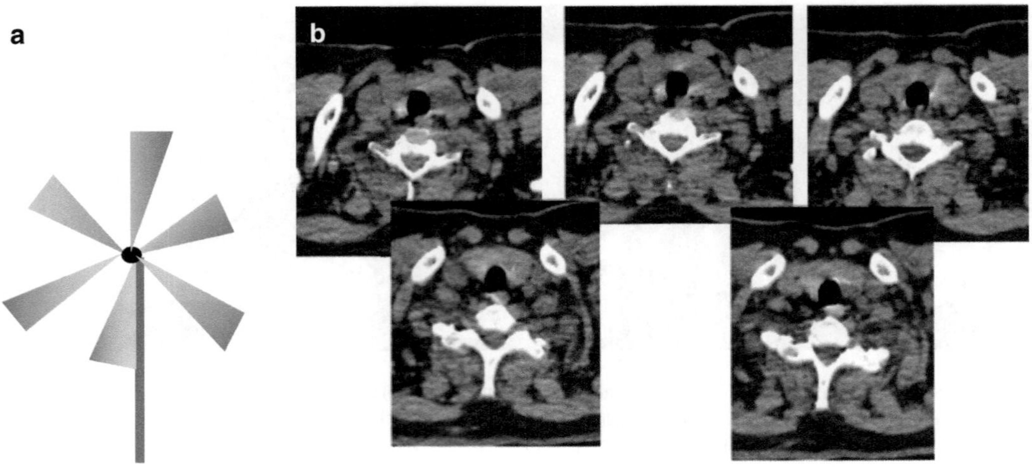

Fig. 22.9 (**a**) Windmill artefacts. These are swirling, fan-like motion artefacts, shown in a case under investigation. Serial sections of the trachea (**b**) show a windmill artefact which is changing its position as the scan shifts downwards

Summing up, artefacts can degrade images and impact the interpretation. They can occur due to human-related issues, physics and machine-related issues. It is important to recognize them. Every effort should be made to either eliminate or minimize their impact on the image.

References

1. Liu D, Cai X, Che X, Ma Y, Fu Y, Li L. Visibility and image quality of peripheral pulmonary arteries in pulmonary embolism patients using free-breathing combined with a high-threshold bolus-triggering technique in CT pulmonary angiography. J Int Med Res. 2020;48(8):300060520939326. https://doi.org/10.1177/0300060520939326. PMID: 32814489; PMCID: PMC7444127.
2. Boas FE, Fleischmann D. CT artifacts: causes and reduction techniques. Imaging Med. 2012;4(2):229–40.
3. Barrett JF, Keat N. Artifacts in CT: recognition and avoidance. Radiographics. 2004;24(6):1679–91.
4. Triche BL, Nelson Jr JT, McGill NS, Porter KK, Sanyal R, Tessler FN, McConathy JE, Gauntt DM, Yester MV, Singh SP. Recognizing and minimizing artifacts at CT, MRI, US, and molecular imaging. Radiographics. 2019;39(4):1017–8. https://doi.org/10.1148/rg.2019180022. Pubmed.
5. Mayo-Smith WW, Hara AK, Mahesh M, Sahani DV, Pavlicek W. How I do it: managing radiation dose in CT. Radiology. 2014;273(3):657–72. Radiological Society of North America Inc. https://doi.org/10.1148/radiol.14132328.
6. Mithun S, Jha AK, Panchal K, et al. A rare cause of tube arcing artifact seen in computed tomography image of a positron emission tomography/computed tomography scanner. Indian J Radiol Imaging. 2016;26(1):153–5. https://doi.org/10.4103/0971-3026.178368. PMID: 27081241; PMCID: PMC4813068.
7. Botz B, Glick Y, Murphy A, et al. Windmill artifact. Radiopaedia.org. Accessed 17 May 2024. https://doi.org/10.53347/rID-72190.
8. Brown KM, Žabic S. Method for reducing windmill artifacts in multislice CT images. In: Proc. SPIE 7961, Medical Imaging 2011: Physics of Medical Imaging, 79611; 2011. https://doi.org/10.1117/12.877437.

23 CT Protocols

Abstract

Computed tomography is a versatile imaging technique frequently used for the purpose of detection, diagnosis and management of pathologies hidden within the confines of the body. When setting up a protocol, the clinical indication for scanning is the first thing to know. The technician as well as the radiologist must go through the clinical data, the previous records, if any and if need be, have a discussion with the referring clinician prior to scanning. The information gathered should enable choosing from the available protocols and modifying or planning a suitable study for that patient. The scan parameters should be fed into the console on the workstation and everything should be in place before the patient is wheeled into the gantry room.

In this chapter, we will look at some of the parameters and protocols available in order to perform a high-quality CT scan.

Keywords

CT protocols · Parameters · Protocols · Diseases · Organs

There are various protocols available to study both anatomy and pathology while performing a CT scan. Most protocols are common to all institutions and many are modified depending upon the clinical situation and local preferences.

23.1 Basic Preparation for CT Examination

We will begin by discussing the process of scanning starting from the arrival of the request for CT examination.

Firstly, the technologist must read the request form carefully and understand the clinical situation which needs to be addressed by the CT examination. Previous records, if any, must be looked at before commencing the study. This is both to prevent unnecessary scanning and to suggest modality changes for that patient. Once the reason for scanning and the expectations from the investigation are understood, the patient's biometrics as well as the protocol for scanning are uploaded into the system. The scanner is now ready to take images.

23.2 Positioning of the Patient

- The patient is positioned on the motorized table with either the head or the feet first, to enter the gantry. The direction of entry into the gantry can be modified depending upon local factors, such as ease of positioning, length of the supporting tubes if attached to the patient, the position of the ventilator attached to a patient with severe breathing issues and trauma patients on a life support system. The technologist must, however, remember to

R. Gothi, *Radiographic and Imaging Techniques for Radiology Residents and Technologists*,
https://doi.org/10.1007/978-981-96-4816-0_23

make corresponding changes in the altered position on the console, or else, there will be issues later with regard to labelling the left and right side of the patient. Mistakes, if any, must be recognized early or will entail making corrections after the scanning is over.

- Irrespective of the position of the patient, the technologist must be able to continuously monitor the vital parameters and observe the patient for any possible issues arising during the study.
- The next step is to ensure that the patient is correctly centred inside the gantry. This is done with the help of laser lights present on the X-ray side of the gantry. The midline of the patient's body from the glabella to the symphysis pubis should coincide with the table midline as well as with the "Z" plane of the laser rays. The height of the table should also be adjusted so that the horizontal laser beam passes through middle of the patient's side. The radiation dose and noise is reduced in a well centred patient.
- Before the procedure commences, the patient should be instructed to stay still. Breathing instruction should be given and rehearsed. The patient should be reassured and informed about the inbuilt two way microphone through which the breathing instructions will be given before the scan begins as well as for communication with the technologist, in case of any problem.
- A dry run should be performed to ensure smooth movement of the table with the patient's body part not touching the inner walls of the gantry aperture. The dry run is particularly useful in children as it alleviates their fear of the investigation to a considerable extent.
- All tubings should be checked. An adequate amount of contrast must be prefilled in one syringe and saline in the other syringe if using a dual-headed pressure injector. All emergency preparations must be handy to manage any adverse event happening while the patient is in the CT room. The "code blue" phone number should be displayed in bold letters in the scanning as well as in the console room.

23.3 Breathing Technique

- All non-contrast and contrast-enhanced chest scans are first performed by asking the patient to take a deep breath and hold it. Often during this manoeuvre, the patient pulls the diaphragms upwards into the chest, rather than pushing them down into the abdomen. This prevents adequate expansion of the lower lobes. To circumvent this issue, the patient can be taught "diaphragmatic breathing". This is performed by asking the patient to push the diaphragms downwards into the abdomen while taking a deep breath and to hold on in this position for a few seconds. The abdomen protrudes out because of the downward movement of the diaphragms resulting in raised intraabdominal pressure. Diaphragmatic breath-hold images show good expansion of the lower lobes. Holding breath is also easier in diaphragmatic breathing as compared to holding breath in the usually performed deep inspiration.

  Before commencing the scan, the following steps are performed:

  1. The patient is made to lie down comfortably on the couch.
  2. The shoulders should be relaxed and at a lower level than the ears.
  3. The patient is asked to inhale deeply or perform diaphragmatic breathing. He/she can feel the abdomen expanding and the flanks bulging in diaphragmatic breathing.
  4. Breath is held for about 15–20 s.
  5. The chest should stay still.
  6. Following the inspiratory phase, the patient is allowed to relax.
  7. If an expiratory phase is planned, then the patient is asked to exhale slowly through the lips and feel the abdomen being sucked inwards.
  8. The patient should be made to practice this manoeuvre a few times before commencing the expiratory scan.

- If the patient is breathless or cannot follow breathing instructions (for example, children and sick adults), then switch off the voice command in the CT console and let the patient breathe freely. In this technique, also called the "free breathing technique", no breathing instructions are to be given to the patient.

1. The patient is made to lie down comfortably with the shoulder lower than the ears.
2. Observe the breathing pattern.
3. Do not give any breathing instructions.
4. Do a quick scan by reducing the exposure time and increasing the pitch.

This method works well most of the time, even while performing CT pulmonary angiogram (CTPA) because there is very little effect of breathing on the main pulmonary arteries and its central branches. However, it is worth remembering that the free-breathing technique might produce "bird-wing-like artefacts" in the distal branches of the pulmonary arteries. These artefacts may obscure small subpleural thrombi, if present.

- **Essentials Which Should Always be Available in a CT Suite:**

  The CT scan room should be equipped with life support systems such as oxygen, suction apparatus, a defibrillator, pulse oximeter and all the drugs needed to manage contrast reaction.

  The patient should be kept warm and monitored continuously during the study.

  - **Post Scanning:**

    Once the scan is over, go through the study for technical quality, completeness and any requirement for additional scanning. One of the personnel should also reach out to the patient immediately after the scan is over and check for the patient's well-being.

23.4 Commonly Used Protocols for Various CT Studies

An imaging protocol is a planned manner of performing a study, which should be easily replicated by all CT technicians. It requires the selection of a scanning technique appropriate for that clinical situation.

The role of the radiologist is to evaluate the clinical data and determine the best way of addressing the clinical issue. The technologist, in collaboration with the radiologist, should then select the most appropriate scanning parameters keeping in mind the patient's age, weight, volume of intravenous contrast needed, speed of injection and the most appropriate way to provide a diagnostic study using only the required amount of radiation.

It is worth remembering that no prescribed protocol is sacrosanct. They are subject to modification whenever the situation demands. Situations change with types of CT scanners, information based on current literature and departmental expertise.

23.5 Some of the Commonly Used Protocols

23.5.1 Head

These include non-contrast studies, contrast-enhanced scans, angiograms, perfusion studies and cerebral venograms.

- **Non-contrast CT(NCCT) of the head.**

  Indications:

  (a) *To evaluate head injuries for the presence of any intracranial bleed.* In the hyperacute phase, ongoing fresh bleeding may be isodense to the brain parenchyma but can be suspected if a whorl sign of isodensity is seen within a dense clot. Intracranial haematomas when clotted have a higher HU value as compared to the adjoining cerebrospinal fluid (CSF) spaces and brain parenchyma. They again become isodense in the subacute phase and slightly hypodense in the chronic phase. Don't forget to look for fractures of the skull, facial bones, mandible, nasal bones and any pathology of the TM joints and temporal bones. Occipital bone fractures often extend into the temporal bones. If the mastoid air cells appear opaque, add temporal bone imaging protocol to look for any fractures and involvement of the ossicular chain.

(b) *To evaluate acute stroke*. NCCT is generally the first line of investigation for a patient admitted with stroke-like symptoms. It rules out intracranial bleeding and can also detect obvious signs of ischaemia as well as stroke mimics. However, its main role is to detect bleed. MRI is certainly a better investigation in the evaluation of stroke patients and many centres prefer MRI over CT scans as the initial imaging modality.
(c) *Evaluation of skull deformities*: Both congenital and acquired skull deformities may need a CT scan to assess abnormalities, such as early fusion of sutures, called "craniosynostosis". This is a requirement for surgical planning.
(d) *Non-specific but troublesome symptoms*. These include headache, giddiness, dizziness, vertigo, altered mental status and dementia, where NCCT might be the initial and sometimes the only study needed. However, since NCCT is insufficient to rule out subtle parenchymal abnormalities, MRI should also be considered in these cases, if the clinical suspicion of an abnormality being present, is strong.
(e) *Follow up of patients*, especially to look for changes in the size of bleed, development or change in size of hydrocephalus, midline shift and post-op complications.
(f) *For detection of any calcification*. NCCT is also indicated if there is suspicion of a metallic foreign body embedded in the orbit.

Technique:

(a) Before commencing the study, as far as possible, all metallic objects, including those on the patient's person, should be removed from the scanning field. The patient should lie on the scanning table in a supine position with the arms by the side and in the head first position. The head should be placed in the head holder and fixed so that it does not move during the exposure. Using the vertical light of the laser beam, try to position the glabella, the tip of the nose and the chin in alignment with the "Z" axis of the table. Tucking in the chin helps avoid dentures and irradiating the ocular lenses. This position is preferable to the neutral position where the orbitomeatal line is perpendicular to the tabletop. The side light of the laser beam corresponds to the horizontal plane which should be used to position the head in the centre of the gantry. By using the laser beams, the patient can be appropriately centred.
(b) A lateral scout film should be obtained to plan the extent of the study and decide the degree of angulation of the tube if needed. Angulation is needed in the sequential axial mode and not in the helical mode.
(c) Scanning should be planned to extend from the C2–C3 vertebra to the vertex. The reason for including the C2–C3 vertebra is to ensure that any upper cervical spine injury or abnormality is not missed. Sometimes patients with dizziness or vertigo, may have an upper cervical spine pathology.
(d) Scanning can be performed by both helical and axial/sequential (stop-shoot and proceed), methods. A helical scan can be used for fast scanning of restless patients. Sequential scans, by tilting the tube help avoid radiation to the lenses in the orbits. Artefacts due to dentures, if any, and beam hardening artefacts, seen in the posterior fossa, are also reduced by tilting the tube.
(e) The scan parameters are chosen from the technical protocols provided by the vendor. The kVp can be adjusted and reduced from 120 kVp to 100. For a child, a paediatric protocol can be selected.
(f) The slice thickness should be more than the table feed so that the slices overlap. (This means that the pitch will be lesser than the slice thickness.)
(g) Multiplanar reconstructions of the images in axial, coronal and sagittal planes should be performed to ensure nothing is overlooked.

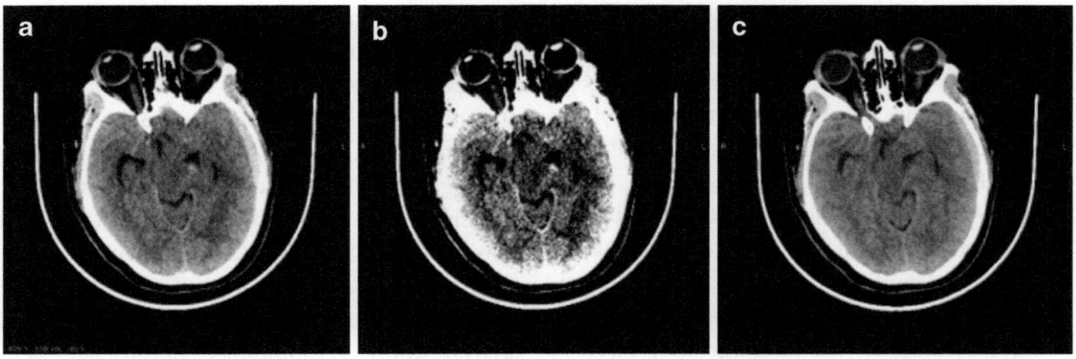

Fig. 23.1 NCCT windows for evaluation of stroke and intracranial haemorrhage: (**a**) normal brain window width and window level (100/40) for gray/white matter lesions, (**b**) stroke window (to accentuate the gray-white differentiation for detection of strokes (WW 40, WL 30) and (**c**) "subdural" window for distinguishing peripheral blood from bone (WW, 150 HU WL 30 HU)

(h) Images should be viewed in brain, bone, stroke, 3D and soft tissue windows (Fig. 23.1).

- **Contrast-Enhanced CT Scan of the Head (CECT)**:

  Indications:

  (a) For evaluating space-occupying lesions such as inflammatory or malignant diseases affecting the brain or meninges.

  (b) To evaluate the vascularity of tumours and vascular malformations.

  Technique:

  (a) Before beginning the study, cannulate a vein in the cubital fossa or dorsum of the wrist, using an appropriate sized, preferably 18–20 gauge cannula.

  (b) Obtain an NCCT as described above. This helps in detecting non-enhancing causes of increased density, such as calcification or acute bleeding in the parenchymal and extra parenchymal regions of the brain.

  (c) Then, perform the CECT.

  (d) Use non-ionic contrast agent, approximately 1 cc/kg body weight for children and about 50 cc for adults.

  (e) The injection can be given manually or by a pressure injector.

  (f) Follow the contrast bolus with a saline chase of 10–30 ccs, at the same rate which was used for IV contrast administration.

  (g) The injection rate can be kept between 3 and 4 cc/s. Scanning time is protocolled as per the indication for the CT scan.

  (h) For parenchymal evaluation, a delayed scan after 5 to 10 minutes may be appropriate as many lesions retain contrast enhancement due to the break in the blood–brain barrier. These lesions become more obvious in the delayed images.

- **CT Angiogram of the Brain (CTA)**:

  Indications:

  (a) Evaluation of patients with stroke to detect any vascular cause, such as occlusion due to stenosis, vasculitis, dissection, arterial or venous thrombosis and vascular malformations.

  (b) In patients with severe thunderclap headaches, raising a suspicion of subarachnoid haemorrhage.

  (c) To elucidate the vascular supply of an intracranial lesion.

  (d) For planning interventional procedures.

- **Stroke Protocol**

  Technique:

  This protocol should include the brain, neck and upper chest.

  (a) **Scout views** are obtained in lateral and AP projections. The AP projection should extend from the vertex, inferiorly till the level of the carina. Delayed scans are obtained to cover the left atrial appendage

(LAA), which helps in excluding a thrombus within it. This is because in the early scans, there may be poor filling of the entire LAA, and high density of the contrast may mask a small thrombus in the base of the LAA.

(b) **An NCCT** of the head is first obtained to look for features of stroke, including bleed, midline shift, vessel wall calcification and stroke mimics, if any.

(c) **Coming to CT Angiogram (CTA)**: A four-phase study is planned. The first and the last phases cover the upper chest (including the LAA), neck and head. The second and third phases extend from the skull base till the vertex. A bolus tracker is kept in the distal arch of the aorta and the trigger set at 80–100 HU. 50–70 ccs of Iodine 350 contrast is injected intravenously at the rate of 4–5 mL per second followed by a saline chase and scanning performed caudocranially.

A CT perfusion can also be performed immediately after the fourth phase using the CT perfusion protocol. There will be sufficient contrast in the arteries and veins of the brain at this time for performing CT perfusion. Thereafter, a preliminary evaluation of the images is performed followed by multiplanar reconstruction and shaded surface display (SSD) of the vessels. The reason for performing the four-phase study is to evaluate the neck vessels of both vertebral and carotid systems. It gives an idea about the presence of collaterals, if any, in the delayed phases. If collaterals are seen and well-formed, it indicates a good chance of significant recovery. The first phase is predominantly the early arterial phase demonstrating arteries of the neck and intracranial arterial circulation till the vertex. The second and third phases show both arteries and veins including the dural venous sinuses. The fourth phase shows the internal jugular veins, any delayed arterial filling and presence or absence of a thrombus in the LAA. A vertebral steal can also be inferred from the delayed phase, if the vertebral artery, unopacified in the early phases, fills in the delayed images (Fig. 23.2).

(a) **CT perfusion protocol**: CT perfusion [1] is usually performed as an initial technique. Some of its applications include the evaluation of acute stroke, chronic stroke, exclusion of vasospasm mimicking organic vascular occlusion, detection of ischaemic areas in patients with head injuries and brain tumour evaluation. The CT perfusion protocol, which is distinct from the conventional brain protocol, is chosen. It includes an NCCT followed by post-contrast 16–17 continuous passes through either the MCA territory alone or the whole brain. The contrast dose needed is 50 ccs of iodine 350 mg/mL. The injection rate is 4–5 cc/s followed by 25–30 ccs of saline injected at the same rate as the IV contrast. Scanning starts automatically. It takes a minute or two for the

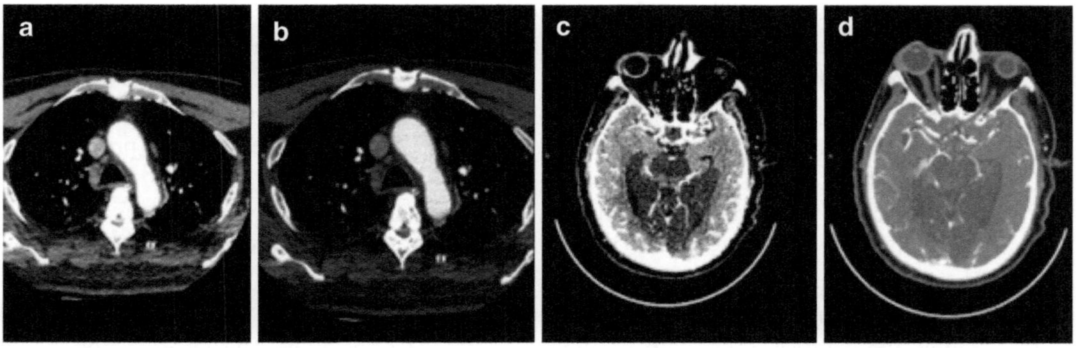

Fig. 23.2 CT brain angiogram from the aortic arch upwards. (**a**) Note the high density of the IV contrast which can mask a thrombus, if present, within the vessel. (**b**) Window width is increased to examine the presence of any thrombus, within the aorta. (**c**) Base image of intracranial arteries. (**d**) MIP image of Circle of Willis

perfusion study to get over. The initial few passes may not show contrast within the vessels. The protocol automatically chooses an intracranial artery and a vein when they become visible. It creates a time-intensity curve by plotting graphs showing the artery (in green and vein (in red), and calculates the cerebral blood flow, the cerebral blood volume and the mean transit time as the blood flows from the artery to the vein. The images are displayed in colour maps. The entire base set of CT images can also be downloaded separately to study the collateral circulation.

(b) **CT venography protocol for cerebral venous thrombosis**: A non-contract CT scan (NCCT) scan should be performed initially. This will enable the detection of intracerebral haematoma and sometimes, especially in the early phases of the disease, a hyperdense clot in the dural venous sinus, producing a "cord sign". Following NCCT, a contrast study is performed extending from the vertex down to the upper cervical spine, which will include the superior sagittal sinus at the vertex and the internal jugular vein in the upper cervical spine. 1 cc/kg body weight of iodinated contrast, having 300 mg/mL iodine, should be enough. The injection rate can be kept between 3 and 4 cc/s depending upon the vein used and the needle size chosen. The scan delay should be 45–50 s. A wider window width (250–280 HU) and a higher window level (approximately 120–140 HU), MPRs and MIP projections should be used for adequate delineation of the cortical veins and dural venous sinuses.

- **CT of face and paranasal sinuses**

  Indications:

  (a) Examination of the paranasal sinuses and nasal cavity for evidence and extent of sinonasal pathology.
  (b) Determination of the presence and extent of polyposis.
  (c) For any bone destruction or fracture.
  (d) For deviation of bony nasal septum.
  (e) Cases of epistaxis.
  (f) Preoperative evaluation for FESS.
  (g) In patients with trauma to the face.
  (h) Prior to facial reconstruction.

  Technique:

  (a) Most CT scans of the face and paranasal sinuses are non-contrast scans.
  (b) A lateral scanogram is obtained with the patient in a supine head-first position.
  (c) The scan field for paranasal sinuses extends from above the frontal sinuses till the inferior edge of the alveolar process of maxilla. This is because sometimes the maxillary sinuses extend into the alveolar bone. Also, an infected tooth projecting into the maxillary sinus, hence responsible maxillary sinusitis, can be evaluated.
  (d) A helical/axial scan is performed in axial plane in the caudocranial direction with the scanning being perpendicular to the hard palate.
  (e) The slice thickness is 0.6 mm and the interslice gap, 5 mm, which reduces the radiation dose to the patient. The midline should pass through the glabella.
  (f) The field of view should be adequate enough to include the paranasal sinuses and adjoining brain parenchyma. Approximately 22 cm coverage should suffice [2].
  (g) Multiplanar images are obtained in axial, coronal and sagittal planes. In addition, a 3D reconstruction in various planes should be obtained for evaluation of facial bones [3].
  (h) Images are displayed in bone (WW 2000 WL 100) and soft tissue windows(WW 350 WL 30).
  (i) IV contrast is needed in patients having vascular lesions, tumours, nasal bleeding and for surgical mapping in such cases. An NCCT scan should be obtained first. About 50 ccs of non-ionic contrast having a strength of 300–350 mg/mL iodine is injected at a rate of approximately 4 cc/s. For patients where the vascular anatomy has to be studied, scanning should commence as soon as the IV contrast injection is over. In other cases, par-

ticularly those having tumours, a delayed scan after 3–5 min might also be needed. This allows adequate contrast enhancement of the lesion.

(j) If the face is to be examined, especially to correct deformities, as well as in cases of polytrauma, the entire skull from vertex to the chin should be included in the scan (Figs. 23.3, 23.4, and 23.5).

- **CT of temporal bones:**

  Indications:

  (a) To evaluate congenital anomalies of the ear.

  (b) Evaluation for any cause of vertigo, sensory or conductive hearing loss.

  (c) Evaluation of ear discharge.

  (d) Preop assessment for cochlear implant.

  Technique:

  (a) A scout film is obtained in the sagittal plane.

  (b) The head should be positioned as symmetrically as possible using the laser cross-hair beam. The vertical line should pass through the glabella, nose and chin. The horizontal beam should be at the level of the external auditory canals.

  (c) The field of view should extend from above the tegmen tympani till below the mastoid process in the supero-inferior direction and from the level of the anterior wall of the sella till the anterior border of the foramen magnum in the anteroposterior direction.

  (d) High-resolution helical scan is performed in the caudocranial direction.

  (e) The slice thickness is 0.6 mm. The axial images are obtained with an interslice gap of 3 mm. Coronal and sagittal reconstructions are obtained at 5 mm intervals.

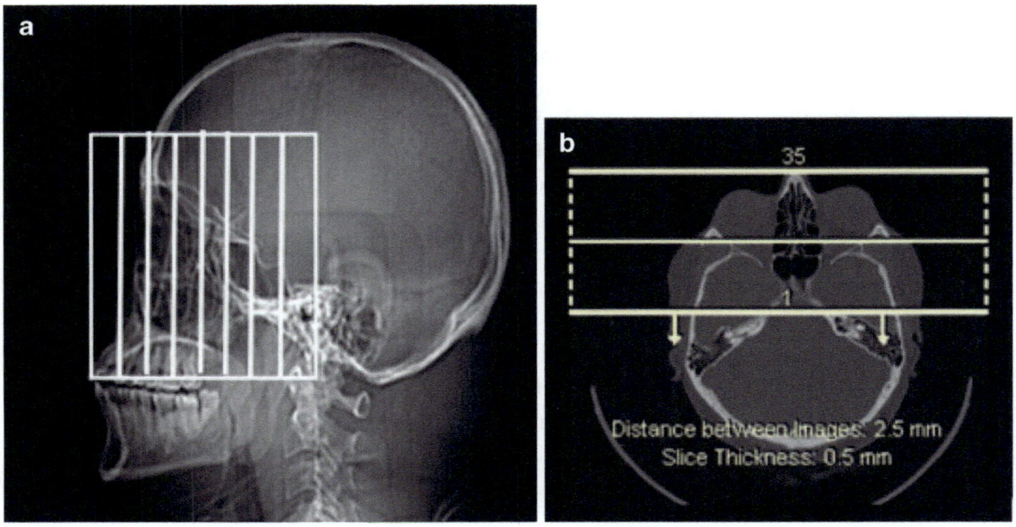

Fig. 23.3 Lateral scout film (topogram) showing scan lines perpendicular to the hard palate (**a**), and extending from in front of the hard palate till behind the clivus (**b**)

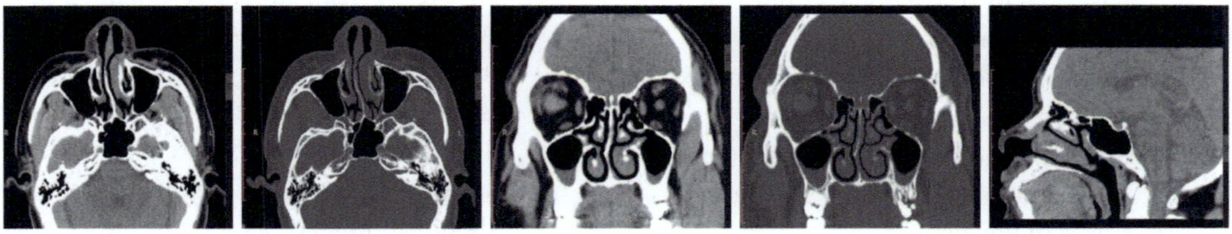

Fig. 23.4 Images of the paranasal sinuses in axial, coronal and sagittal planes, displayed in soft tissue and bone windows

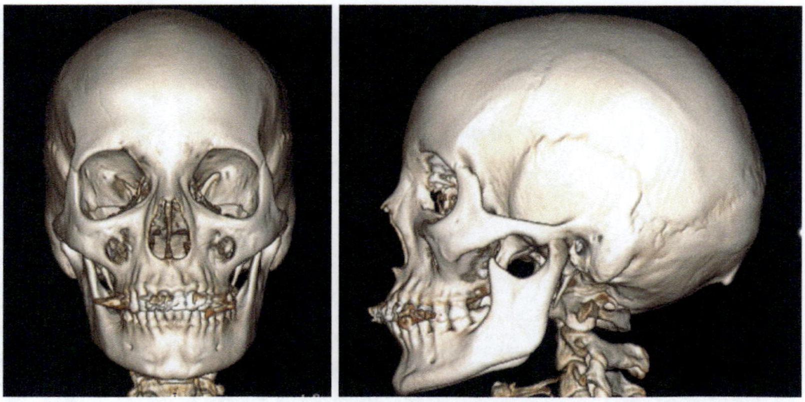

Fig. 23.5 3D reconstruction of the facial bones for the detection of fractures. The reconstruction is also needed in cases of trauma to the face

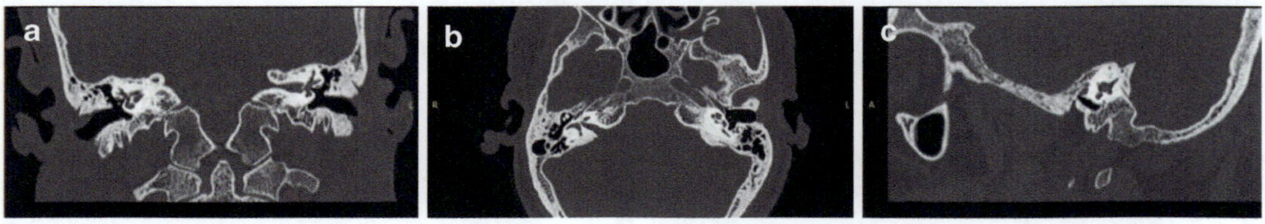

Fig. 23.6 Coronal (**a**), axial (**b**) and sagittal (**c**) views of the temporal bone

(f) Using the cross-hair of the multiplanar reconstruction software, the images can also be manipulated to demonstrate Stenver's and Poschl view.

The images are displayed in high-resolution bone window setting. Use bone algorithm with a window setting of high WW (4000 HU) and high WL (700 HU). This window setting will enable obtaining sharp images of the small and thin bones, constituting the temporoparietal region, including the ossicular chain. The scan should conclude with imaging of the posterior and middle cranial fossa, using a brain CT algorithm, to exclude any adjoining intracranial pathology such as abscess or venous sinus involvement.

(g) In patients suspected to have a mass lesion, infection or any congenital anomaly, an additional NCCT/CECT may be considered for ruling out any associated intracranial abnormality, including its extent (Figs. 23.6, 23.7, 23.8, 23.9, and 23.10).An MRI may be considered for studying the labyrinthine structures, the 7th and 8th cranial nerves, and the adjoining brainstem and for studying vascular lesions, including tumors and cholesteatomas.

- **CT Cisternography for CSF Rhinorrhoea**

Intermittent or continuous watery discharge from nose, especially in the upright position, could be leaking CSF and is called CSF rhinorrhoea. Both CT and MRI may be needed to detect the site of CSF rhinorrhoea. High-resolution CT shows bony defect in the base of the anterior and middle cranial fossa very clearly while MRI demonstrates the presence of fluid-CSF, in the nose and sinuses as well as any herniation of the brain parenchyma through the defect associated with the CSF rhinorrhoea.

CT Technique:

(a) The scan should be performed at the time of active discharge.
(b) Obtain an NCCT of the paranasal sinus. Place cotton plugs in the nasal vestibule to absorb the nasal discharge.

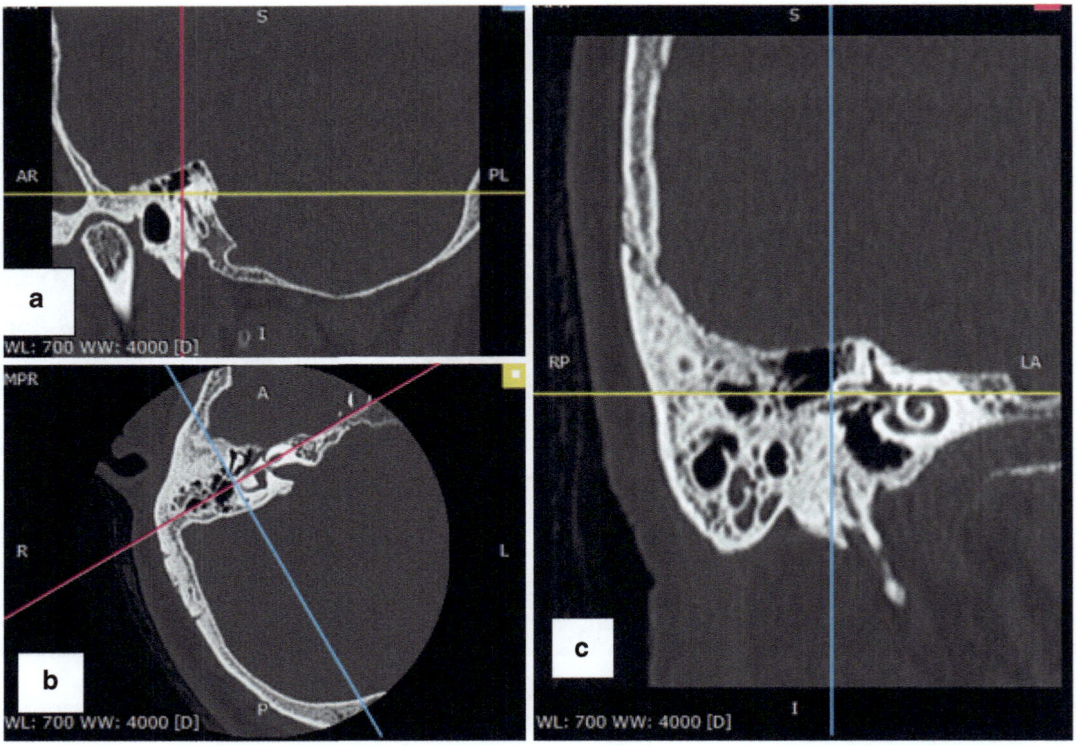

Fig. 23.7 (**a–c**) Using the cross hairs of MPR, and reconstructing along the long axis of the petrous bone (**a**, **b**), Stenver's view (**c**) can be created. The Stenver's view is used to study round and oval windows as well as to see the turns of cochlear implant electrodes

(c) Look for any defect in the bony structures located between the brain and the nasal passage, such as in the roof of the orbit, the frontal and sphenoid sinuses, the cribriform plate, the floor of the sella and any other bony defect in the floor of the anterior or middle cranial fossa.
(d) Look for fluid collection in the paranasal sinuses and note their HU value in the non contrast scans. This value acts as a baseline which will be needed for comparison with the scan obtained after intrathecal injection of non-ionic iodinated contrast medium.
(e) Next, a lumbar puncture is performed in the lateral decubitus position for administering intrathecal contrast.
(f) Approximately 10 mL of non-ionic contrast having 300 mg Iodine/mL is slowly injected under fluoroscopic guidance.
(g) The patient is placed in a prone Trendelenburg position for about 10 min to allow contrast to reach the basal cisterns.
(h) In those few minutes, the intrathecal contrast, enters the cranium, mixes with the CSF and spreads all over the skull base, leaking into the nasal cavity, if there is a bony defect.
(i) Scan the paranasal sinuses in the supine position from the alveolar margin of the maxilla till the top of the frontal sinus. If the CSF leak is not demonstrable, rescan the same area in the prone position.
(j) The scanning field should extend from the nose anteriorly to the clivus posteriorly, so that the entire area from where the CSF leak is possible is covered in the scan. Also include the nasal plugs in the scan. An increase in their density after contrast administration, also helps in confirming the CSF leak.

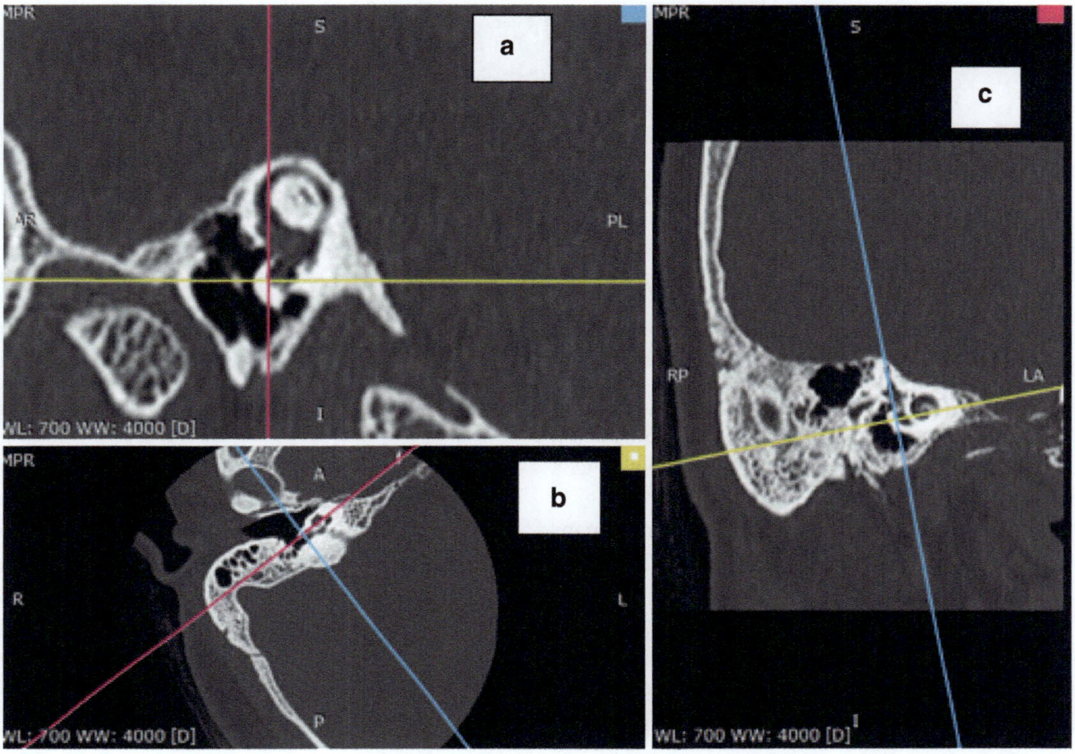

Fig. 23.8 (**a**–**c**) Poschl's view seen in (**a**) is created from Stenver's view. Using MPR (**b**) first reconstruct the Stenver's view (**c**), from which the Poschl's view can be created. Reconstructions perpendicular to the Stenver's view yields the Poschl's view

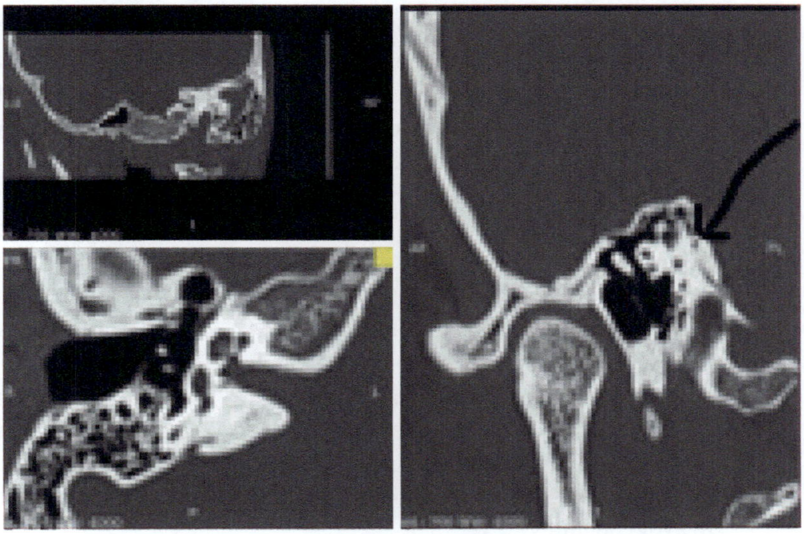

Fig. 23.9 Poschl view—This view is used to study the integrity of SSC (**a**) and also to evaluate the vestibular aqueduct (arrow in Fig. 23.9)

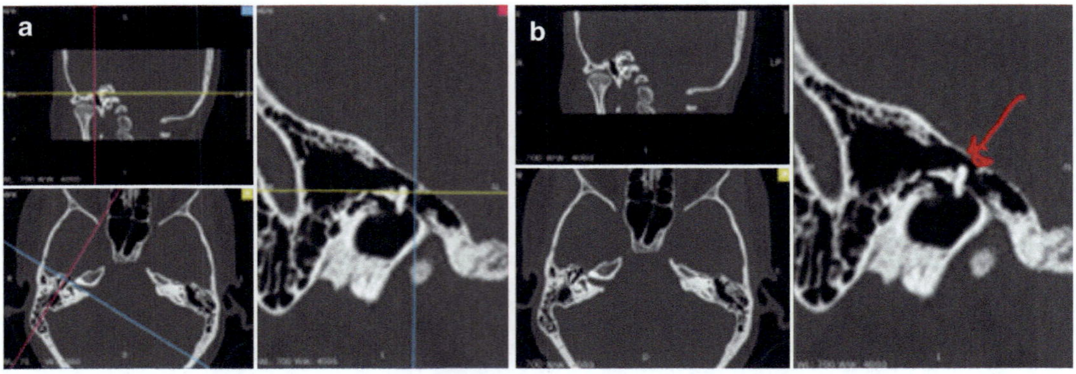

Fig. 23.10 (**a**, **b**): How to acquire a molar tooth view from Stenver's view (**a**). Molar tooth (arrow) in (**b**). This view is another way of looking at the relationship of the incus and malleolus. The more commonly used view is the axial view which shows the "ice cream cone" relationship of the malleolus with the incus

(k) Compare the pre and post-contrast scans and check for difference, if any, in the HU value of any fluid present in the nose or sinuses in the pre and post-contrast scans. The increase in HU value confirms the CSF leak. Examine the bone carefully to determine the site of the CSF leak.

- **Protocol for Evaluation of Oral Cavity and Floor of Mouth Lesion**

  Indications:

  (a) Evaluation of oral cancers for any bony involvement, extension of tumour across the midline, presence of nodes or vascular invasion.
  (b) Evaluation of inflammatory lesions to determine their location, extension, bony and vascular involvement.
  (c) Examination of soft tissue and vascular lesions of the face and mouth.
  (d) Evaluation of oro-dental lesions.
  (e) Salivary gland examination.

  CT Technique:

  (a) Obtain a two-plane scanogram with the patient in the supine position and the OM line perpendicular to the tabletop. Plan the study based on the clinical diagnosis for the results expected of this study.
  (b) Remove artificial dentures, if possible. If not, angle the gantry as much as possible to avoid dentures.
  (c) Puffed cheek technique: This is done to detect small lesions affecting the mucosa of the oral cavity, that is the buccal and gingival mucosa [4]. Ask the patient to puff out the cheeks with the lips pursed and stay still for a few moments. The breathing should be held while performing this technique [5].
  (d) Another method is to scan with the mouth opened with the tongue extended. This method reduces dental artefacts and improves the analysis of oral cancers [6].
  (e) Inject 50 ccs of non-ionic contrast having 300 mg/mL Iodine followed by 30 ccs of saline at 4 mL/s.
  (f) The scan field should extend from the upper margin of the alveolar process of the maxilla to the hyoid bone in the vertical direction and from the lips to the cervical spine in the AP diameter. In this way, the floor of the mouth, the nodes in the upper neck and the pharynx will be covered by the scan.
  (g) Scan in helical mode.
  (h) The direction of scanning is craniocaudal.
  (i) The scan thickness is usually 2.5–5.0 mm and the reconstruction for bone and soft tissue windows is between 0.625 mm and 1.2 mm, respectively.

(j) The reconstructed images should be both perpendicular and parallel to the hard palate [7].

- **CT Scan for Head and Neck Pathologies:**
  Indications:
  (a) Tumours of head and neck, including nasopharyngeal, laryngeal and pharyngeal tumours.
  (b) Investigation of change in voice.
  (c) To ascertain the presence and evaluation of nodes in the neck.
  (d) Evaluation of abscess or other inflammatory lesions affecting the head and neck.
  (e) Evaluation of thyroid or parathyroid lesions.
  (f) Evaluation of blood vessels and vascular lesions.
  Technique:
  (a) The field of view should extend from the base of the skull to the aortic arch. This will cover the nasopharynx, oral cavity, all soft tissues, cartilage and bones of the neck and detect any extension of the disease into the superior mediastinum. IV contrast administration may be needed if a tumour, infection or any mass is suspected.
- **CT Scan of the Larynx and Vocal Cords:**
  Indications:
  (a) Change in voice.
  (b) Difficulty in breathing.
  (c) H/o haemoptysis.
  (d) Pain and swelling in the neck region.
  (e) Difficulty in swallowing.
  (f) To look for nodes, vascular involvement and any destruction of the thyroid cartilage by a laryngeal mass.
  Technique:
  (a) The patient is in supine, head-first position and breathes in quiet respiration.
  (b) Axial scans are obtained in the helical mode.
  (c) The scan field should extend from the floor of the mouth till the aortic arch. This is to evaluate neck vessels and the presence of nodes at various stations in the mediastinum.
  (d) About 50–70 ccs of non-ionic contrast having an iodine content of 300 mg/mL is injected at 4 mL per second followed by a 30 mL saline chase at the same rate.
  (e) Scanning is in the cranio-caudal direction and starts at 45 s.
  (f) To reevaluate during phonation [8], use a small field of view and scan in the axial plane, parallel to the vocal cords from the level of the hyoid bone to the lower edge of the cricoid cartilage. Scanning should be during the period of phonation (patient saying “eee”).
- **CT Scan for Parathyroid Adenoma:**
  Indication:
  (a) Evaluation of cases of hyperparathyroidism for any evidence of parathyroid hyperplasia or adenoma.
  Technique:

1. Patient lies supine, head first, on the table.
2. Make the patient pull the shoulders down. This can be done by using something like a towel, a small rolled up sheet or a bandage that is wrapped around the feet and grabbed by both hands. Alternatively, the patient can stretch out both arms and keep the hands behind the lower back.
3. The radiation dose has to be increased because of the thickness of the shoulders, otherwise the photon starvation effect will be seen in this region and the area will look dark. Increase the kVp and mAs to 120 and 250, respectively. In thin and small patients, 100 kVp should be sufficient.
4. Perform a three-phase scan which includes plain, arterial (25 s) and venous phase at 60 s from the level of the mandible till the aortic arch. By using this technique, the chances of missing an ectopically located parathyroid nodule [9] is minimized.
5. A 4D CT can also be performed. In this, a parenchymal phase, acquired at 90 s, is added to study the enhancement pattern

of a suspicious nodule. The change in HU value of a nodule over the time, from the initial non-contrast scan to the additional parenchymal phase is studied [10, 11]. It is of use when the observations are unequivocal in an isotope scan and also helps in determining the functionally active gland among multiple parathyroid nodules.

6. A parathyroid nodule can be low in density as compared to the thyroid gland in both early and delayed phases. It also shows rapid enhancement and rapid washout.
7. Use contrast volume of 1 cc per kg, injected at a rate of 4 mL/s followed by 30 mL saline chaser at 5 mL/s.
8. Acquire 0.625 mm thin sections at 2 mm interval.

23.5.2 CT Scan of the Chest

Indications for non-cardiovascular pathologies:

(a) For chronic chest symptoms, such as cough, expectoration, shortness of breath and haemoptysis.
(b) Evaluation of an acute episode showing no abnormality in a chest X-ray.
(c) Investigation of congenital anomalies of the chest,
(d) Chest trauma.
(e) Pain in chest,
(f) Fever of unknown cause,
(g) In cases of malignancies to evaluate primary and secondary lesions.

Protocols for non-cardiovascular chest pathologies:

(a) Non-contrast CT.
(b) Contrast-enhanced CT.
(c) Low-dose CT.
(d) HRCT chest.
(e) CT pulmonary angiography.
(f) CT venography.
(g) Haemoptysis protocol.
(h) Virtual bronchoscopy.
(i) 3D CT for chest wall.
(j) CT perfusion [12].

Indication for cardiovascular pathologies:

(a) Chest pain of uncertain origin.
(b) Triple rule out.
(c) Triple rule out with lower limb venogram.
(d) CT coronary angiography.
(e) CT pulmonary angiography for congenital heart diseases in children.

Protocols for cardiovascular pathologies:

(a) Only cardiac calcium scoring.
(b) CT coronary angiography.
(c) CT scan for TAVR.
(d) Aortogram.
(e) Triple rule out and lower limb venogram.

- **Protocols for non-cardiovascular chest CT:**
  (a) All patients are scanned in supine position with the head-first, using the helical mode. The axial, "shoot-stop-step-shoot" mode can be used for HRCT chest of limited area of the chest. However, as high-resolution images can be created from the data set obtained by volumetric scanning, performing only HRCT is no longer needed. The present scans are called noncontrast scans (NCCT).
  (b) The patient should be correctly centred so that the midline of the chest corresponds with the isocentre of the gantry. Improper positioning can lead to increased radiation dose, artefacts and abnormal appearance of the chest size in the scanogram.
  (c) Ensure that the arms are above the head before taking the scanogram. This is because if the arms are by the sides, the machine miscalculates the body size and delivers a higher radiation dose, despite repositioning the arms later on.
  (d) For the above reason, as far as possible, fold the arms above the head before scanning starts.
  (e) The scanning field extends from the lower neck till the upper abdomen. This covers the lung apices as well as the posterior segments of the lower lobes which extend into the upper abdomen, behind the hepatic and splenic shadows. The

adrenals are also covered if there is a suspicion of bronchogenic carcinoma.

(f) The X-ray beam thickness is kept under 5 mm. The kV varies with the patient size, ranging from 80 kV for children, 100 kV for normal built patients and 120 kV for larger patients.

(g) Patients are also studied in the prone position, when it is necessary to differentiate between gravitational (dependant) pulmonary oedema and basal subpleural fibrosis.

(h) Scans are normally performed after a deep breath. Simultaneously, the patient is asked to distend the abdomen and stay still for a few seconds during which the scanning is on (diaphragmatic breathing).

(i) If the patient is unable to take a deep breath, scanning can also be done during quiet breathing.

(j) Scans are also performed during expiration to detect any air trapping, which happens when segmental or subsegmental bronchi are occluded.

Non-contrast CT scans (NCCT). Scans can be performed without the use of intravenous contrast. These scans are sufficient in to detect most parenchymal lung lesions. They can also detect most anatomical abnormalities affecting the mediastinal structures, pleura and pericardium as well as calcium deposition in the coronary arteries.

Low-dose CT scans are appropriate for lung cancer screening and in detecting parenchymal lung lesions. 5 mm contiguous scans are obtained in axial plane. 1.2 mm thick images are derived from these slices and evaluated in mediastinal (WW 400, WL 40) and lung windows (WW 1500, WL −400).

High-resolution CT scans (HRCT). These are meant to evaluate the interstitium or the lattice framework of the lung parenchyma. The slice thickness is kept at 1.2 mm for reconstructing images which are displayed using high-spatial resolution algorithm (bone window algorithm). If slices are very thin, the noise in the image increases because there are lesser number of X-ray photons to produce the image. Too thick slices incorporate more soft tissue within them, than needed, resulting in partial volume averaging effect. The WW is kept between 1400 and 1700 HU and the WL between −400 and −600.

IV contrast-enhanced CT scans. These are often requested to evaluate mediastinal pathology including nodes, lesions involving the lungs, pleural or pericardium. Non-ionic contrast having 300 mg Iodine/ml is administrated intravenously at 4 mL/s. The contrast dose is approximately 1 mL/kg body weight. It is followed by saline chase using 30 mL saline which is injected at the same or slightly higher rate to flush the contrast out of the veins. Images are obtained between 45 and 60 s following completion of contrast injection. This gives sufficient time for uptake of contrast by the nodes or any lesion in the chest. It is always better to obtain a low-dose NCCT first. Sometimes that may be enough and the study can be terminated. Initially obtained low-dose NCCTs can also shows parenchymal cavitatory lesions, nodes and masses, which help in focussing on those areas during contrast study.

CT pulmonary angiogram. This investigation is commonly asked for in patients who have sudden onset of shortness of breath, to rule out pulmonary thromboembolism. An NCCT scan is first obtained to look for parenchymal or pleural causes of shortness of breath. The NCCT can also detect a calcified chronic thrombus and vessel wall haematoma. Thereafter, 1 mL/kg body weight of Iodine 300–350 is injected through an 18G cannula, preferably inserted in the antecubital fossa. (A low dose of contrast, such as 50 mL, can also be administered [13] with the bolus tracker kept in the main pulmonary artery or right atrium and triggered at 250 HU.) The injection rate should be kept between 3 and 4.5 mL/s. The contrast scan is followed by a saline chase of 30 mL injected at the same rate to wash out contrast from the SVC. It is better to inject contrast through the left arm. This is because, as compared to injection from the right side, contrast injected from the left side has to take a longer route to reach the pulmonary artery. This allows for some dilution of contrast with the unmixed blood and lowers the high-density streak artefact produced by the contrast present in the SVC. The scan can be timed as a single study or can be multiphasic. Scans can be obtained by timing bolus or bolus tracking techniques. In a timing bolus, the scanning can start 6–7 s after completion of a rapid injection that is around 12–15 s after commening the injection,using an injection rate of 3.5–4.0 mL/s. In a bolus tracking scan, the bolus tracker can be in the right atrium or main pulmonary artery. It can also be kept in the left atrium especially when the injection speed is slower due to a thinner needle being used or if a small vein has been cannulated. The scan is initiated in the craniocaudal direction [12] and triggered when an HU value of 100 is reached in the area chosen for bolus tracking. Scanning can also be initiated in the caudocranial direction, especially in patients who are unable to hold their breath. The images taken in the caudocranial direction are less affected by streak artefacts which emanate from the SVC due to blood mixing with high-density contrast. However, streak artefacts do not affect the diagnosis, hence craniocaudal scanning can be performed as a matter of protocol. Some equipments provide a multiphasic protocol in which at least one phase will be free of streak artefacts. Breathing could be quiet respiration or, in sick patients, free breathing can be allowed. Deep inspiration followed by breath holding is not recommended as unopacified blood may enter the pulmonary vessels and mimic a thrombus.

Haemoptysis protocol: This protocol is used to elucidate the cause of haemoptysis, such as a pseudoaneurysm of the pulmonary artery, dilated bronchial arteries supplying an area of bronchiectasis or a cavity, a vascular mass or a vascular malformation. In this protocol, a low-dose plain scan is first obtained to evaluate the lung parenchyma for evidence of any focal ground glass haze (which may be seen in intraparenchymal bleed), any mass lesion, bronchiectasis, cavity or abnormal collection of vessels. Following the plain scan, a contrast-enhanced scan using an Iodine concentration of preferably 350 mg/mL, is obtained. About 1 cc/kg body weight of contrast is needed for the study. The bolus tracker is placed in the proximal descending aorta at the same level as the carina. Contrast is injected at a slightly slower speed of 3.5 mL/s. This allows adequate concentration of contrast in the pulmonary artery and its peripheral branches, as well as in the thoracic aorta. The descending aorta is well opacified and bronchial arteries, arising from it, fill up well. Saline chaser is avoided, otherwise the contrast in the peripheral vessels can get diluted or washed out. By using this protocol, the pulmonary artery and its branches, the pulmonary veins, aorta and its branches can be adequately evaluated.

The scan length should extend from above the thoracic inlet to the upper abdomen in order not to miss out on any ectopic collateral arterial supply to the diseased lung parenchyma.

Virtual bronchoscopy: This is the endoluminal study of the trachea and bronchi. It uses a software which provides a luminal view of the airways. The initial scan can be NCCT or CECT, obtained using the standard chest protocol. The data can then be reconstructed using the virtual bronchoscopy software.

- **Protocols for cardiovascular chest CT:**

  Triple rule out: This technique is used to evaluate the pulmonary artery and its branches, the thoracic aorta including the aortic root as well as the arch vessels and coronary arteries. The technique envisages the use of a triple rule-out ECG gated protocol. ECG gating should be set up before scanning. The scan should be done in a fasting state, if the patient is stable. However, in an emergency, fasting is not necessary. A tablet of nitroglycerine should be placed beneath the tongue, 10 min before starting the scan. The heart rate should be close to 70 beats per minute for adequate coronary artery evaluation. An NCCT scan should be obtained first for calcium scoring followed by IV contrast enhanced scan, using 1 mL/kg body weight of Iodine 350–370. The bolus tracker should be kept in the descending aorta near the carina. The patient should be asked to hold breath during scanning. The scan will show the pulmonary arteries, aorta and the coronary arteries. If the entire aorta is also to be examined, plan the scan right at the beginning, covering an area extending from the apex of the chest to the inguinal region. A delayed scan at 120 s from the beginning of injection may be considered if evaluation of the IVC, pelvic and lower limb veins has also been requested.

Coronary CT protocol: This study is best suited for excluding coronary artery occlusion and anomalous origin of the coronary arteries, especially in young individuals presenting with atypical pain or sudden onset of breathlessness. It is also performed as a screening test and in post-treatment patients to confirm the patency of stents and grafts The study requires planning. The procedure should be explained to the patient. The clinical record should be checked for any history of difficulty in breathing, especially any history of bronchial asthma, medicines being used, pulse rate and blood pressure status. If the heart rate is high, it needs to be brought done to 70 or below, either by oral metoprolol (50–100 mg about 2 h prior to scanning) or 2.5–5 mg injected slowly intravenously. The dose can be repeated with an additional 5 mg administration after 5 min and repeated till a maximum of 15 mg has been administered. In patients having bronchial asthma, the administration of beta blockers must be confirmed by the cardiologist. If the heart rate is less than 65 and the patient is young with non-specific signs and symptoms, a prospective study should be considered which gives a lower radiation dose. However, no functional study can be obtained in a prospective scan. If the heart rate is above 70, it is better to perform a retrospective scan. In the retrospective study, unlike in the prospective study, the radiation is continuously on, hence the higher radiation dose. Image reconstruction can be made either during mid-diastole if the heart rate is high (40% of R-R interval) or near the end-diastole, if the heart rate is low (70% of R-R interval). A functional study can be performed in a retrospective gated study, which is an advantage of this type of study. Upon reaching the imaging department and all records as well as the heart rate checked, the patient is asked to relax in the waiting room. One of the members of the radiology team should meet and reassure the patient. The procedure starts with non-contrast administered calcium scoring. If the Agatston score used for determining the severity of calcium score is 0, there is minimal or very low risk of significant coronary artery disease. The risk rises with the elevation of the calcium score. Following calcium scoring, the protocol for contrast study is set up. The heart rate should be approximately 60–70 beats per minute. A few minutes (approximately 5–10 min) before beginning the scan, a tablet of nitroglycerine is given to the patient with instruction to keep it beneath the tongue. On the planning workstation, the scanning field of view is adjusted so that it covers the entire cardiac shadow from the level of the carina, till below the diaphragm (so that both the proximal ascending aorta and base of the heart are included in the study). The scanning area is rectangular and is shifted slightly to the left of the midline, to have the aortic root in the centre of the scan field. Using bolus tracking with the tracker kept in the descending aorta (at the same level as the carina), scanning is commenced as soon as the threshold value of contrast-laden blood reaches 80–100 HU (varies with the machine being used). The patients are asked to hold their breath during the scanning. About 80–90 mL of IV contrast, having 350 mg Iodine/mL is injected at the rate of 5–6 mL/s. The needle should be preferably 18 gauge. The site of injection should be the antecubital vein. A large vein of the dorsum would also do if the antecubital vein is small in calibre. As soon as the study is completed, the images should be evaluated and if necessary, followed by a venous phase of the entire chest. The data obtained is reconstructed on the workstation as per standard coronary angiogram software preinstalled in the workstation.

Trans arterial aortic valve replacement (TAVR): This is a technique used to replace the diseased aortic valve through an arterial route. It consists of two parts [14].

The first part includes an initial calcium scoring for coronary arteries and evaluation of the aortic valve and annulus for the presence of calcium deposition. Excessive calcium deposition in the aortic valve or annulus may influence the decision of whether to carry on with the procedure or go for surgery. Thereafter, an ECG-gated retrospective contrast study with the bolus tracking kept in the proximal descending aorta, as in the coronary artery study, is carried out. The aortic root should be well-opacified. The sino-tubular junction is then evaluated in detail at the workstation either manually or by using TAVR/TAVI software.

The second part consists of a repeat aortogram extending from the aortic arch to the femoral arteries. This is to determine the feasibility of introducing the TAVI device through the femoral artery route and to be prepared for any obstacle higher up in the aorta. This second part can also be planned with the first part by deploying a protocol that covers the entire area from the neck to the groin.

23.5.3 CT Scan of the Abdomen (Gastrointestinal and Urinary Tracts)

Indications: Here are a few indications for which a CT scan of the abdomen can be requested. The list is by no means exhaustive.

(a) Fever of unknown origin.
(b) Pain abdomen.
(c) Altered bowel movement.
(d) Mass in the abdomen.
(e) Abdominal trauma.
(f) GI bleeding.
(g) Investigation for weight loss.
(h) Urinary tract abnormality.
(i) Renal donor assessment.

Protocols for CT scans of the abdomen:

(a) Non-contrast CT scan using a high pitch ratio and thick slices (say about 7.5 mm), especially if the clinical details are not clear.
(b) Contrast-enhanced CT scan.
(c) CT angiography in cases of abdominal trauma, GI bleeding and to study vascular anatomy for abdominal pain.
(d) CT enterography for small bowel lesions.
(e) CT colonography for large bowel lesions.
(f) CT urography to evaluate the renal outflow tract.
(g) Multiphasic CT for abdominal trauma, liver tumour, masses in the abdomen, pancreatic pathology and urinary tract masses.
(h) Renal transplant donor and recipient protocol.

Technique for CT abdomen:

Before taking in a patient, check the clinical records which implies checking both current and previous records. This will give an idea about what to expect and what needs to be seen in a CT scan.

(a) The scans are performed in the supine position in the feet or head-first position.
(b) The area covered should extend from above the diaphragms till the level of the lesser trochanter. This will cover the lower chest and the perineum including all structures exiting the pelvic floor.
(c) Scanning is performed with the breath-hold technique. The patients are asked to hold their breath till the scan is completed.

Non-contrast CT of the abdomen: Usually requested for evaluation of the urinary tract, confirmation of perforation or as a follow-up study. Always check previous records. No preparation is needed for NCCT. Sometimes, oral positive or neutral contrast may be needed. The radiologist can decide about this after perusing the clinical records. Oral positive contrast is usually needed in post-operative cases, especially to rule out any anastomotic leak.

Contrast-enhanced CT: In this study, intravenous contrast is administered, depending upon the weight of the patient. Usually, 1.0 mL/kg body weight is adequate. The injection rate can be kept between 3.5 and 4.5 mL/s for an adult. If the vein is thin or the patient is a child, the injection rate can be reduced to as low as 1 mL/s. The study should commence either from the delayed arterial phase, which is approximately 35 s from the beginning of the injection or from the venous phase, which is approximately between 60 and 70 s after IV contrast administration. Oral contrast may or may not be needed. If the radiologist deems it necessary, it is best to give a neutral contrast which will allow evaluation of the stomach and small bowel wall enhancement as well as demonstrate the presence of any enhancing intraluminal lesion. In cases of acute abdomen, small or large bowel obstruction (where the bowel loops are already fluid-filled) and in cases of trauma, oral contrast need not be given. Before giving IV contrast, it is worthwhile to know the state of renal function. However, this is not necessary for polytrauma patients, patients presenting with acute abdomen including intestinal obstruction and patients who have with them a recent normal kidney function test report.

CT abdominal angiography. An initial non-contrast (NCCT) scan may be obtained to evaluate any density which can get mistaken for blood. Also, if a bowel wall appears dense in NCCT, it is a helpful sign of intestinal ischaemia [15]. The NCCT is followed by an early arterial phase which can either be timed by bolus tracking method or by timing the bolus at 15–20 s after commencing injection. The contrast is injected at the rate of 4.5 mL/s. The bolus trigger can be set at 100 HU at the level of the coeliac trunk. 1 cc per kg body weight of iodinated contrast medium, preferably 350 mg/mL strength can be administered to adults. For children, both injection rate and contrast dose should be adjusted. Smaller amounts of contrast, slower injection rate and low kVp should be considered in children. Many machines have paediatric protocols which can be deployed. The scan plane should extend from above the diaphragm till the level of the lesser trochanter. A late arterial phase as well as a venous phase may occasionally be needed after the early arterial phase study. The images should always be monitored by the on-call radiologist. The role of orally administered neutral contrast is controversial. It is not needed in most cases of CT angiography. This is because it delays the performance of study, till the patient finishes drinking the oral contrast. It can also dilute the iodinated contrast which has leaked out into the lumen from the bowel wall, making detection of active intraluminal bleeding difficult to appreciate [16]. In patients with occult blood in stools or inflammatory bowel disease, CT enterography may be considered to distend the bowel loops and get a better view of the presence or absence of mucosal enhancement. However, since there is no control over the rate of flow of oral contrast in the small bowel loops, it results in non-uniform dilatation of the bowel loops. Also, pathological bowel loops generally manifest themselves by dilating, retaining fluid within them or thickening their walls. CT enterography, therefore, is not satisfying in many situations. On the other hand, since gastric pathologies are more likely to present themselves, oral neutral contrast (approximately 250 cc of water or mannitol) can be given when the patient is on the table just before scanning. Similarly, the colon can be distended rectally with approximately 500–750 ccs of water or positive contrast (or as much as the patient tolerates), for better visualization of the more common recto-signoid and colonic lesions.

CT enterography: For this study, the patient should be off solids for at least 4 h. This prevents mistaking food bolus for intraluminal lesions and the presence of gas in large amounts in the bowel lumen. However, since most food bolus have air bubbles trapped within them, there is usually no problem in identifying them. There is no restriction on water intake before scanning. Upon reaching the department, a dose of 20 mg Metoclopramide (5 mg/mL) is administered intravenously. This hastens peristalsis and rapid onward movement of oral contrast within a few minutes. Alternatively it can also be given orally in a tablet form. The orally administered drug hastens peristalsis within an hour. Thereafter, 1.5 L of neutral fluid containing mannitol is given to the patient to drink within 45 min [17]. After having had the fluid, the patient is taken up for the study. About 250 mL of oral mannitol or water is given on the table to distend the stomach. This is immediately followed by an intravenous injection of 20 mg Buscoupan which results in a reduction of peristaltic activity, slows down further bowel movement had helps keep the fluid-filled bowel loops distended. Following this, approximately 1–1.5 cc/kg body iodinated contrast is administered intravenously and whole abdominal scanning is performed in the venous phase. This technique improves the visibility of mucosal enhancement and the detection of small intestinal lesions. However, the drawback of this study is the uncertainty regarding distension of all small bowel loops [18]. Some patients are unable to drink the large volumes of fluid in 45 min, resulting in inadequate distension of the bowel loops. These are some limitations for obtaining a good quality study in every case.

CT colonography: In this study, air or CO_2 is insufflated into the colon in order to detect small sessile or pedunculated or ulcerating colonic lesions. The patient needs to come after adequate preparation of the large bowel. The preparation starts 3 days before the study. The patient takes a low-residue diet and avoids solids, which includes substances producing roughage, seeds and meat products. Other than fruit juices which can cause gaseous distension, there is no restriction on fluid intake. About 250 mL of iodinated contrast is also given 3 days before the study, to allow faecal tagging with the high-density contrast. A day before the study, only a liquid diet and a laxative are prescribed to clear the colon. On the day of the study, fluid is avoided for 4 hrs before the study begins. The study is performed by introducing a flexible tube into the rectum through which air is insufflated with the help of a blood pressure pump. The quantity of air introduced is as much as the patient can tolerate. An injection of Buscoupan can be given intravenously just prior to the study, in order to reduce peristaltic activity. Images of the abdomen are obtained in supine followed by prone positions. Further images in decubitus position are decided after evaluating the first two sets of images.

CT Urography: For this procedure, permit the patient to void urine about an hour before commencing the study. An overdistended bladder makes the patient uncomfortable and can lead to movement artefacts caused by the discomfort of controlling the urge to micturate. An overfilled bladder also dilutes the intravenously administered iodinated contrast, thereby reducing the density of contrast in the bladder.

Start the study by obtaining a low-dose non-contrast scan of the abdomen from the level of the diaphragms to the lesser trochanter of the femurs. This is to detect any radiopaque calculus, foreign body or any unexpected pathology in the abdomen. Thereafter, inject 1 mL/kg body weight of iodinated contrast having 300 mg/mL iodine. Take a nephrographic phase image of the renal area at 90 s and then wait for about 5–9 min for the urographic phase. It helps to roll the patient on the table once or twice during these 9 min. This enables proper mixing of contrast with the urine present in the bladder. A prone study may be needed if the anteriorly located calyces are not fully opacified or if there is evidence of hydronephrosis or delayed excretion of contrast. The patient can also be taken off the table and made to walk around or sit outside in the waiting area for the urographic phase. Sitting upright or walking helps in a drainage of contrast from the calyces into the ureters.

23.5.4 Multiphasic Intravenous Contrast Study of the Abdomen

This is performed in cases of abdominal trauma, liver, pancreatic, urinary tract pathology and GI bleeding. The preparation of patients varies from case to case. Patients presenting in the emergency with a history of trauma or bleeding do not need any preparation including providing results of renal function tests. Other non-emergency patients are usually asked to avoid solids for at least 4 h. Fluids, especially water, are not restricted in any case. Using a low-dose, high-pitch technique, a plain scan of the abdomen and pelvis is first obtained. This gives an idea about the presence of iso to hyperdense peritoneal fluid, which could be blood in the peritoneal cavity, exudate, urine, bile or ascites due to any coexisting cause. It can also demonstrate the presence of any radiopaque shadow, free peritoneal air and distortion of the normal anatomical appearance of solid organs and hollow viscus. Usually, no oral contrast is administered in acute cases. Following the non-contrast study, a multiphasic intravenous contrast-enhanced study is performed. This study includes an early arterial phase using bolus tracking. The bolus tracker is placed at the level of the celiac trunk. When the HU value reaches 100, scanning is triggered. Using a low kV improves visualization of the contrast enhancement. The next phase is late arterial at 35–40 s, followed by portal venous phase at 60–70 s and parenchymal phase, if necessary, at 90–100 s. The scanning protocol can be modified on a case-to-case basis and the preference of the radiologist as well as the institution.

In trauma and abdominal bleeding, multiphasic scanning of the whole abdomen is recommended. This is because it can show active bleeding which appears dense in the early phase and dilutes or washes off in the later phases. It can show the source of bleeding, the cause of bleeding and the presence of any AV shunting. The delayed scans can show the urinary tract and any extravasation of contrast from the urinary system.

In liver lesions, such as during evaluation for hepatocellular carcinoma (HCC), the early and late arterial scans should cover only the liver (the scan length can be judged from the initial NCCT). This is because most HCCs show arterial supply by the hepatic artery in early phases with rapid AV shunting by the late arterial or venous phase. The portal venous phase can cover the entire abdomen. The early arterial phase helps delineate a vascular lesion (which most HCCs are) receiving hepatic arterial supply. It may also show rapid washout into the hepatic veins—indicating rapid arteriovenous shunting. The venous phase helps delineate any portal or hepatic vein thrombus.

For demonstration of liver metastasis, early arterial phase CT is performed if a hypervascular metastasis such as from a melanoma or a neuroendocrine tumour is suspected. Or else, late arterial, venous and delayed phases are sufficient as most deposits are less vascular than HCC and often hypovascular.

For liver haemangiomas or fibronodular hyperplasia, a delayed arterial followed by venous and parenchymal phases should be obtained.

In liver transplant cases, the early arterial phase is necessary especially if the donor liver is being studied. If a liver abscess is suspected, then a single venous phase at 60 s is sufficient.

For pancreatic pathology, begin with a late arterial phase at 35–40 s post-injection, covering the area from the diaphragms to the iliac crest. The pancreas enhances best in the late arterial phase. The entire abdomen is subsequently covered at 60 s during the portal venous phase. Why is the early arterial phase not recommended/performed in cases of acute pancreatitis? This is because in the early arterial phase, contrast remains is mainly within blood vessels and is yet to enter the pancreatic parenchyma. Hence, unless there is an ultrasound or prior CT scan which shows an aneurysm, a pancreatic neuroendocrine tumour or a pancreatic carcinoma, the early arterial phase adds little to the diagnosis and management. There is no need to give any oral contrast and no need to fast, especially in cases of acute pancreatitis. However, if a tumour is suspected, oral neutral contrast may be administered to distend the stomach and duodenum. The need for testing for renal function is questionable in acute pancreatitis as IV contrast will be given in every case to detect areas of pancreatic necrosis and vascular complications (Figs. 23.11, 23.12, and 23.13).

Evaluation of the urinary tract for haematuria. A plain CT KUB scan is first obtained, followed by early arterial phase at 25 s covering only the upper abdomen (if a renal mass is known to be present). In these cases, the next phase is the late arterial phase, at 35 s which is also the renal cortical phase. This is followed by the corticomedullary phase which corresponds with the portal venous phase(60 s) and a nephrographic phase, which is the parenchymal phase(90 s). These phases are limited to the kidney narea. The final phase is the urographic phase, taken at approximately 5–9 min after initial injection of IV contrast. Most renal tumours will show early arterial enhancement due to rapid AV shunting and will become hypodense in the later phases. The same protocol can be tailored for bladder tumours. (Add to the above phase, a cystographic phase after 10 min to opacify the bladder lumen if there is suspicion of a urothelial tumour of the bladder). The patient may be asked to roll on the table for proper mixing of contrast with the urine. This will enable detection of any non-dependant bladder lesion, especially those arising from the anterior non-dependant wall (Fig. 23.14).

Once done, examine all structures including, liver, renal vessels, IVC, bones and lung bases before concluding the study (Figs. 23.15 and 23.16).

Renal transplant donor protocol. The purpose of this protocol is to ensure that donor has two healthy kidneys so that donating one of the

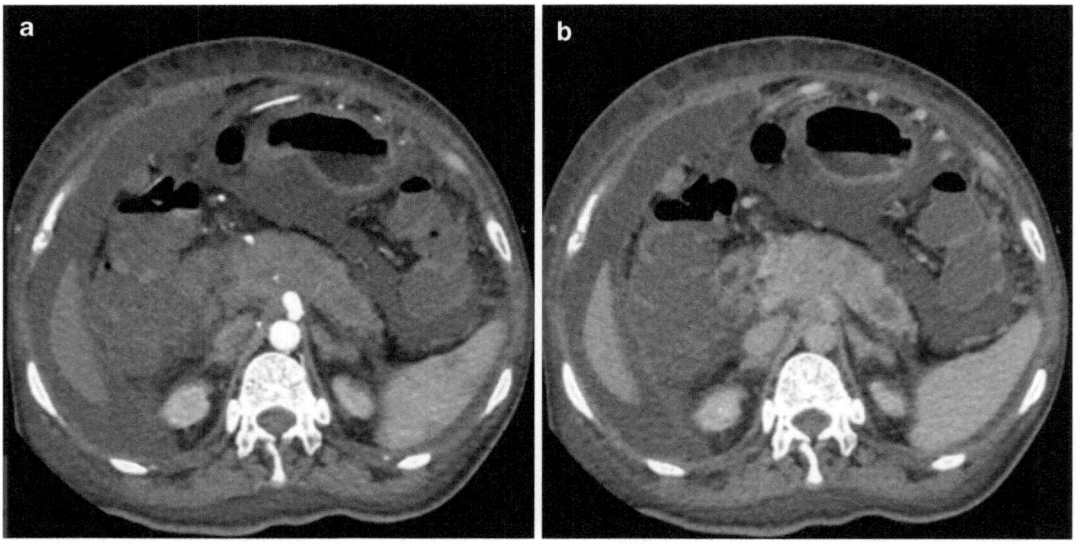

Fig. 23.11 Early arterial (**a**) and later arterial (**b**) phases. Note the lack of enhancement of the pancreas in the early arterial phase because most of the contrast is still in the arteries

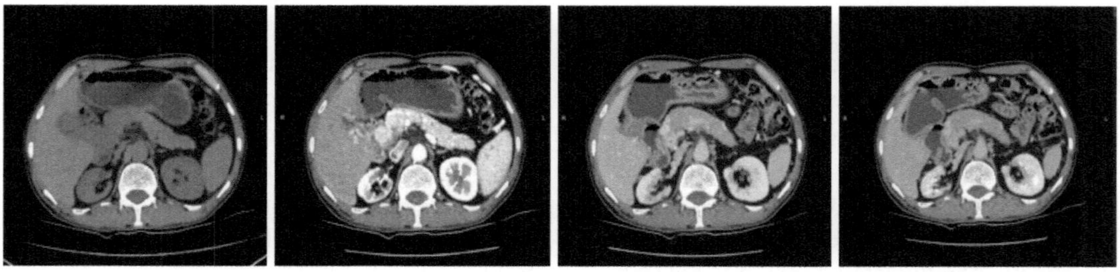

Fig. 23.12 Appearance of pancreas (from left to right) in non-contrast, delayed arterial, venous and parenchymal phase

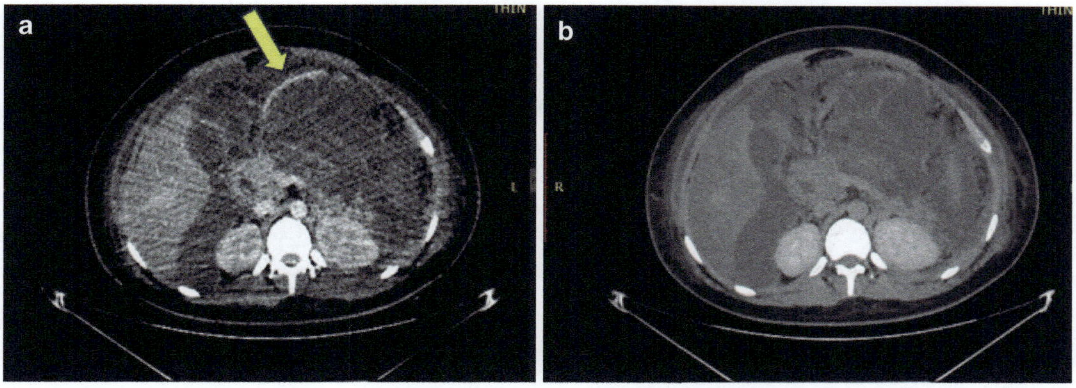

Fig. 23.13 Late arterial (**a**) and venous (**b**) phase of a case of acute pancreatitis. Note that only the head is enhanced in (**a**). The rest of the pancreas has been replaced by a necrotic mass which is elevating a proximal jejunal vein (arrow). Also, note the presence of streak artefacts in the arterial phase, caused by arms being kept near the patient's body. This artefact can be avoided by elevating the arms above the head. If that is not possible, keep something like a thick folded bedsheet between the arm and the torso

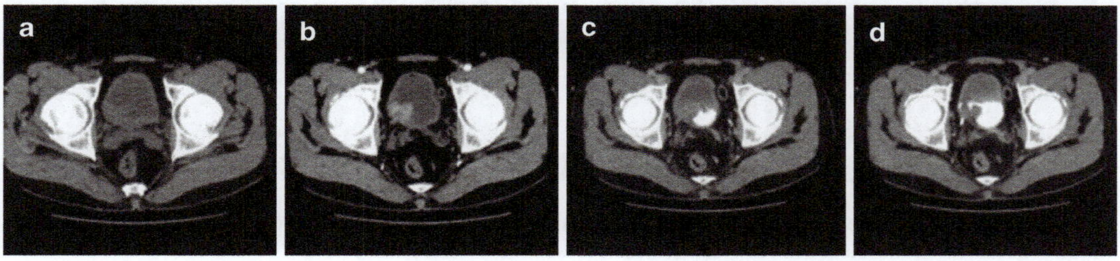

Fig. 23.14 Bladder protocol: (**a**) NCCT of the pelvis for exclusion of calculus, calcification or blood (**b**), arterial phase. Note the enhancement of bladder mass. No other enhancing lesion is seen in the bladder, (**c**) venous phase to evaluate the rest of the abdominal organs and (**d**) urographic phase. Note the obstructed distal right ureter with hold up of contrast within it. Since this patient was not rolled on the table before urographic phase scanning, there is layering of the high-density contrast towards the bladder base

healthy kidneys does not impact the life of the donor. The donor protocol is also meant to study the vascular anatomy of the kidneys for surgical planning. The CT sequence includes: NCCT for any calculus disease. Small calculi can be accepted but large and staghorn calculus need to be removed first. This is followed by the arterial phase at 25 seconds, and a nephrographic phase between 90 and 100 s. For these phases, the scan length should can be planned using the NCCT images. The scan should extend from the level of the coeliac trunk to the iliac crest, so as not to miss the unusual sites of origin of accessory renal arteries and muliple draining renal veins. Finally, a urographic phase around 5–9 min should be obtained. The images are thereafter post-processed. This includes 3D reconstruction showing the renal arteries and veins, MIP and curved MPR for the urinary outflow tract.

For the arterial phase, the triggering bolus is kept at the level of the coeliac axis. The bolus is triggered when the HU value reaches 100. This is followed by a delayed arterial phase at 35–40 s to delineate the corticomedullary junction. Next, a nephrographic phase at 90 s should be obtained which is the best sequence to exclude the presence of any hypoechoic or non-enhancing renal mass and to delineate location and number of renal veins. The scan in all these phases extends from above the renal artery to the iliac crest. This

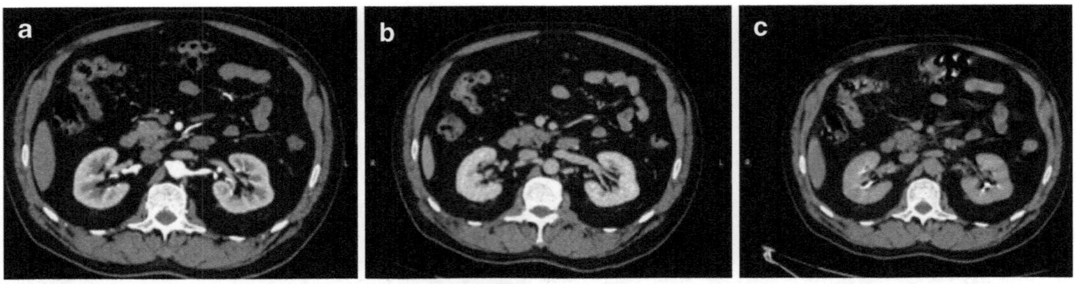

Fig. 23.15 Examples of appearance of the kidneys during the various phases of transit of intravenous contrast through the renal parenchyma: (**a**) Corticomedullary (delayed arterial), (**b**) Nephrographic (venous) phase and (**c**) Urographic phase

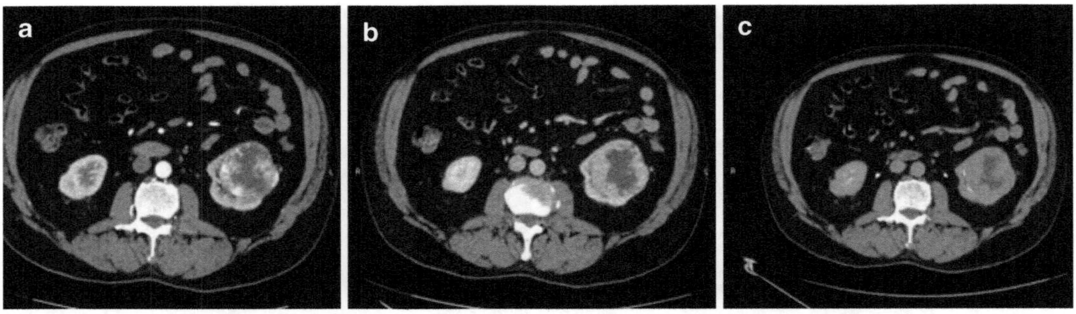

Fig. 23.16 Case of a left renal mass in delayed arterial (**a**), venous (**b**) and urographic phase (**c**). Note that the maximum enhancement of this clear cell renal cell carcinoma, is in the arterial phase

enables detecting any accessory renal artery arising from anywhere else in the abdominal aorta, as mentioned above.

The report should include not only findings pertaining to the urinary tract but also the description of any other abnormality in the abdomen and pelvis. Measurements to be given include the number, length and width of the main renal artery at distal, middle and proximal levels. Besides the usual images, multiplanar and 3D reconstructions, should also be provided to the surgeon to plan the transplant surgery.

Transplant imaging recipient evaluation: The site of anastomosis, that is, the recipient iliac vessels need to be assessed to determine the feasibility of suturing the donor vessels to the recipient's external iliac vessels. The anastomotic site should be an atherosclerotic calcific-free arterial segment with a patent external iliac vein and inferior vena cava. Also, worth excluding is the presence of any other intraabdominal and pelvis pathology which might complicate the surgical plan and decision to transplant the kidney in the chosen area. Large kidneys as in polycystic disease, may not leave adequate space for the transplant. Vascular anomalies affecting the iliacs, IVC and aorta may have to be addressed first, before considering the transplantation.

23.6 Imaging Protocol for CTA for Non-traumatic Aortic Conditions, Angiography of the Upper and Lower Limbs

Indications: These include aortic dissections, aneurysms, following trauma to the extremities, occlusive vascular disease, precomputation scanning angiograms and congenital vascular malformations.

CT technique

The iodinated contrast used should have a high concentration of iodine, that is between 350 and 400 mg iodine/mL. The volume of contrast is between 1 and 2 mL/kg body weight. The speed of injection can be kept at 4–5 mL/s. Both scanning at a slower speed (<3 ms/s) and scanning at very high speeds such as 5–6 cc/s may result in completion of the even before the contrast reaches the area of interest. A 4–5 mL/second timing is usually sufficient to get good arterial phase enhancement. If along with the arteriography the central venous system study is also being considered, add a delay of 35–45 s for the contrast to fill the lumen of the veins. Prior to arteriography, a plain scan of the part being examined should be obtained, especially in diabetic patients, smokers and patients with high BMI. This helps identify calcified plaques in the vessel walls, for it might be difficult to differentiate calcification from contrast in densely opacified vessels, particularly in the small peripheral arteries, unless a dual-energy CT scanner is being used.

CT angiography of upper limb vessels. The arm being investigated can either be raised above the head or kept by the side. 1–2 mL/kg body weight of iodine 350 mg/mL contrast is injected through the opposite limb vein. The bolus tracker should be kept in the ascending aorta and scanning triggered when the HU value reaches 100. Scanning should be performed in the craniocaudal direction from the level of the lower cervical spine till the tip of the fingers.

CT venography of the deep veins of the chest. This is often requested when the AV fistula of a chronic kidney disease patient is not working well. The scan can start as soon as the IV contrast, usually iodine 300 mg/mL has been administered. A dose, say of 50 ccs contrast, is enough to see the central systemic veins of the axilla and mediastinum.

CT aortogram for aortic dissection: 1–2 mL/kg body weight of 350 mg/mL iodinated contrast is used. It is preferable to use ECG gating as this reduces image degradation caused by cardiac movement artefacts and allows better visualization of the coronary arteries which can get involved in an ascending aortic dissection. The bolus tracker is kept on the proximal descending aorta. Contrast should be injected from the right arm, as an injection from the left arm, may result in the presence of high-density contrast in the left brachiocephalic vein which can obscure the arch vessels. The scan is triggered when the HU value reaches 100. The area covered extends from the root of the neck to the groin.

CT angiography of the lower limb arteries: Using the same technique as described above for CT abdominal aortography, use a larger volume of contrast, approximately 1.5 mL/kg body weight and scan from the level of the mid aorta (above the iliac bifurcation) till the level of the toes. Take another run to detect collateral flow or delayed filling of vessels due to partial obstruction.

CT abdominal and lower limb venography: To get good opacification of the lower limb veins, use a stocking covering up to the thigh. Inject about 50 mL of contrast through the veins in the dorsum of the foot. Scanning is then performed caudocranially from the feet to the lower chest. This will include the leg veins and IVC. A saline chase is given to push the contrast upwards from the leg veins. The other option is to use the same technique as used for lower limb angiograms with a delay of 120–150 s post-IV contrast injection.

CT angiography for Multiorgan trauma. In a patient with severe trauma involving multiple organs, the undermentioned protocol can be tried.

CT Technique

1. Plan the scan length to extend to cover the entire thorax and abdomen from the thoracic inlet till the lesser trochanters.

2. Inject 100 cc 350 mg iodine through antecubital vein at 4 mL/s followed by a 30 mL saline chase at the same rate.
3. A delayed scan may be obtained if considered necessary.
4. The arms should be above the head.
5. No oral contrast is needed.
6. There is no need to obtain KFT in life-threatening situations.

CT Examination of Bones and Joints.

Indications: CT is mainly needed to evaluate bone trauma, tumours and for interventional procedures.

CT Technique

(a) Always check previous records and examine the patient for the site of complaint. Obtain the history for better evaluation and programming of the study.
(b) The limb being examined should be immobilized in in true anatomical position, if possible. This is because true anatomical position allows quick interpretation of the images.
(c) Scans should be performed in helical mode using bone and soft tissue algorithms.
(d) The scan thickness should be 0.6 mm for bone windows and 1.2 mm for soft tissue evaluation. The pitch should be increased to reduce exposure.
(e) The windows settings for bone should be 2000 WW and 300 WL. For soft tissues, the window width will be 400 and the window level 40.
(f) The images should be reconstructed in true axial, coronal and sagittal positions for both bones and soft tissues. This means that the reconstructions should be parallel and perpendicular to the area of interest (similar to the two views which are obtained at right angles while performing radiography of bones and joints). 3D reconstructions should be obtained and displayed in AP, PA and both lateral positions. An oblique position can also be provided if the abnormality is better demonstrated in this view.
(g) If there is a presence of metallic implants, use metallic artefacts reduction sequence (MARS).
(h) IV contrast is usually not needed. However, in cases of trauma, especially in fractures around the knee joint, the popliteal artery can be injured and will need evaluation.
(i) Filming should include the most obvious abnormality in both bone and soft tissue window settings along with multiplanar and 3D images (Figs. 23.17, 23.18, 23.19, 23.20, 23.21, and 23.22).

CT Scans of the Shoulder

- The arm should be positioned with the shoulder in neutral position. It should not be rotated internally or externally.

The scan should begin from above the shoulder to include the entire scapula. The scan field should include the adjoining soft tissues.

In case of any metal being present, use metal-reducing software.

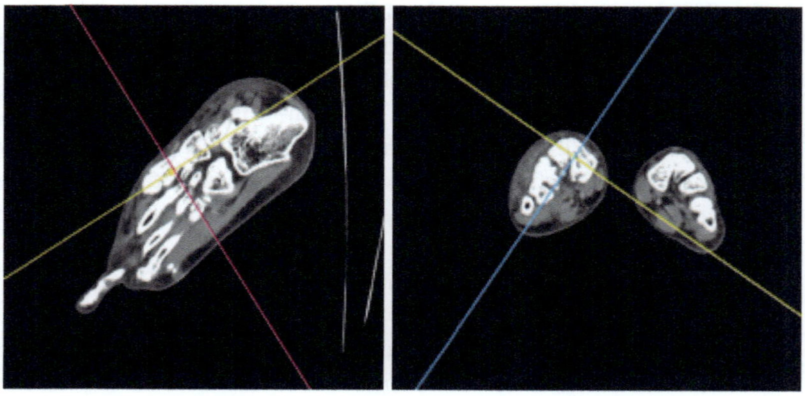

Fig. 23.17 Image reconstruction of the foot in two planes at right angles to one another

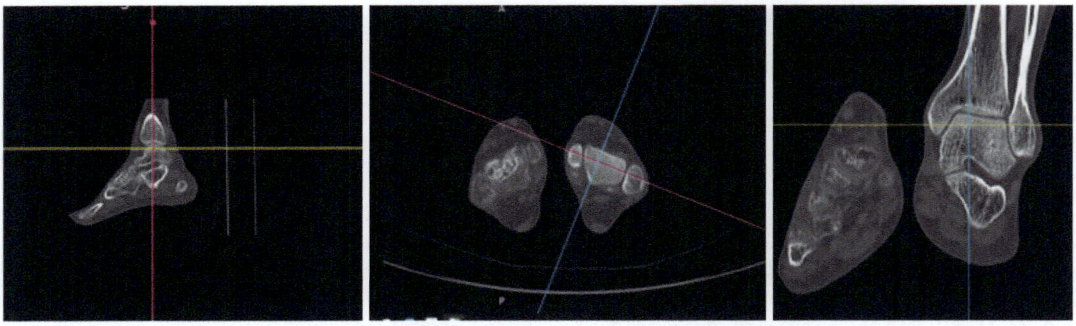

Fig. 23.18 Cross hair for obtaining reformative images for ankle mortice

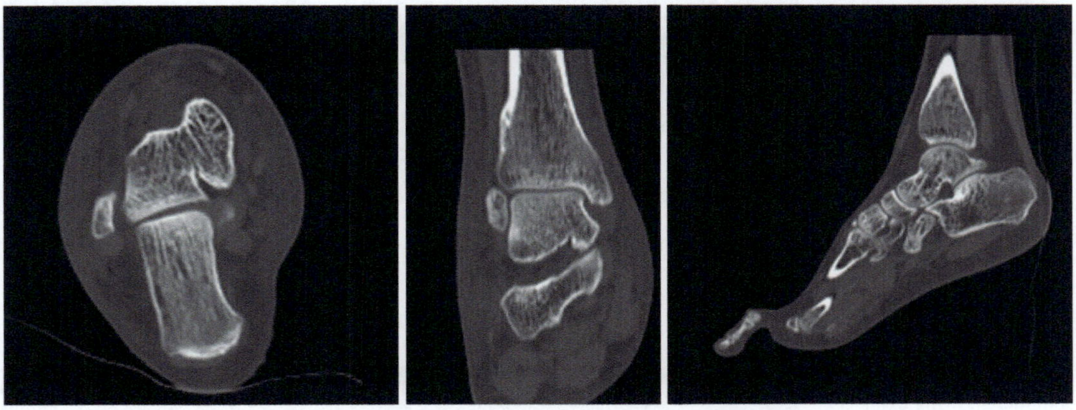

Fig. 23.19 Reconstructed images of the ankle joint and calcaneum

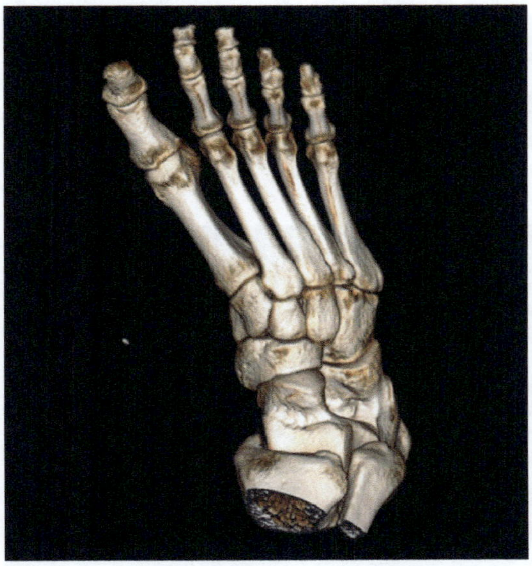

Fig. 23.20 3D reconstruction of the foot

Reconstruct in all planes and make a 3D image in AP, PA and both lateral and "Y" views (Figs. 23.23, 23.24, and 23.25).

23.7 Paediatric Protocols

- **Paediatric Brain CT Protocols**:
  NCCT: This protocol is the same as in adults. The radiation dose can be reduced by following the vendor's protocol which is based on the weight of the patient.
  CECT: Same protocol as is used for NCCT. The contrast dose depends on the weight and injection rate on the needle size. The scan delay can be up to 90 secs as it takes time for the contrast to enter the brain paren-

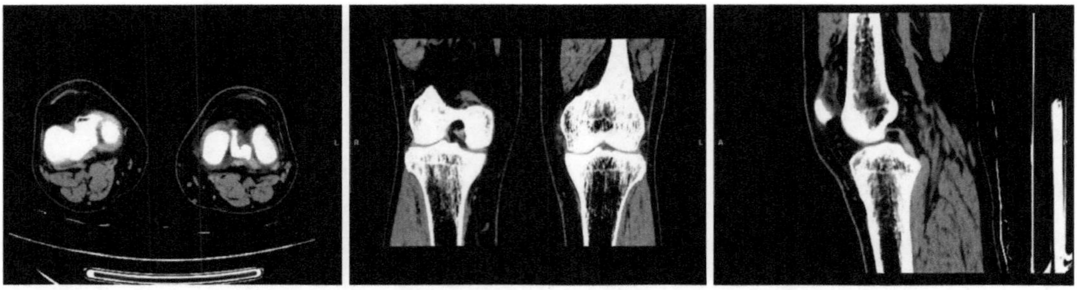

Fig. 23.21 CT scan of the knee joint showing soft tissues in axial, coronal and sagittal planes

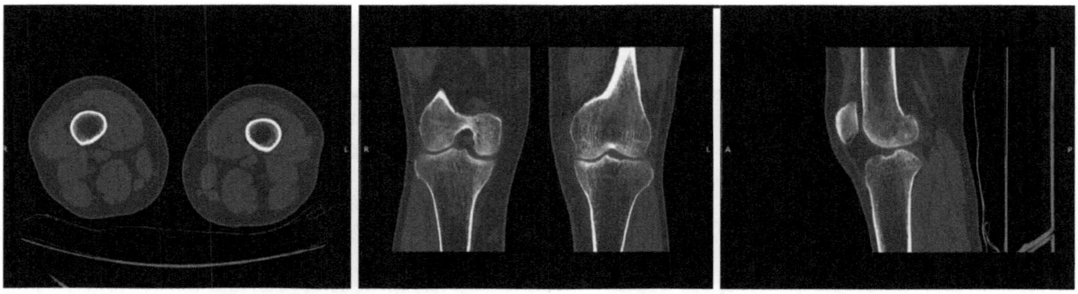

Fig. 23.22 CT scans of the knee joint shown in bone window setting

Fig. 23.23 Scans of the shoulder showing axial and coronal views obtained in soft tissue windows

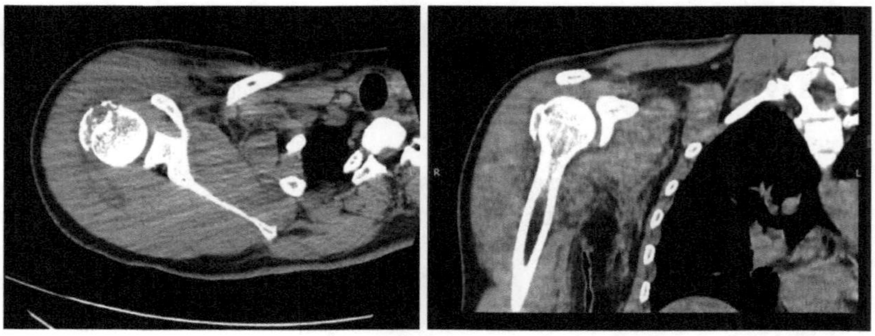

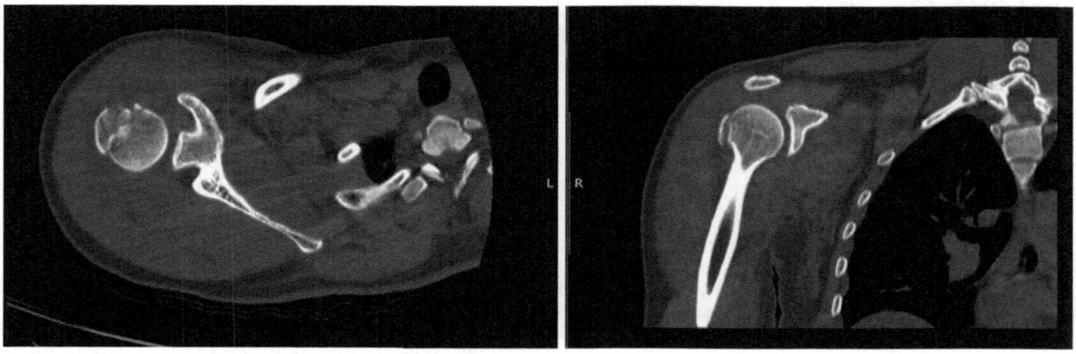

Fig. 23.24 Axial and coronal scan of shoulder obtained in bone window

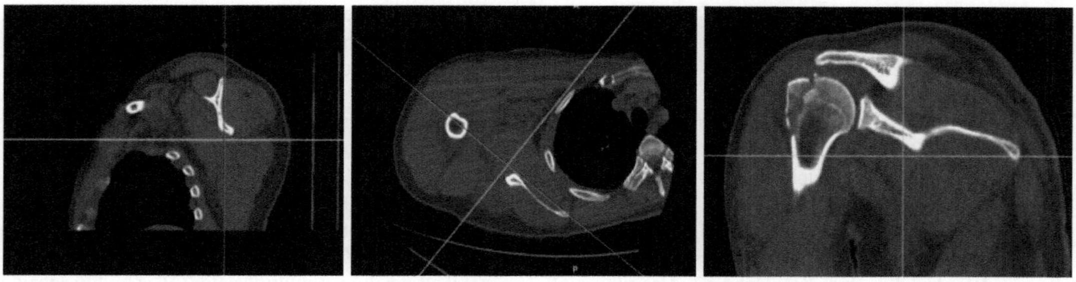

Fig. 23.25 Grashey view reconstructed using MPR

chyma. Contrast usually stays for a longer time in a lesion, since there is a break in the blood–brain barrier. If the scan is performed early, the contrast will still be in the vessels and may not opacify either the parenchyma or any lesion within it.

CT thorax:

Depending upon the clinical context, the study could be an NCCT, a CECT for evaluation of any thoracic mass, a lesion with an aberrant vascular supply, a vascular lesion or a pulmonary angiogram for evaluation of congenital heart disease.

The CECT of the thorax is done in the same way as in adults. The contrast used is iodine 300 mg/mL and the injection rate is determined by the needle size. Since small needles are used in children, under 10 years and most often the needles are inserted in the dorsum of the hand, the rate will vary from 1 mL/s. for a 24 G needle to 2 mL/s for a 22 G needle and 3 mL/s. for a 20 G needle. A manual injection can also be given if need be. The rate of manual injection will be approximately 1 mL/min.

The amount of contrast used depends on the body weight. Between 1 and 1.5 mL/kg is usually sufficient.

The scan delay for the CECT thorax will be 60 s.

CT pulmonary angiogram for congenital heart diseases:

Before performing a pulmonary angiogram for congenital heart disease, obtain all relevant details including any history of previous surgery.

1.5 mL/kg body weight of Iodine 350 mg, IV contrast should be used. The injection can be given by an automatic pressure injector, the injection rated depending upon the needle size.

A fast manual injection can also be given.

Scanning should start as soon as the injection is over.

Obtain two runs covering an area extending from the neck to the upper abdomen.

The protocols described above are based on the author's experience and work well. However, they are not sacrosanct. They are subject to modification and improvement based on local experience, availability of more advanced machines and newer refinement in techniques.

References

1. Heit Jeremy J, Wintermark M. Perfusion computed tomography for the evaluation of acute ischemic stroke: strengths and pitfalls. Stroke. 2016;47(4):1153–8. https://doi.org/10.1161/STROKEAHA.116.011873.
2. Cashman EC, Macmahon PJ, Smyth D. Computed tomography scans of paranasal sinuses before functional endoscopic sinus surgery. World J Radiol. 2011;3(8):199–204. https://doi.org/10.4329/wjr.v3.i8.199. PMID: 22022638; PMCID: PMC3198264.
3. Macori F, Murphy A, Yap J, et al. CT paranasal sinus (protocol). Radiopaedia.org. Accessed 29 May 2024. https://doi.org/10.53347/rID-92692.
4. Tibrewala S, Roplekar S, Varma R. Computed tomography evaluation of oral cavity and oropharyngeal cancers. Int J Otorhinolaryngol Clin. 2013;5:51–62.
5. Law CP, Chandra RV, Hoang JK, Phal PM. Imaging the oral cavity: key concepts for the radiologist. Br J Radiol. 2011;84(1006):944–57. https://doi.

org/10.1259/bjr/70520972. PMID: 21933981; PMCID: PMC3473765.
6. https://www.sciencedirect.com/science/article/pii/S1368837519301356.
7. Maraghelli D, Pietragalla M, Calistri L, Barbato L, Locatello LG, Orlandi M, Landini N, Lo Casto A, Nardi C. Techniques, tricks, and stratagems of oral cavity computed tomography and magnetic resonance imaging. Appl Sci. 2022;12:1473. https://doi.org/10.3390/app12031473.
8. Kim BS, Ahn KJ, Park YH, Hahn ST. Usefulness of laryngeal phonation CT in the diagnosis of vocal cord paralysis. AJR Am J Roentgenol. 2008;190(5):1376–9. https://doi.org/10.2214/AJR.07.2778.
9. Bahl M, Sepahdari AR, Sosa JA, et al. Parathyroid adenomas and hyperplasia on four-dimensional CT scans: three patterns of enhancement relative to the thyroid gland justify a three-phase protocol. Radiology. 2015;277:454–62.
10. Nagano SYM, Bitencourt AGV, Torres IDCG, Porto GCLM. Four-dimensional computed tomography protocol for preoperative evaluation of the parathyroid glands and its correlations with other imaging methods: a pictorial essay. Radiol Bras. 2021;54(3):193–7. https://doi.org/10.1590/0100-3984.2020.0056. PMID: 34108767; PMCID: PMC8177685.
11. Hoang JK, Sung W-k, Bahl M, Douglas Phillips C. How to perform parathyroid 4D CT: tips and traps for technique and interpretation. Radiology. 2014;270(1):15–24.
12. Bhalla AS, Das A, Naranje P, Irodi A, Raj V, Goyal A. Imaging protocols for CT chest: a recommendation. Indian J Radiol Imaging. 2019;29(3):236–46. https://doi.org/10.4103/ijri.IJRI_34_19. Epub 2019 Oct 30. PMID: 31741590; PMCID: PMC6857267.
13. Trad HS, Boasquevisque GS, Giacometti TR, Trad CY, Zoghbi Neto OS, Trad CS. Pulmonary 64-MDCT angiography with 50 mL of iodinated contrast material in an unselected patient population: a feasible protocol. Radiol Bras. 2016;49(2):75–8. https://doi.org/10.1590/0100-3984.2014.0115. PMID: 27141128; PMCID: PMC4851474.
14. Blanke P, Weir-McCall J, Achenbach S, et al. Computed tomography imaging in the context of transcatheter aortic valve implantation (TAVI)/transcatheter aortic valve replacement (TAVR): an expert consensus document of the Society of Cardiovascular Computed Tomography. J Am Coll Cardiol Img. 2019;12(1):1–24. https://doi.org/10.1016/j.jcmg.2018.12.003.
15. Geffroy Y, Boulay-Coletta I, Jullès M-C, Nakache S, Taourel P, Zins M. Increased unenhanced bowel-wall attenuation at multidetector CT is highly specific of ischemia complicating small-bowel obstruction. Radiology. 2014;270(1):159–67.
16. Sengupta N, Kastenberg DM, Bruining DH, Latorre M, Leighton JA, Brook OR, Wells ML, Guglielmo FF, Naringrekar HV, Gee MS, Soto JA, Park SH, Yoo DC, Ramalingam V, Huete A, Khandelwal A, Gupta A, Allen BC, Anderson MA, Dane BR, Sokhandon F, Grand DJ, Tse JR, Fidler JL. The role of imaging for GI bleeding: ACG and SAR consensus recommendations. Radiology. 2024;310(3):e232298. https://doi.org/10.1148/radiol.232298. PMID: 38441091.
17. Ilangovan R, Burling D, George A, Gupta A, Marshall M, Taylor SA. CT enterography: review of technique and practical tips. Br J Radiol. 2012;85(1015):876–86. https://doi.org/10.1259/bjr/27973476. Epub 2012 May 2. PMID: 22553291; PMCID: PMC3474054.
18. Boudiaf M, Jaff A, Soyer P, Bouhnik Y, Hamzi L, Rymer R. Small-bowel diseases: prospective evaluation of multi-detector row helical CT enteroclysis in 107 consecutive patients. Radiology. 2004;233(2):338–44. https://doi.org/10.1148/radiol.2332030308. Epub 2004 Sep 30. PMID: 15459329.

Further Reading

CT protocols from Radiology Assistant.
CT protocols from CTis US.

24 Guide to Patient Safety in the Radiology Department

Abstract

The radiology department uses radiation and contrast medium for diagnosis of various diseases. Both can be potentially harmful to the patient. It is therefore essential to know their harmful effects and how to minimize and manage the risks without adversely affecting their beneficial effect.

Keywords

Risks with x-rays · Harmful effect of contrast · Minimizing harmful effects of radiation and contrast medium

X-rays and iodinated contrast medium are essential for the detection and diagnosis of various diseases. Contrast medium is routinely used while performing radiography and imaging studies.

In this chapter, we will briefly discuss the side effects of x-rays and iodinated contrast medium. We will also discuss how to minimize the side effects and what measures should be taken in case of an adverse event.

24.1 Harmful Effects of Radiation

X-rays are ionizing radiation. Ionizing radiation has no threshold and can affect the DNA and cell membranes causing harmful effect, called "Stochastic effect". These effects can be caused even by low level of radiation dose. Their effect may manifest years later as cancer. They can produce genetic mutations which are inheritable and their effect may be seen in later generations. Since these harmful effects are not visible immediately, x-rays tend to used indiscriminately. There is another effect called "deterministic effect", which is visible and manifests early. It is caused by high radiation exposure. These effects are seen in cancer patients treated with radiation. They manifest as nausea, erythema, loss of hairs, brittle nails and development of skin and bone cancers as well as fibrosis in the radiation field. They are also seen in medical professionals, especially in interventional radiologists, who are exposed to long-term radiation during continuous fluoroscopy.

Since the use of x-rays in diagnosis is essential and is increasing with the increasing use of CT scans, it is essential to know how to use the radiation judiciously. The principle of ALARA (as low as reasonably achievable) must be firmly adhered to. The benefit of radiation dose should be balanced by ensuring that by only a minimal radiation exposure is used to produce diagnostic quality images (as high as reasonably achievable—AHARA) [1].

General Recommendations

- Always ask for previous records. The patient may be carrying their previous record which is

R. Gothi, *Radiographic and Imaging Techniques for Radiology Residents and Technologists*,
https://doi.org/10.1007/978-981-96-4816-0_24

not asked for by the clinician. They may have left the record at home, thinking that the studies are probably old hence not useful anymore. If the patient has visited the hospital previously, check the hospital records. An x-ray or a CT scan done a few days back may be good enough to skip an investigation using the same imaging modality.
- The clinician should request the most appropriate imaging studies and radiographic views. The radiation technologist must talk to the patient, examine the region affected, which helps in deciding additional useful views. Many times, clinicians are busy and may have unwittingly made some mistake or asked for a view which will not help. The technologist must not hesitate to check with the clinician and then perform the most appropriate radiograph.
- Take care of positioning and radiation factors. Make sure that the x-ray does not have to be repeated due to technical reasons.
- The technologist must ensure proper coned down views.
- There should be no one else when radiation is on. If an attendant needs to be present, make sure to provide a lead shield and try to keep the person away from direct radiation exposure.
- The technologist and radiologist must stay behind the protective lead shield during radiation exposure and should wear a lead apron, thyroid guard while performing fluoroscopy.
- Make sure that the patient is not pregnant. Radiation during the first trimester should be avoided as the maximum cell division takes place at this time. At other times, during pregnancy, avoid performing X-rays which need high radiation dose, such as X-rays lumbosacral spine.
- In non-pregnant patients, for studies requiring radiation of the lower abdomen and pelvis, use the "10 day rule" which is the first 10 days from the day of onset of the menstruation., during which radiation may be given. However, this rule is not applicable to every woman. It may also be better to check with the patient and, if necessary, perform a pregnancy test before doing an X-ray.

24.2 Recommendations for CT Scans

The risk of medical radiation to the health of a person is considered very small [2]. This does not mean indiscriminate use of radiation. Clinicians, radiologist as well as the technicians should work in tandem to obtain an optimal quality study, using low exposure factors.

The effective radiation dose given in a CT scan is far less than the dose needed to produce "deterministic effect". However, stochastic effect can be produced because it does not have a minimum threshold. Therefore, care should be taken in deciding which patient needs a CT and in which patient an alternative examination such as MRI and USG will be equally appropriate. Nevertheless, if CT is to be done, one must strive for as low a radiation dose as possible to arrive at a diagnosis.

Radiation in CT Scans Can Be Reduced as Follows

- Reduce either kVp or mAs or both.
- Keep an eye on the CTDI vol and DLP which is displayed on the monitor as soon as the exposure factors are selected [1].
- Reduce scan length. Avoid over-scanning.
- Reduce the width of the scanning area by collimating the beam.
- Increase the pitch ratio to 1.0, in follow-up studies as well as where multiplanar reconstructions are not necessary.
- Centre the patient correctly. It reduces the radiation dose.
- Use AEC, that is automatic exposure control (also called automatic tube current modulation). In this technique, the radiation dose is adjusted automatically while scanning, based on the patient size and thickness of the body part as it appears from different angles. For example, the chest at the shoulder level appears thinner when it is exposed by a beam from 12'o clock position. AEC chooses a lower radiation dose in this position of the x-ray beam. However, when the beam is at 3'o clock position, it has to pass through a greater thickness at the shoulder level. The AEC

increases the radiation dose in this position.

- Use iterative reconstruction instead of filtered back progression. In iterative reconstruction, the noise in the image is reduced in both standard and low-dose protocols.
- Modifications of iterative reconstructions, such as adaptive statistical iterative reconstruction(ASIR) and especially model-based iterative reconstruction (MBIR) provide adequate image quality at low-dose CT. They can be used in paediatric population and urinary tract evaluation for calculus disease.
- Use low-dose protocols for non-contrast CT of the thorax. Modify protocols in order to obtain adequate quality images at low dose [3, 4]. Low-dose CT is used in cancer screening and has been employed during Covid 19 pandemic. It gives satisfactory lung, bone and soft tissue images by using smoothening or edge-enhancing filters.
- Low-dose CT can also be employed where the difference in contrast density between adjoining tissues is high. CT scans of the paranasal sinuses and bones can be obtained using a low-dose protocol.
- For paediatric patients, use paediatric age/weight-specific protocols provided by the vendor.
- Scanning rapidly, especially in small children also reduces radiation dose [5].
- Shields for eyes, thyroid, breasts and gonads are also available. The use of radiation-protective shields for the eyes, thorax, gonads and breasts must be considered [6]. However, the issue with them is that radiation dose may actually increase, important information may be obscured and scans may have to be repeated, which will raise the radiation dose.

24.3 Contrast Mediums Used in Imaging

Contrast medium is frequently used in conventional radiology, CT scan and MRI.

- **Conventional radiology and CT scans**: Barium sulphate is used primarily in the study of the gastro intestinal tract. Intravenous iodinated contrast medium is used both in conventional radiology as well as in CT scans.

Barium sulphate: Barium is available in liquid form and is administered orally to study the upper GI and small bowel. It can also be administered per-rectally to evaluate the colon. **Iodinated contrast medium can be ionic and non-ionic**. Iodinated contrast is meant for intravenous use but can also be used for performing RGU, MCU, HSG, fistulogram and sinogram. It can be given orally while performing upper or lower GI studies in neonates and in patients with suspected post-operative intestinal anastomotic leaks. In cases of large intestinal obstruction, instead of barium, it can be safely given orally. Transit of this contrast till the rectum supports the choice of conservative management in suspected cases of intestinal obstruction. Barium should not be given orally to study colonic obstruction as it can get impacted at the site of obstruction and might spill over into the peritoneal cavity during corrective surgery. When evaluating tracheoesophageal fistula (TOF) in newborns, it is best not to give any oral contrast. Using an NG tube and observing the position of its distal end should suffice. If it enters the stomach, either there is no fistula or at worse it could be an "H" type of fistula. If it folds over itself in the thorax, it indicates the presence of a blind ending upper oesophageal pouch. In these cases, if the stomach contains air, it means that there is communication of the distal end of oesophagus with the trachea with an atretic segment in between the two ends of the oesophagus. If contrast study has to be done to diagnose an "H" type of fistula, both small quantities of barium and non-ionic contrast can be used. The latter is preferable because if it enters the lung fields either through the fistula or by aspiration, it is less likely to cause chemical pneumonitis,. However, carefully administered small quantities of diluted barium can be given as its contrast density is better than that of the water-soluble non-ionic contrast. Barium given in small quantities is safe and unlikely to cause any serious problem even if it enters the lung parenchyma. Complications which can occur with barium sulphate are few and rare. Large volume of barium, if aspirated into the lung fields, however, can cause acute respiratory distress. Small quantities may rarely cause chemical pneumonia or granuloma formation. Barium can cause a drug reaction which is generally mild and in the form of nausea or skin rash. It can also cause temporary constipation. Hydration of patients after a barium meal study and taking immediate supportive and corrective measures in cases of flooding the lung parenchyma by aspiration is essential. Spillage into the peritoneal cavity needs to be conveyed to the surgical team for further management. Irrespective of which type of contrast is being given to the patient, there should be no complacency on part of the radiology team.

Injectable contrasts: Iodinated contrasts, especially non-ionic and Gadolinium based contrasts are generally safe but can be associated with reactions [7]. Iodinated contrast can be ionic and non- ionic. The use of ionic contrast has reduced considerably on account of greater side effects associated with it. These side effects can be minor, like nausea, skin rash, vomiting, moderate or severe like angioneurotic oedema, difficulty in breathing or anaphylactic shock. It is still used as a positive oral contrast in CT scans and for performing, fistulograms, sinograms, RGU and MCUG studies in conventional radiography.

The risk of reaction with non-ionic contrast is much smaller. Hence, it is the preferred intravenous contrast medium.

The use of iodinated contrast medium is restricted in patients with renal insufficiency. The risk is uncertain but needs to be kept in mind as there is an increased chance of developing acute kidney injury [8]. Patients of AKI or those with eGFR <30, must be prophylactically hydrated [8]. If the eGFR is less than 60, or large volumes of contrast are to be injected, it is preferable to use Visipaque (iodixanol) which is an iso-osmolar contrast with osmolality similar to blood. When osmolality or concentration of ions is similar between intravenous (IV) contrast like Visipaque and blood, there is diminished risk of withdrawal of fluid from the tissues into the blood stream. This factor reduces contrast-induced nephropathy and adverse effects as compared to other low osmolar contrast medium such as Omnipaque (iohexol) which has a higher osmolality than blood. However, Visipaque has greater viscosity than Omnipaque. This results in difficulty in injecting the contrast especially if the veins are small. Hence, it is preferable to use Visipaque for intraarterial studies required in patients with contrast-induced nephropathy (CIN) [9]. Amongst low osmolar contrasts, iohexol is considered safer than iopamidol as far as contrast-induced nephropathy goes [10].

A Word About Dosimeters:

Dosimeters are devices worn by radiation workers to measure the radiation exposure during the course of their professional work. These are of two types—either film badge dosimeter or thermoluminiscent dosimeter (TLD) badges.

- **Film badge**: A film badge contains a silver-coated photographic film [11] within a metallic or plastic holder. Upon exposure to radiation, the film darkens to varying degrees depending upon the type of exposure (x-rays, gamma rays). The silver coating may be of different thickness to identify low and high energy radiation. The film holder may also contain beam attenuation filters of different materials, such as copper, aluminium or lead on both sides of the holder to identify different types of radiation. Film badges, though still in use, may be affected by heat, moisture and light. They are also less accurate and need processing time which may cause delay in reading out the exposure data. A film badge is cheaper and does not require any specialized equipment to deduce the absorbed radiation energy.
- **TLD badges**: In these badges, radiation energy is stored in nickel-coated aluminium cards containing chips made of either lithium

fluoride or calcium sulphate with dysprosium. The card containing the chip is enclosed within a plastic casing [12]. Upon heating this chip in a TLD reader, the stored energy is released in the form of light. The output of the emitted light corresponds to the extent of radiation exposure. A TLD badge is more accurate than a film badge, less affected by moisture and more sensitive in detecting low-energy exposures. It can measure radiation dose ranging from 0.01 to 10.0 mGy [13]. It is costlier and needs special equipment for reading the radiation exposure [14].

These badges are worn at the chest level over clothes and beneath lead aprons for estimating the radiation dose to the body. They can also be worn outside the lead apron for evaluation dose to the extremities, thyroid gland and eyes.

References

1. Maldjian PD, Goldman AR. Reducing radiation dose in body CT: a primer on dose metrics and key CT technical parameters. Am J Roentgenol. 2013;200(4):741–7.
2. McCollough CH, Primak AN, Braun N, Kofler J, Yu L, Christner J. Strategies for reducing radiation dose in CT. Radiol Clin North Am. 2009;47(1):27–40. https://doi.org/10.1016/j.rcl.2008.10.006. PMID: 19195532; PMCID: PMC2743386.
3. Mayo-Smith WW, Hara AK, Mahesh M, Sahani DV, Pavlicek W. How I do it: managing radiation dose in CT. Radiology. 2014;273(3):657–72.
4. Joyce S, O'Connor OJ, Maher MM, McEntee MF. Strategies for dose reduction with specific clinical indications during computed tomography. Radiography. 2020;26(Supplement 2):S62–8.
5. Gottumukkala RV, Kalra MK, Tabari A, Otrakji A, Gee MS. Advanced CT techniques for decreasing radiation dose, reducing sedation requirements, and optimizing image quality in children. Radiographics. 2019;39(3):709–26.
6. Antypas EJ, Sokhandon F, Farah M, Emerson S, Bis KG, Tien H, Mezwa D. A comprehensive approach to CT radiation dose reduction: one institution's experience. Am J Roentgenol. 2011;197(4):935–40.
7. Beckett KR, Moriarity AK, Langer JM. Safe use of contrast media: what the radiologist needs to know. Radiographics. 2015;35(6):1738–50.
8. Davenport MS, Perazella MA, Yee J, Dillman JR, Fine D, McDonald RJ, Rodby RA, Wang CL, Weinreb JC. Use of intravenous iodinated contrast Media in Patients with kidney disease: consensus statements from the American College of Radiology and the National Kidney Foundation. Radiology. 2020;294(3):660–8.
9. Heinrich MC, Häberle L, Müller V, Bautz W, Uder M. Nephrotoxicity of iso-osmolar iodixanol compared with nonionic low-osmolar contrast media: meta-analysis of randomized controlled trials. Radiology. 2009;250(1):68–86.
10. Solomon R, Dumouchel W. Contrast media and nephropathy: findings from systematic analysis and Food and Drug Administration reports on iodixanol, iohexol, and other ionic and nonionic contrast media. Invest Radiol. 2006;41(8):651–60.
11. Pardue LA, Goldstein N, Wollan EO. Photographic film as a pocket radiation dosimeter. At Energy Biophys Biol Med. 1948;1(5):169. PMID 18878757.
12. Goel A, Wilczek M, Murphy A, et al. Thermoluminescent dosimeter. Reference article, Radiopaedia.org. Accessed 8 Aug 2024. https://doi.org/10.53347/rID-36761.
13. Huda W. Review of radiologic physics. isbn: 9780781785693. https://books.google.co.uk/books?vid=ISBN9780781785693.
14. https://www.epa.gov/radiation/radiation-dosimetry.

Further Reading

https://www.iaea.org/resources/rpop/health-professionals/radiology/pregnant-women#1.

https://www.cdc.gov/radiation-health/about/health-effects-of-radiation.html.

https://www.iaea.org/resources/rpop/health-professionals/radiology/pregnant-women.

Part III

MRI (Magnetic Resonance Imaging)

25 MRI: Some Basic Facts

Abstract

Magnetic resonance imaging is a technique that produces images based on the presence of hydrogen protons within fluids, fat and other soft tissues in the body. Using a powerful magnet, gradient and radiofrequency coils, signals are generated from the predetermined regions of the body and slices are selected from these areas which are then displayed as cross-sectional images. MRI can display a variety of images of the same body section by tweaking the many parameters provided in the operator console. Concentration of hydrogen protons, the presence of other magnetic susceptible protons, the direction and speed of blood flow and the effect of contrast administration on various tissues contained in that region, affect the appearance of the images when different MRI parameters are employed. For example, by altering the relationship of T1 and T2 relaxation time, acquiring proton density images, obtaining susceptibility-weighted images, diffusion and ADC maps(produced by the extent of Brownian motion in the tissues), fat and blood flow imaging, diffusion tensor imaging and by MR spectroscopy, a range of images conveying a variety of information can be obtained from the same selected slices. In this chapter, we will look at the MRI equipment, understand how to prepare the MRI suite, safety issues and questions often asked.

Keywords

MRI · Signals · Spin echo · Hydrogen proton · DTI · Spectroscopy · SWI sequence · Blood flow

25.1 MRI Hardware

The MRI machine consists of a magnet which can have a field strength (B_0) ranging from an ultralow strength of a 0.055 T portable brain scanner [1] to a 7 T whole-body scanner. The "T" stands for Tesla, which is a measure of magnetic field strength. In practice, the magnet commonly used is either of a 1.5 T or a 3 T field strength. Magnets can be closed or open. Closed magnets are cylindrical in shape and have mid-field, high field or ultra-high field strength that ranges from 1.5 to 3 to 7 Tesla (T). The open magnets are of mostly low-field strength such as a 0.2T magnet, but high-field strength open MRI systems are also available. Open magnets are composed of two horizontal plates with an open area between them. This reduces claustrophobia, making the MRI machine more patient friendly.

MRI magnets can be of different types. They can be permanent, resistive or superconductive types. Most MRI machines in use have superconductive type of magnets, which we will discuss here.

R. Gothi, *Radiographic and Imaging Techniques for Radiology Residents and Technologists*,
https://doi.org/10.1007/978-981-96-4816-0_25

There are four main components of an MRI system [2]. These are the MRI gantry, gradient coils, RF coils and computer systems.

The MRI gantry is a tunnel-shaped structure with a central bore through which the table slides in and out during the scanning.

The gantry houses the following structures.

1. The main magnet: This is a superconductive magnet. It is formed by a superconducting coil of wires made of Niobium Titanium alloy, which is wrapped around a fibreglass cylinder. **It is the outermost layer of coils**. The strength of the magnet depends upon the number of turns of wires in the coil and the amount of current running through it. The coil is cooled to such an extent (almost 0°) that it does not give any resistance to the passage of large electric currents through it. The cooling is done by surrounding the coil with cryogenic gas (refrigerated liquefied gas), usually liquid helium, which brings down the temperature of the coil to below −293 °C or 4 °K. The liquid helium is permanently sealed within the magnet so that it does not escape into the atmosphere. The magnetic field created by the main magnet is in the Z axis and is denoted by the value "B_0".
2. Shim Coils: These are coils which **homogenize** the main magnetic field by steading the main magnetic coil. They are located between the main magnet and the gradient coil. They can be either passive or active shims. Passive shims are small triangular-shaped objects made of sheet metal or pellets of ferromagnetic material, placed in the bore of the MRI machine. They help to passively homogenize the magnetic field. Active shims are coils that have their own electrical supply. They produce magnetic fields when current passes through them. This enables manipulation and thus, actively homogenizing the magnetic field. They can be copper coils (resistive coils) and can also be made of a superconducting material.
3. Gradient coils:-.The gradient coils are located between the shim coil and the RF coils. They are made of copper windings or copper strips embedded in various patterns, such as fingerprints on a cylinder. There are three sets of gradient coils, located in the "x" "y" and "z" axis at right angles to one another. The coils in the x and y axes have a saddle-shaped design while the coil in the z-axis has a circular design [3]. Each set of coils has its power amplifier which results in coils from one end of the magnet to the other having different strengths. On applying an electric current to the gradient coils, thereby varying the strength of the magnetic field from one end of the coil to the other, the precessional frequency of the hydrogen atoms along the length of various axes is changed. In other words, the electric current will create a gradient of different magnetic field strengths at different points along the length (z axis) of the main magnetic coil. This change in precessional frequency of the hydrogen atom is in the form of a slope—a gradient—in the magnetic field strength along all axes. Hence, these coils are called gradient coils. The change in gradient along the X, Y and Z axes results in spatial encoding of the MR signals (that is, localizing the source from which the signals are emerging).
4. Radiofrequency (RF) coils [4]. These are the innermost layers of coils. They can be "transmit-only", "receive only "or "transmit-receive" types of coils. They generate an alternating magnetic field called the "B1" field at right angles to the z axis of the main magnetic field, that is in the x–y plane. If a hydrogen proton is processing at the same rate as the RF pulse sent out by the RF coil, this proton will flip at a right angle to the "z-axis" in which it was earlier processing and will then give a signal which will be received by the RF coil. This signal will also be the slice selection signal. RF coils are important for maintaining image quality, signal uniformity and improved signal-to-noise ratio [4]. RF coils can also be surface coils, phased array coils or volume coils which can be used in addition to the coils within the gantry. The reader is referred to reference [4] for further information regarding the RF coils (Fig. 25.1).

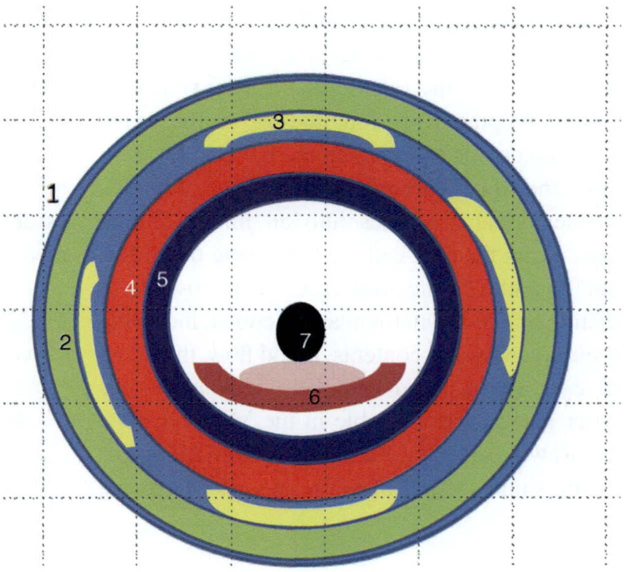

Fig. 25.1 Components of the MRI gantry. The outer shell of the gantry (1). Main magnetic coil (2). Shim coils (3). Gradient coils (4). RF coils (5). MR couch (6). Patient (7)

The computer systems used in MRI consists of a central processing unit and a data storage unit. They are used for the acquisition and storage of data.

The MRI table is hydraulically driven and made of MRI-compatible material (carbon fibre, plastics, fibre-glass and non-ferromagnetic materials).

Comparison of 1.5 T with 3 T magnet. A 3 T magnet is twice as powerful as a 1.5 T magnet. The image quality, especially of the brain, spine and musculoskeletal system, is better shown in a 3 T MRI. This is because the stronger the magnet, the better the signal received from the area under study. The slice thickness of a 3 T MRI can be thinner than that acquired by a 1.5 T MRI. The artefacts due to patient movement are reduced. However, as compared to the 1.5 T MRI, the 3 T MRI is noisier and more unsafe in the presence of metallic foreign bodies. This means that in the presence of a metallic foreign body, a 1.5 T MRI would be better and safer. Also, the specific absorption rate of 3 T is more than 1.5 T. This means that there is increased heat generation during scans using a 3 T scanner, which may cause local burns.

25.2 Principles of MRI Imaging

The human body is made up of many tiny magnets which present as fluid molecules in the body. These tiny magnets have positively charged hydrogen protons. They are normally revolving and moving in a state of disarray and therefore cancel out each other's signals. When the patient is placed inside the strong magnetic field (B_0) of the MRI machine, these protons are forced to align with the "z" axis of the main magnet (that is, the hydrogen protons align and precess in the same direction along the length of the magnetic tunnel/gantry). This alignment of the tiny magnets forms a magnetic vector (force) called "longitudinal magnetization" (LM). On applying a radiofrequency (RF) pulse to the longitudinal alignment, the magnetization tilts into the transverse plane. This means that the LM decreases and the "transverse magnetization" (TM) increases. Upon switching off the RF current, the protons start wobbling back to their original resting phase, resulting in the regaining of LM and reduction of TM. The protons finally realign with the Z axis. By using different pulse sequences and noting the time taken for all the protons with different energy levels, to realign with the Z axis and regain the LM (T1 time) as well as the time taken (T2) for the release of the energy gained during flipping from longitudinal to the transverse plane, the receivers in the RF coil can convert the data through a series of complex mathematical processes into an image of that area. From the data gathered, by using the different T1 and T2 relaxation times, it is possible to distinguish most anatomical structures, including their fat and water contents, blood flow, the effect of contrast on them and their response to the other parameters available in the MRI machine. In this way, several different types of MRI images of the same section of the body can be created [5].

25.3 Preparation of MRI Suite

The MRI suite should have 4 zones. These are [6] as follows:

1. Zone 1: The entrance. This is a common area.
2. Zone 2: This is the reception area. It should have a changing room and lockers for the patients to store their valuables including credit cards, phones, any metallic wearables, wallets, etc. It should have a toilet and a space where the patient can be searched for any inadvertently left-out metal object on their person.
3. Zone 3: This is the post-screening waiting area, where the patient waits before entering the MRI room. This zone can be included in Zone 2.
4. Zone 4: This is the MRI scanner room.

The purpose of this division is to ensure the safety of the patient. The MR magnet being very powerful can attract ferromagnetic substances which can harm the patient as well as the members of the medical team present in the MRI suite, to the extent of endangering their life.

25.4 Safety Issues in MRI

The MRI magnet can pose safety issues to the patients, attendants, technical staff and other health workers in the vicinity of the MRI machine. Therefore, to prevent mishaps, it is essential to take precautions and institute safety measures.

1. All personnel in zones 3 and 4 should be well versed with safety-related protocols and this should be documented. The MRI personnel should be graded into levels 1 and 2 based on their experience and level of knowledge. A supervisor, who will be ultimately responsible for the overall safety-related issues, must also be present in the MRI area.
2. There should be adequate security measures in case of fire, electrical short-circuiting or any other untoward incidents.
3. There should be ferromagnetic detectors which are not the same as the usual metal detectors. They should supplement a thorough physical examination.
4. Enquire for any history of foreign body penetration or implants in the body. In the latter situation, find out the MR compatibility of the implanted foreign object.
5. MRI personnel should preferably be out of the scanning room while the scanning is on.

25.5 Questions Often Asked by Patients, Attendants and Referring Doctors

1. Is fasting necessary for MRI? In most cases, fasting is **not needed**. However, in some situations, fasting may be required. These include:-
   (a) **Abdominal MRI**: This is because food and fluid can interfere with imaging, particularly of the bowel loops and pancreas.
   (b) **MRI with Sedation**: Approximately 4 h of fasting is sufficient to reduce the risk of complications. If the patient feels thirsty, sips of water can be allowed.

(c) **Contrast MRI**: Other than institutional preference, no fasting is required. For non-contrast MRI brain, spine, joints, or soft tissue imaging, fasting is not necessary.

2. Can MR contrast be administered to a pregnant patient? MR contrast should be avoided unless it is likely to change the management. The effect of GBCA on the foetus (Gadolinium-based contrast agents) is not fully known [7].
3. Any safety issues for a pregnant person? Non-contrast MRI can be performed in pregnant patients, if essential.
4. Can MRI be performed in the presence of dental implants? MRI is safe, as dental implants are made of either ceramic or titanium which is a non-ferromagnetic material [8].
5. Can ECG leads, pulse oximeters and medical implants cause burns at the site of contact with the body? Yes, they can [9].
6. What can be the other effects of metal implants? They can move, if loosely fixed, heat up (though this is an unlikely complication) and cause image degradation (the real problem). Other than image degradation, the rest of the problems, such as heating and instability of the implant, are negligible [10].
7. What should be done when the patient has either old implants or implants whose magnetic susceptibility, hence safety status is unknown? Take the help of MHRA (Medicines and Healthcare products Regulatory Agency) guideline [11].

References

1. Liu Y, Leong ATL, Zhao Y, et al. A low-cost and shielding-free ultra-low-field brain MRI scanner. Nat Commun. 2021;12:7238. https://doi.org/10.1038/s41467-021-27317-1.
2. Serai SD, Ho ML, Artunduaga M, Chan SS, Chavhan GB. Components of a magnetic resonance imaging system and their relationship to safety and image quality. Pediatr Radiol. 2021;51(5):716–23. https://doi.org/10.1007/s00247-020-04894-9. Epub 2021 Apr 19. PMID: 33871725.
3. Hidalgo-Tabon SS. Theory of gradient coil design methods for magnetic resonance imaging. Concepts Magn Reson A. 2001;36A:223–42.
4. Kwok WE. Basic principles of and practical guide to clinical MRI radiofrequency coils. Radiographics. 2022;42(3):898–918. https://doi.org/10.1148/rg.210110. Epub 2022 Apr 8. PMID: 35394887.
5. Berger A. Magnetic resonance imaging. BMJ. 2002;324(7328):35. https://doi.org/10.1136/bmj.324.7328.35. PMID: 11777806; PMCID: PMC1121941.
6. https://www.acr.org/-/media/ACR/Files/Radiology-Safety/MR-Safety/Manual-on-MR-Safety.pdf.
7. https://www.acr.org/-/media/ACR/Files/Clinical-Resources/Contrast_Media.pdf.
8. Kim YH, Choi M, Kim JW. Are titanium implants actually safe for magnetic resonance imaging examinations? Arch Plast Surg. 2019;46(1):96–7. https://doi.org/10.5999/aps.2018.01466. Epub 2019 Jan 15. PMID: 30685951; PMCID: PMC6369045.
9. https://www.fda.gov/Radiation-EmittingProducts/RadiationEmittingProductsandProcedures/MedicalImaging/MRI/ucm482765.htm.
10. Csernátony Z, Zhang L, Kristóf T, Csámer L, Kovács AE, et al. Metal implants and MRI: a mythbuster study. Glob Imaging Insights. 2021;6:2021. https://doi.org/10.15761/GII.1000215.
11. https://www.gov.uk/government/organisations/medicines-and-healthcare-products-regulatory-agency.

26 Acronyms and Artefacts in MRI: A Beginners Guide

Abstract

There are many symbols, terms and abbreviations used in MRI. These may be confounding to the beginner. In order to familiarize the new entrants in this field, an attempt is made to introduce them to the commonly used acronyms and abbreviations. Hopefully, this will prepare the student to quickly and confidently negotiate this complex minefield and soon blend into the day to day working in the MRI department.

Keywords

MRI acronyms · Spin echo · Gradient echo · Relaxation time · MR sequences · MRS · MR artefacts

There are several words, acronyms and abbreviations used daily while performing and reporting MRI scans.

The student should sooner than later become familiar with these terms. Here is a list of commonly used terms with an explanation. Interested readers are advised to look up references provided at the end of the chapter [1–3].

26.1 ADC Maps

The apparent diffuse coefficient (ADC) tells us if the protons in the water molecule are moving or if their movement is restrained. When the movement is restrained, a dark signal caused by the restricted diffusion (movement) is seen in the suspected region in the ADC image. On the other hand, when there is no restriction of movement, the affected area produces a bright signal in the ADC map. This is called the "T2 shine-through" effect. Restricted diffusion is seen in lesions that have tightly packed cells or viscid fluid. Examples are lymphoma and abscesses.

Active Shielding. Magnetic fields called "fringe fields" are present outside the MRI suite. These may interfere with image production and are, therefore, undesirable. To eliminate the interference from these magnetic fields, active shielding is applied. This is done by using coils, located around the magnetic coil in the gantry. These coils can be located in the cryostat which maintains the temperature of the magnet. They can also be outside the MRI gantry on either side of the gantry aperture.

R. Gothi, *Radiographic and Imaging Techniques for Radiology Residents and Technologists*, https://doi.org/10.1007/978-981-96-4816-0_26

26.1.1 Analogue to Digital Convert

This means converting an ordinary electrical signal into a digital format for storage and displaying images on a computer.

Aliasing: When the field of view used for obtaining an image is smaller than the image itself, the left-out portion of the image, falling outside the boundaries of the field of view, wraps itself on the opposite side of the image. The artefactual wrapping of the image on the opposite side of the image results in what is called a "wrap around" artefact. The remedy is to enlarge the field of view, in order to accommodate the entire image obtained by the MRI sequence.

"B" Values: The symbol (B_0) is used in MRI to denote the field strength of the main magnet and is measured in Tesla. A 1.5 Tesla MRI, therefore, denotes having a B value of 1.5T [4]. The **B**1 symbol denotes the magnetic field applied by the RF coil at a right angle to $\mathbf{B_0}$. The strength of **B1** magnetic field is much less as compared to the strength, $\mathbf{B_0}$, of the main magnetic field. B1 magnetic field results in deviation of the magnetic moment from the resting "Z"-axis into the X and Y directions.

b Values: The lowercase symbol "b" is used in diffusion-weighted images (DWI) and indicates the magnetic field strength applied by the diffusion gradients. These values can be 0, 800, 1000, 1500 or even 2000. As the b value increases, there is increased restriction of the Brownian motion of water molecules. Thus, a b value of "0" is like a T2-weighted image. If at b values of 1000 or 1500, in a DWI sequence, high signals are seen, These will not be from water but from some tissues having severely restricted motion of water molecules. These tissues could be infarcts, blood products, solid tumours, abscesses or necrotic tumours.

Bandwidth: This means a range of frequencies contained in a signal.

26.2 BLADE (Propeller)

The classic MRI scan takes time. Therefore, there is always a chance of the production of motion-related artefacts. To limit these artefacts, certain advanced sequences are applied. BLADE (PROPELLER) is one such sequence which is frequently used to lessen motion-related artefacts. Because T2W sequences take longer, BLADE is used in T2 W sequences. It can also be used in T1W, FLAIR and DWI sequences and can be applied in all planes and all body regions.

26.2.1 Black/Dark Blood Imaging

These are sequences meant to subdue signals from flowing blood. By doing this, signals from static tissues either within the lumen of a vessel or arising/related to the vessel walls can be highlighted. In this sequence, blood appears black due to suppression of its MR signals. The adjoining stationary vessel walls, myocardium and Gadolinium contrast and clots appear brighter than the blood flowing through the lumen. A black blood sequence can be a spin echo technique (HASTE) or a Spoiled GRE (SPGR) sequence. Spin echo sequences depict flowing blood as a signal void (black). Because the spins are exposed to 90- and 180-degree RF pulses, vascular imaging using spin echo is called "black blood" imaging. If there is an intraluminal thrombus, the signal void, in the FSE T2 W sequence, is replaced by a bright signal. The SPGR sequence needs to be supplemented by additional methods, in order to obtain uniform suppression of the dark signals of the blood. Black blood sequence is used in cardiac MRI and angiography.

26.2.2 BOLD (Blood Oxygen Level-Dependent) Sequence

This is a sequence used in functional MRI to visualize the increase in oxygen requirement by brain tissue in response to various activities. Whenever there is an increased requirement of oxygen, by active neuronal tissues, the blood supply to that region increases to supplement the additional requirement of oxygen to that region. This leads to an increase in oxyhaemoglobin level while the deoxyhaemoglobin level decreases. (It is this change in oxyhaemoglobin/deoxyhaemoglobin ratio, which is used to study

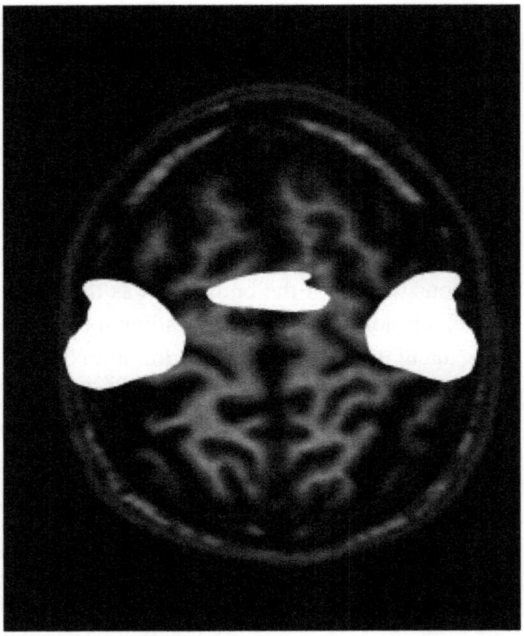

Fig. 26.1 MRI scan showing increased activity in the posterior frontal regions, demonstrated by "BOLD" technique

the effect of activity on the brain parenchyma). The reduction in deoxygenated haemoglobin levels results in a diminished magnetic susceptibility effect. This leads to modification of the MR signal from dark to bright. To detect this subtle change in MR signals, a gradient echo-based echoplanar imaging sequence (EPI) is used. BOLD sequence is also used during awake surgery to spare areas which are associated with various important activities. The active areas are colour-coded and superimposed on the brain image for viewing by the neurosurgeon (Fig. 26.1).

26.2.3 Bright Blood Sequences

Both spoiled and balanced GRE sequences can produce bright blood images.

The spoiled gradient sequence does this by highlighting the differences in T1 shortening time (T1 relaxation time) between various tissues. Blood has a shorter T1 relaxation time. Hence, it appears bright.

Balanced sequence, unlike in a spoiled GRE sequence, maintains T2 effect. The resulting images make the flowing blood appear bright.

The main use of bright blood sequence is in cardiology where it is also used for functional studies. It can also be used in other areas, such as in the abdomen, to show the flowing blood appearing as bright signals within the blood vessels.

26.2.4 Chemical Shift

This imaging technique is used to study the chemical composition of a tissue. It takes advantage of the slight difference in the radiofrequency pulse between the protons in fat and protons in water molecules, which are present in the intracellular space.

Water protons have a higher resonant frequency than fat. Protons within fat molecules precess 150 Hz/Tesla slower than the protons in water molecules. By using different TEs, separation of water from fat protons can be achieved. In this way, in- and opposed-phase images as well as the four-point Dixon techniques images can be derived.

- **In and Opposed-Phase Sequence**: This technique helps identify the presence of intracellular fat as both fat and water have different resonating frequencies. In the in-phase image, by using a long TE, both water and fat resonant frequencies are in phase. This produces a combined image of water and fat protons. Hence, there is no signal dropout (that is, no signal loss from the fat-containing area). However, in the opposed-phase image, when the timing TE (short TE) is shortened such, that when the fat signals are at zero (nulled) and the images are acquired at that time, there is signal loss from the fat and a dark India ink effect (black margins) is seen in the fat-containing molecules in the images. The TE values in the "in and opposed images" are different in 1.5 T and 3 T magnets. The TE of in-phase echo is 4.6 ms at 1.5 T and 2.3 ms at 3 T (means preservation of all signal, no dropout!). The TE of out-of-phase (OP) echo is 2.3 m at 1.5 T and 1.15 ms at 3 T.

The reverse of this chemical shift happens in the presence of iron in the liver. The in-phase images appear dark as compared to the OP images.

- **Dixon Techniques**: This is another chemical shift-based technique. The technique incorporates the in- and out-of-phase sequences as well as water-only and fat-only images. This means we get four types of images, by using this technique. Hence, conventional in-phase and out-of-phase techniques are not needed separately when the Dixon technique is being employed.

(For the details of these sequences, one may refer to any textbook of MRI physics [3] **(A, B)).**

26.3 CISS (Constructive Interference in Steady State) Technique

This comprises of two 3D, fully refocused balanced sequence which run in succession. By slightly varying the excitation pulse, the spins are kept in phase and artefact-free images with a high signal-to-noise ratio are obtained. The CISS sequence is used to study complex areas such as the temporal bone. Since this sequence is relatively insensitive to CSF flow, it is used in anatomical areas surrounded by CSF, such as in temporal bone imaging to study the 7th and 8th cranial nerves in the region of the cerebellopontine (CP) angle. It can also be used to study the ventricles and cystic lesions in the spine. The limitation of this study is that the acquisition time is long.

26.3.1 Coherence

This means that all spinning protons are lined up in the same direction and spin at the same speed and in the same direction.

26.3.2 Contrast MRI Scans

These are performed by injecting Gadolinium chelate, an extracellular contrast media and using a spoiled gradient sequence to obtain images. Gadolinium is a heavy metal ion and a paramagnetic substance which appears bright in the T1W sequence. It is toxic to the kidneys and deposits in various tissues of the body, such as the brain. Hence, it is administered after binding it to a chelating agent which makes the Gadolinium chelate (e.g. gadopentetate dimeglumine) stable and prevents the release of the Gadolinium ion in the body. The reaction of Gadolinium ion with body tissue is consequently minimized. The Gd chelate is excreted out of the body through the kidneys. The administration of Gadolinium makes the flowing blood produce bright signals in the T1 W sequences. During Gadolinium administration, it is important to suppress the T1 bright signals arising from the surrounding fatty tissue. The fat signals are suppressed (masked) by fat saturation techniques. A dose of 0.1–0.2 mmol/kg Gadolinium chelate, injected intravenously, is considered sufficient. The timing of peak arterial enhancement is 2–3 s of the total 15–20 s of scanning time. By using a technique called keyhole imaging, the temporal resolution of MRA can be fine-tuned in order to separate arteries from veins.

Although, extracellular, Gadolinium-based contrast can also be excreted by the hepatobiliary system. These contrast agents (GBCA) are called hepatobiliary contrast media and include Multihance (gadobenate dimeglumine) and Eovist (gadoxetate sodium).

Gadolinium-based contrast can also be given orally. These can produce bright, dark or biphasic signals. The biphasic (bright on T1 and dark on T2W sequence) signals are also produced by manganese-containing ions besides Gadolinium chelates and iron particles.

Another type of MR contrast medium, called, superparamagnetic contrast, is iron oxide-based particles which are taken up by Kupffer cells. The images appear dark on T1 and T2 W sequences.

26.4 Contrast-to-Noise Ratio

It is a ratio between the signal intensity contributed by different tissues divided by the background electronic noise. The greater the noise, the more the negative effect on the final image.

Diffusion-weighted imaging (DWI) sequence and apparent diffusion coefficient (ADC) maps/values: DWI is the study of Brownian motion of particles. Brownian motion is a random motion or a movement of particles in any direction and at any speed. It is akin to the diffusion of a drop of ink in water. Hence, the sequence is called diffusion-weighted sequence.

1. The DWI sequence acquires images with gradients in three planes, namely the phase, readout and slice selection planes. The images are combined to produce a final DWI. DWI works by highlighting the presence of water molecules which are trapped and unable to move freely within their milieu. These trapped molecules provide bright signals. The molecules which move have a loss of signal. To generate a diffusion-weighted image, magnetic gradients are applied to the spin echo EPI sequence. The timing and strength of the magnetic gradient applied is called the "b" value. The "b" value can be 0, 800, 1500, etc. A "b0" value is a T2 W image and shows no diffusion weighting. As the "b" value increases, the mobile protons lose their signals, while the fixed protons retain their bright signals and show T2W effect. Thus, at higher b values, fixed protons in infarcts, abscesses and tumours emit bright signals. These bright signals need to be matched with the ADC values. The DWI differs from the FLAIR sequence, as the former shows restricted diffusion while the latter shows vasogenic oedema due to its long TR.
2. ADC: The apparent diffusion coefficient reflects the restricted speed of movement of protons within a lesion. If the lesion is fluidic, as would happen at "b0", the speed of Brownian motion of fluid molecules will be high, resulting in a high ADC value (called "T2 shine-through effect"). In solid areas, where the movement is restricted, the speed of moving protons (i.e. the ADC value) will be low. When the ADC values are low, the lesion appears dark in the ADC map. The ADC value of a tissue is measured in mm^2/s.
3. The DWI sequence uses single or multishot spin echo echoplanar imaging. A non-echoplanar imaging, that is a fast spin echo sequence, can also be used when a lesion is adjacent to or within a bone. Since all these are fast sequences, and the images are captured in seconds to 1–2 minutes, the DWI is insensitive to the movement of patients. However, the image is degraded by noise and, therefore, cannot be substituted for the convention T2 W sequence. There is also image degradation at the sites where there are tissues having different magnetic susceptibility. An example will be the interface between air-filled frontal or mastoid air cells and brain. Here, one can see artefactual high signal intensity (Figs. 26.2 and 26.3).
4. Diffusion Tensor Imaging (DTI): A DWI is independent of the direction of diffusion and is called isotropic diffusion. DTI is the study of the movement of protons in one direction and is a direction-dependent study. This direction-dependent diffusion is called an anisotropic study. The diffusion gradient can be applied craniocaudally, left to right and anterior to posterior to study white matter tracts coursing in these directions. The fibres are colour-coded as per the direction in which they are running. The colour red is for fibres running from left to right, green is for anterior to posterior fibres and craniocaudal fibres are coded blue. DTI tells us about the integrity of fibres.

Diamagnetic substances have paired electrons which repel one another on the application of an external magnetic field. This results in the cancellation of their individual magnetic strength (no magnetic moment or magnetism). They also repel the external magnetic field, which results in the loss of MR signals. Examples of diamagnetic

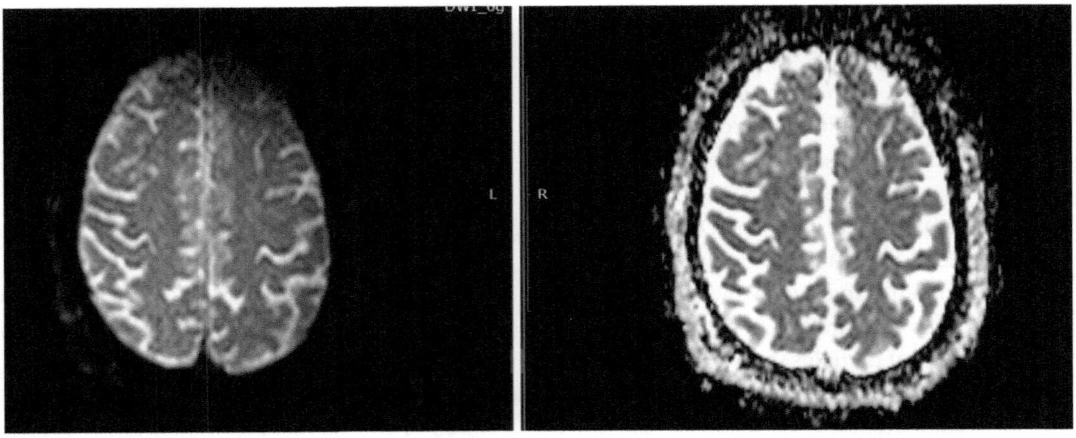

Fig. 26.2 DWI and ADC maps: In normal cases, both the DWI and ADC maps show unrestricted movement of fluid as bright areas

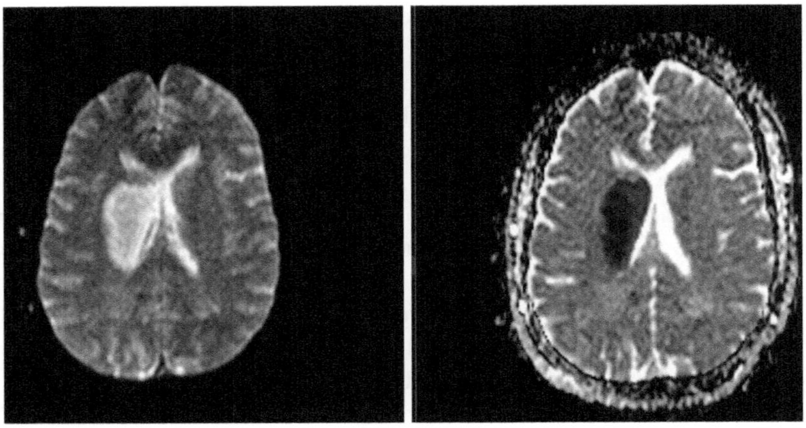

Fig. 26.3 DWI and ADC map in a case of venous infarct: The area of restricted diffusion in the right thalamic and basal ganglia appears bright in the DWI but appears dark in the ADC map

substances include water, barium sulphate and copper. Chemical shift imaging is an example of the diamagnetic effect of fat and water in tissues.

DRIVE (RESTORE/FR-FSE): This is a sequence, used in T2W imaging. In these sequences, the TR is long, say 4000, and an additional 180 degrees followed by a 90-degree pulse is used to "DRIVE/ RESTORE", the residual transverse magnetization back to the transverse magnetization. This results in an improvement of the T2 signal intensity. An example is the use of "DRIVE" sequence to improve the signal intensity of CSF during the evaluation of the spine.

26.5 Fat Suppression Techniques and Fat Fraction Mapping

Fat can be suppressed in both T1 and T2 W imaging. There are various methods used to suppress signals arising from fat. These include fat saturation, inversion recovery (IR) and opposed-phase sequences. The quantity of fat present in the liver can also be measured as a fraction of the total quantity of combined fat and water protons present. This called fat fraction mapping and is abbreviated as **PDFF** (proton density fat fraction).

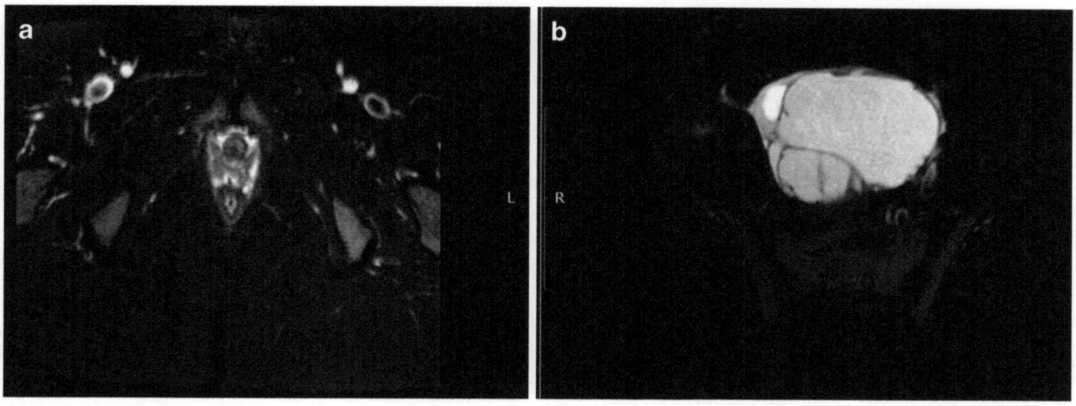

Fig. 26.4 T2 SPAIR sequence. Note that the vessels are visible (**a**) and the fat around the lesion is suppressed. MRI of the pelvis showing an ovarian mass with suppressed fat signals, arising from the adjoining fat containing soft tissues (**b**)

- **Fat saturation** (FS) technique: FS technique is used for large areas and when IV contrast is to be given. It suppresses fat inhomogeneously, (unlike the inversion recovery sequences) (Fig. 26.4).
- Inversion recovery sequence: STIR sequence suppresses fat signals uniformly. However, it also suppresses other bright signals such as those arising from IV Gadolinium.
- In and Opposed fat sequence: This sequence suppresses fat within tissues in the opposed phase. Microscopic fat-containing areas appear dark (India ink effect) in the opposed fat because its signal drops out in this phase. In the in-phase sequence, the signals of fat and water are combined, hence no India ink effect is seen in the in-phase sequence.
- SPAIR (Spectral attenuated inversion recovery) and SPIR sequence [5]: These sequences selectively suppress fat. The inversion time is longer in SPAIR than in SPIR. SPIR sequence is therefore better for the shorter T1-weighted imaging while SPAIR may be used with longer T2W FSE sequences.

26.6 Fast Spin Echo(FSE)/ Turbo Spin Echo (TSE)

In a conventional spin echo technique, after a single 180-degree refocusing pulse, only one echo is generated after a time "TE". This fills just one line of "k" space during that TR period of the pulse sequence. Which makes the process of image acquisition, slow. In the fast spin echo (FSE) or turbo spin echo sequence (TSE), more than one, 180-degree refocusing pulse is applied during the TR period. This generates multiple echoes after a time TE, thereby filling up more "k" spaces within that TR, which this reduces the time taken to produce an image. The number of 180-degree refocusing pulses, applied in FSE/TSE sequence, form an "echo train". The longer the echo train length, the shorter the scan duration. But this happens at the cost of image quality. There can be blurring of the image at the edges. Also because of the rapid refocusing, fat remains high in signal intensity in all sequences.

One of the problems with a FSE technique using a 180-degree refocusing pulse and a long echo train length is that higher RF power is deposited in the area under study. This amount of power almost reaches the maximum specific absorption rate (heat deposition) in the tissue. This limits the coverage of the entire brain. To circumvent these issues, the flip angle can be reduced from 180° to a lesser angle, which although would be at a cost of image degradation (very difficult to perceive, though) will be able to cover the entire brain within the limits of a specific absorption rate.

26.7 Fourier Transform (FT)

The Fourier transformation is a mathematical technique which is used to split a complex sine wave signal, composed of several simple sine waves having different frequencies (bandwidth) and amplitudes into it's components. Doing this allows the study of the components which make the complex sine wave. FT is used in MR spectroscopy to study the presence of various metabolites in a small region of interest. The various peaks (amplitudes) in the MR spectroscopy spectrum represent the relative contributions of particular biologic metabolites to a given region of interest (ROI), each differing slightly in resonance frequency, characterizing their individual chemical structure [6].

26.8 Free Induction Decay

When the spinning vectors are tilted into the horizontal (X-Y) plane by an RF pulse of 90° or any other flip angle, the transverse magnetization so produced, at the ending of the excitation pulse, starts decaying towards zero, over a constant time which is T2 or T2*. This induces a decaying signal in the receiver coil which is called free induction decay. This phenomenon is applied in echoplanar imaging as well as in single-voxel MR spectroscopy.

Frequency This is the number of repetitions of a sinusoidal curve per unit time. The unit for frequency, earlier known as cycles per second, is now known as "hertz".

Frequency-Encoding Gradient: This is a gradient which is applied during the signal readout phase of MR imaging. It causes variations in the Larmour frequencies along the axis of the imaging plane. The differences in Larmour frequencies are read out using "Fourier transform", which enables localization of the frequency (signal) to a specific position along the frequency-encoding axis. This gradient is called the frequency-encoding gradient.

Functional Imaging: The function or performance of different tissues in the body can be studied by various techniques. These include dynamic contrast enhancement (DCE), arterial spin labelling (ASL), blood oxygen level-dependent (BOLD) and intravoxel inherent motion (IVIM).

Gating: This means synchronization of the image generation with the cardiac or respiratory rate in order to minimize the artefactual effect caused by cardiac pulsation or respiratory excursions.

Gradient Moment Nulling: It is a technique where, by altering gradient field strength and timing, it is possible to cancel out/minimize artefactual signals developed as a result of motion. The artefacts could be related to the motion of fluid, patient-related motion, cardiac pulsation or respiratory excursion. "Nulling" improves the quality of the MRI images.

HASTE Sequence (Half-Fourier Acquisition Single-Shot Turbo Spin Echo sequence) also called Single-Shot Fast Spin Echo Sequence—SSFSE) **by other vendors**.

A HASTE/SSFSE sequence is a heavily T2-weighted TSE/FSE sequence using a long TR with a long echo train of 100 or more, 180-degree pulses. In this sequence, fluid appears bright, fat and flowing blood appear dark. As the name suggests, only 50% of the "k" space is filled using half-Fourier technique. This reduces the scan time, but at the cost of reduction in signal-to-noise ratio. The synonyms for HASTE sequence (Siemens) are SSFSE (GE) and FFE, i.e. fast field echo (Philips). HASTE sequence is used in MRCP (magnetic resonance cholangiopancreatography), liver imaging, MR urography and rapid brain imaging in a restless patient. MRCP sequences can be a series of thick slab 2D single-shot fast spin echo (SSFSE) sequences with TE of 150 ms or more, with images acquired at different angles to best display the pancreaticobiliary system. This approach has some limitations. These include overlap by other fluid-filled structures, unreliable SNR and lack of 3D information. However, it is relatively unaffected by patient motion and respiratory irregularities. A heavily T2 W 3D SSFSE acquisition is the preferred technique to evaluate the pancreaticobiliary system. The resultant maximum-intensity projection images delineate the ductal system from various angles, thus improving the detection of intraductal or ductal pathology. The 3D sequence is long (approximately 4–6 min), and hence needs respiratory gating.

In addition to the HASTE sequence, a Balanced Steady-State Free Precession sequence (TRUFISP, BFFE, FIESTA) can also be used to generate the pancreaticobiliary anatomy. This sequence is unaffected by motion artefacts. In a balanced gradient echo sequence, flowing blood appears bright (Fig. 26.5).

Image Acquisition Time: This term is used in both spin echo and gradient echo sequences and implies the time required to gather signals from every part of the slice under examination, in order to construct the image of the slice. It must be noted that the acquisition time to reconstruct an image from a single slice is different from the total time needed to reconstruct an image of an entire volume of the anatomical part, being scanned.

Inhomogeneity of Magnetic Field: Magnetic fields should ideally have homogenous strength throughout the volume being scanned. But due to several factors, which include machine-related issues, body composition (air, bone) and patient-related problems (implants), the field is often non-homogeneous. This affects the image quality, needing as much correction as possible. This is done by using shimming coils, software programmes and removing foreign objects the patient might be wearing. Reduction of air within the bowel loops by using either orally administered Gadolinium contrast or ingesting manganese-containing food substances help mitigate the effect of bowel gas on the MR images.

Isotropy in Imaging: This means that the voxel size in x, y and z axes is equal (the image voxel is a cube and not a rectangle), which results in uniform image quality in all three imaging planes.

k-Space: “k” space is a representation of mathematical data, acquired during scanning, and displayed in the form of a 2D or 3D matrix. This matrix or grid has a horizontal and a

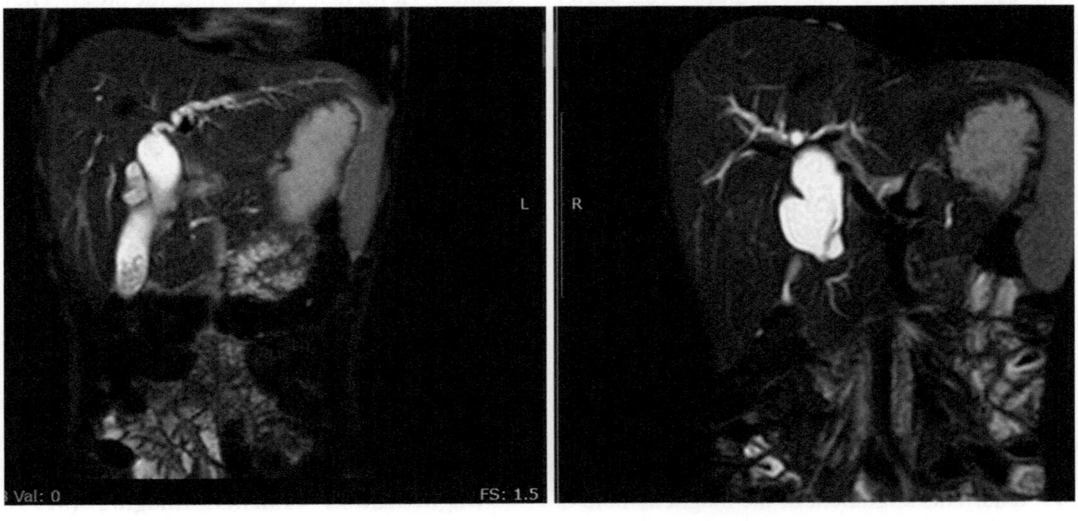

Fig. 26.5 A HASTE sequence is used to produce an MRCP image. Note that the fluid appears bright and flowing blood, in the various abdominal vessels, seen in these images dark

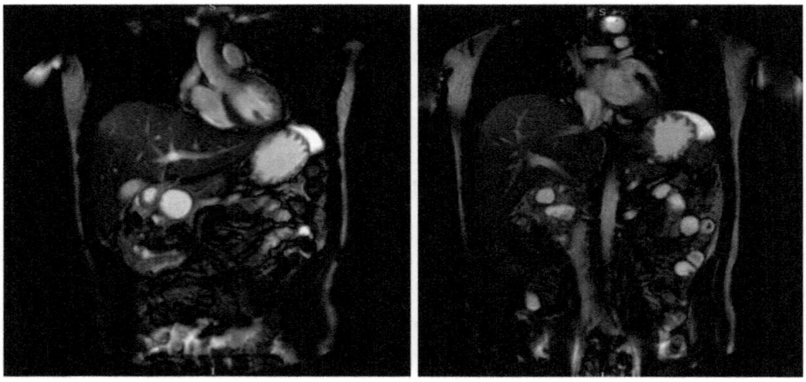

Fig. 26.6 A localizer view obtained by a balanced BFFE, sequence. Note that fluid in stomach, GB, bowel loops and blood in the heart looks bright, in this sequence. Note also that vessels (portal vein, IVC and aorta) also look bright

vertical axis, representing frequency-encoding and phase-encoding directions, respectively. Low-frequency data is in the centre of this grid, while the high-frequency data is in the periphery. The low frequency provides contrast to the image. The "k" space can be filled line by line (as it happens in spin echo sequence and gradient echo sequence). It can be rapidly filled radially, spirally or by partial Fourier sampling. Proper filling of the "k" space is necessary to obtain a good image. Once the "k" space is filled, an MRI image is created.

J Coupling: This is the interaction between the spinning nuclei of different atoms present within a molecule. This interaction or "J coupling" leads to cancelling out of signals during a conventional SE sequence. However, in a fast spin echo sequence, where multiple 180-degree refocusing pulses are applied at short intervals, the realignment of protons is fast and the "J coupling" effect is suppressed. This reduces the dephasing effect of "J coupling". Due to this effect, fat having a short T1 relaxation time recovers fast and appears bright in the FSE sequence.

Larmour Effect: It states that the frequency of precession of the protons in a magnetic field is directly proportional to the magnetic field strength.

Longitudinal Magnetization: When a nucleus is placed in a strong magnetic field, it points in the direction of the magnetic field, the "Z"-axis. This alignment of the magnetic field of the spinning protons within the body with the magnetic field of the main magnet is called longitudinal magnetization. When the spinning proton is tilted horizontally in the X-axis direction by an external magnetic field, it loses its longitudinal magnetization. If this external magnetic field is turned off, the longitudinal magnetization regrows along the Z-axis, which is then called longitudinal relaxation.

Localizer Views: A localizer is like a control or scout obtained in a CT scan. The localizer image is obtained in 3 planes. It can be obtained by a single-shot fast spin echo sequence (SSFSE) or by using a balanced gradient echo sequence. In the SSFSE sequence, flowing blood appears dark while in the balanced sequence, flowing blood appears bright. Both sequences are motion insensitive and have a high signal-to-noise ratio. The localizer views help in planning the study. They are particularly helpful in evaluating the uterus, pelvic floor and rectum. This is because the scan planes can be oriented to align with the longitudinal and transverse axis of these mobile organs (Fig. 26.6).

26.9 Magnetic Field Homogeneity

The MRI data depends on the homogeneity or uniformity of the magnetic field. An inhomogeneous magnetic field produces artefacts in the final image. Therefore, the attempt is always made to homogenize the magnetic field.

Magnetization Transfer Imaging (MTI): Tissues generate MR signals from the hydrogen protons within them. Hydrogen protons can be present as free water protons, protons bound in macromolecules (like protein and fat) as well in the fluidic layer adjoining the macromolecules. The free water protons are responsible for the MR images produced by the usual imaging protocols. In MTI, by applying a specific RF pulse (called MTP—magnetization transfer pulse), the bound macromolecules are saturated, (which is "excited"). These macromolecules transfer their magnetization by a process called "dipole coupling" through the hydrogen protons present in the hydration layer, to the free water protons. When that happens, the contrast difference between the bound macromolecules and free water protons is enhanced, the bound macromolecules appearing darker as compared to the free water protons. This increases the image contrast MTC (magnetization transfer contrast). MTI, therefore, suppresses background signals improving detection of white matter lesions such as MS plaques and small vessels in an MR angiographic study.

Magnetic Field Gradient: Gradient (or slope) implies a change in the magnetic field strength along the (z axis) line of scanning. In MRI, when an electric current is passed through the gradient coils, it results in the creation of a magnetic field differing in strength at different points along the length of the image. The strength of the magnetic field changes from head to toe. This enables the selection of an area of interest for scanning. This type of gradient is called "spatial encoding" (slice selecting) gradient. Once a slice is selected, an image must be created which is done by using frequency- and phase-encoding gradients.

Matrix: It is a two-dimensional structure composed of pixels arranged in rows and columns in frequency- and phase-encoding directions. It is on this framework that the acquired image is displayed. An image matrix could have varying sizes. It could be a 128 (frequency-encoding direction) by 128 sized matrix, (phase-encoding direction) a 256 by 256 or 512 by 512 size matrix. The image matrix is also called the "Field of View" (FOV) within which the image is depicted.

MR Angiography (MRA) Techniques:

MRA can be performed with and without the use of IV Gadolinium.

- **Non-contrast MRI:**
  (a) **Time of Flight (TOF)**:

  Protons in blood just entering into a slice produce bright signals because they have yet not been exposed to the RF pulse, whereas stationary protons in the slice, by repeated application of RF pulse, have insufficient time to recover the longitudinal magnetization, hence appearing dark. This results in the difference of contrast between inflowing blood and stationery tissue and is called "inflow- or flow-related enhancement". The sequence used in TOF image is the spoiled gradient sequence. TOF sequences can be 2D, 3D and MOTSA sequences.

  The **2D sequences** obtain images of blood vessels slice by slice. They cover larger areas and are used for slow-flowing blood such as in veins and peripheral arteries. If only arterial blood flow has to be studied, then venous blood flow is masked by using saturation bands (signal-suppressing bands). These bands expose the incoming venous blood to repeated RF pulses, thus causing signal loss. The 2D sequences are effective where blood flow is in a straight line and in the long channel. But wherever there is a complex flow pattern or turbulence, it causes signal loss.

  The **3D sequences** cover a volume (slab) of tissue, deliver thinner slices, have higher resolution and are used for fast-flowing blood. The drawback is that if larger slabs are covered, the flowing blood has a chance of being saturated under the onslaught of repeated RF pulses with resultant signal intensity reduction. The 3D sequence is highly dependent on the flip angle and TR. Larger flip angles produce greater contrast, to begin with, but which lasts over a short distance. Smaller flip angles give lesser contrast to the flowing blood at the entrance, but the signal lasts over a longer distance. Similarly, with longer TRs, there is better signal in the beginning with lesser contrast over a longer distance, while shorter TRs produce lesser contrast but carry it over a longer distance.

MOTSA acquisition (Multiple overlapping thin slab acquisition/motion-resolved time-resolved angiography). Using multiple thin overlapping slabs which are combined into a single slab, delivers the advantages of both 2D (larger area covered) and 3D (improved resolution). However, band-like artefacts can be seen as the acquisition is a collection of overlapping slabs. MOTSA technique helps overcoming and compensating for motion-related artefacts, such as those produced by movement of blood and patient movement. Hence, wherever there is a possibility of motion-related artefacts, MOTSA technique proves valuable.

(b) **Phase Contrast (PC) Studies:** Phase contrast studies are used to visualize MR signals and detect the direction of flow of blood or CSF [7, 8]. When a spin moves along a gradient from a lower to a higher level (or vice versa), it experiences different field strengths, relative to the stationary tissue. Consequently, the signal intensity and velocity of the spin keep changing. Compared to this, if the spin is stationary, it experiences the same field strength all the time. Thus, blood which flows into a stationary tissue can be differentiated as a bright signal as it remains unsaturated compared to the rest of the tissue. The signals of the stationery protons within the slice are cancelled out because of their immobility and, unlike blood or CSF, they do not cast a bright image. Hence, phase contrast study enables differentiating stationary from moving spins. Phase contrast MR study can also tell the direction and velocity of blood flow. It has two kinds of images, a phase image, which can show moving spins as bright or dark shadows, depending upon the direction of flow, whether it is along or in the opposite direction relative to the flow-encoding gradient. Phase imaging also allows the detection of the velocity of the moving blood by using velocity-encoding gradient (VENC). It can pick up slow and fast flows by adjusting the VENC. Thus, both direction and velocity of blood and CSF flow can be studied by phase contrast technique. The phase contrast sequence also generates a magnitude image which only gives the flow velocity. Phase contrast imaging can be used with both 2D and 3D sequences. It is used both in the study of the flow of blood in blood vessels and heart and also in CSF flow studies in patients with hydrocephalus, especially normal pressure hydrocephalus.

(c) **Dynamic Contrast-Enhanced (DRE) MR Angiography:**

This is a technique, which provides faster image acquisition without reduction of signal-to-noise ratio (SNR). The technique is based on rapid central "k" space sampling which provides information regarding the contrast of the images. The peripheral "k" space provides information regarding spatial resolution and is sampled slowly. This increases the overall speed of sampling.

DCE imaging can cover long areas, obtaining stacks of images, timed at different intervals, thereby providing separate information about arterial and venous phases in a vascular study.

26.10 Perfusion Studies

The word perfusion implies the flow of blood across tissue from the arterial to the venous side. This study is based on the visualization of microvascular blood flow through tissues. It tells us about the size of the microvascular circulation and the time taken to arrive and leave the area of interest [9]. Perfusion studies can be performed both in CT and MR.

- *Perfusion study using GBCA (Gadolinium based contrast agents).* In this study, multiple single-shot echoplanar images are rapidly obtained, typically at intervals of 1 second or less, following the administration of IV Gadolinium-based contrast. This technique utilizes the **T2*** effect of the Gadolinium, which causes spin dephasing and a corresponding signal drop due to local magnetic field inhomogeneities. **In normal tissues**, as Gadolinium remains intravascular and flows through small capillaries, a decrease in signal intensity is observed in **T2*****sequences.* The signal loss is greater in the normal areas which have more contrast-filled capillaries, as compared to regions with fewer capillaries or reduced perfusion. **In regions** such as **tumours, infarcts, or abscesses**, where the **blood-brain barrier (BBB)** is compromised, the microcirculation is disrupted. Gadolinium leaks out of the capillaries into the extravascular space, producing a **T1-shortening effect**. As a result, the abnormal areas may appear bright on **T1-weighted** images. Noteworthy is the fact that even though T2* weighting is being used, the T1 effect from Gadolinium leakage can lead to the brightening of abnormal regions due to the significant accumulation of contrast outside the blood vessels. Thus, in **T2*****sequences* abnormal areas where Gadolinium leaks into the extravascular space can appear brighter against the darker background of the normal tissue.
- *Perfusion studies using Arterial spin labelling (ASL)*: Tissue perfusion can also be measured without using IV Gadolinium contrast by employing the ASL technique [9]. This technique magnetically labels water in the arterial blood using an RF pulse. The tissue through which the magnetically labelled blood is flowing is compared with the control image obtained without labelling the blood. In this way, the amount of blood flow in mL/100 g/min can be quantified. The images obtained by ASL have a low signal-to-noise ratio. Only a single slice is acquired, and scan time is long. ASL provides reliable quantification of cerebral blood flow and is suitable for temporal imaging in functional MRI.

26.11 MR Artefacts

The MRI generates not only high-quality images but artefacts. These are of various types. They can be:

- Motion artefact—caused by breathing or moving. These are also called ghosting artefacts [10–12] (Fig. 26.7).

  Solution: Reassuring the patient, using sequences with shorter acquisition time, using an appropriate coil, performing the scan under sedation, using soft pads between the inner surface of the coil and the patient's skin and the use of immobilizing devices.

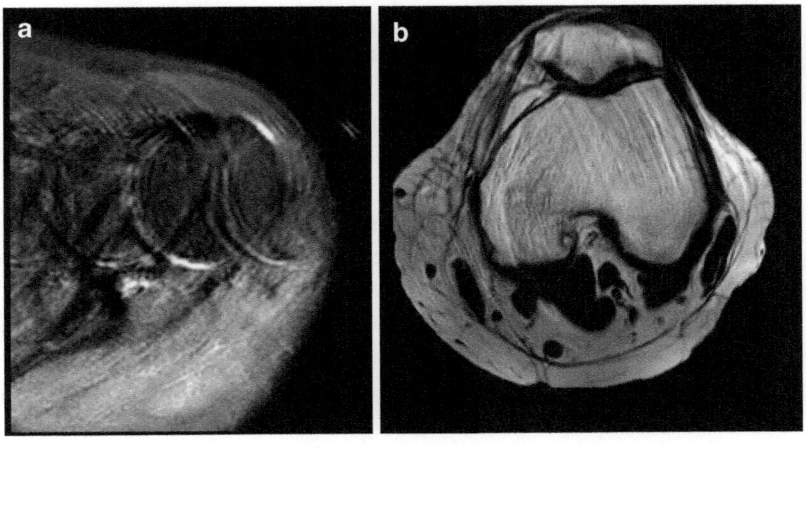

Fig. 26.7 Motion Artefact. Shoulder and Knee (**a**, **b**) MR images of different patients showing motion artefacts

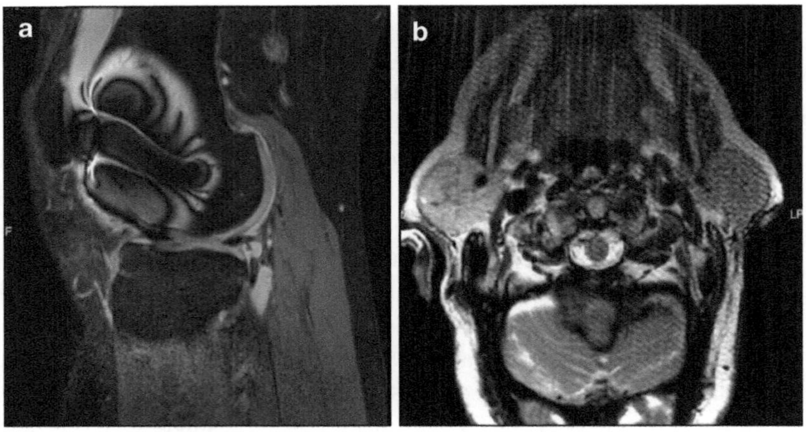

Fig. 26.8 Images demonstrating susceptibility artefact in the post-operative knee (**a**) due to metallic implants and radiofrequency Interference artefacts (**b**) in cervical spine imaging

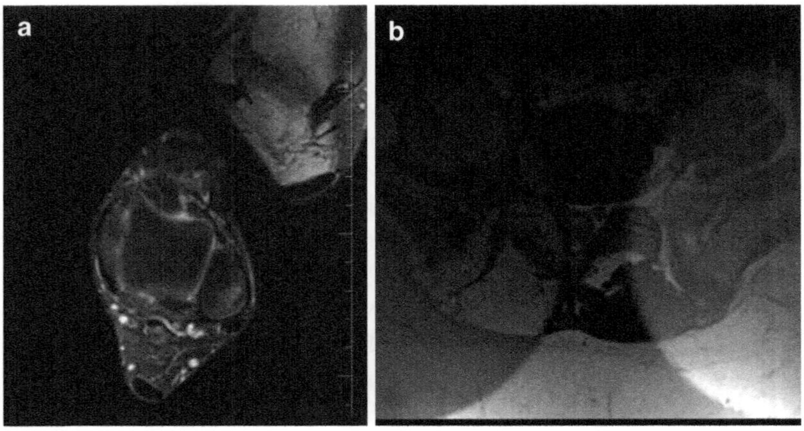

Fig. 26.9 Wrap around artefact. Axial images of ankle (**a**) and lumbar spine (**b**)

- Flow artefacts—as is seen in CSF studies or when a urinary jet enters the bladder.
- Susceptibility-weighted artefact—such as caused by surgical clips (Fig. 26.8).
- Wrap around artefacts (aliasing): This happens when the field of view chosen for scanning is of a smaller dimension as compared to the size of the object. The image of a part of the object, not included in the scanning area, wraps itself to the posterior part of the image (Fig. 26.9).
  Solution: Using a larger FOV, use of oversampling techniques and saturation pulses.
- Parallel imaging artefact: The artefacts in parallel imaging are of the same type as one would see in a normal MRI scan done without using parallel imaging.
- Bounce-point artefact: This is an artefact produced during a T1 inversion recovery sequence (T1 FLAIR sequence). It appears as an artificial black line along the surface of a fluid-soft tissue interface [11]. This black line may be confused with superficial siderosis.
- Zebra artefact: If the arms are by the side of the abdomen but not included in the MRI field of view, they will be exposed to the edge of the MRI field, which will be displayed as a "Zebra stripe" in the centre of a coronal image.
- Chemical shift artefacts: Due to the difference in spinning frequencies of fat and water, a phenomenon called "chemical shift" develops which produces an India ink effect by cancelling out signals from fat at a particular frequency. The advantage of this artefact is that it

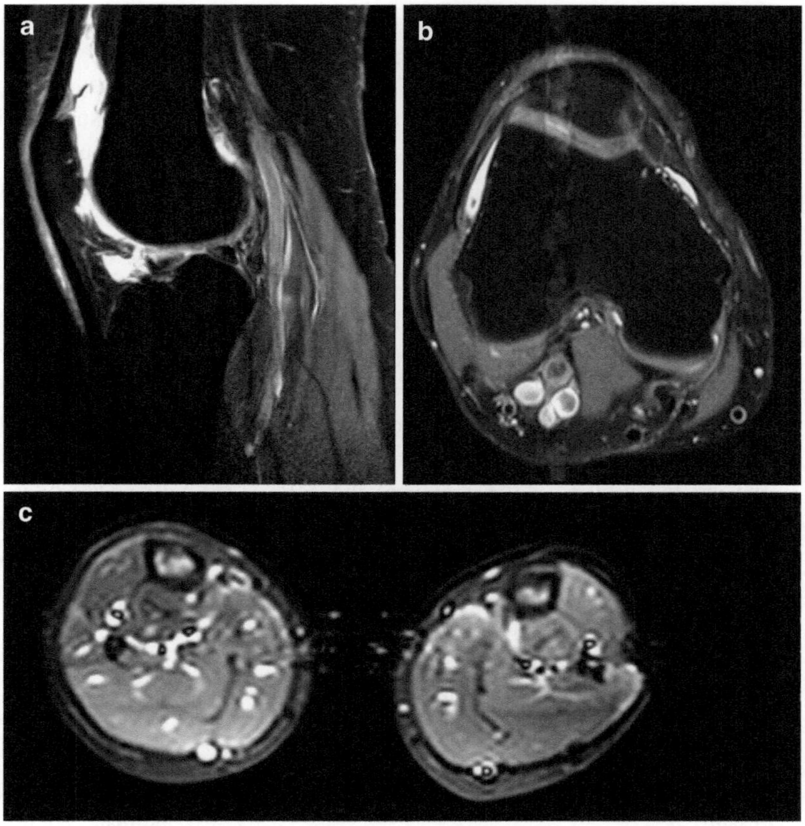

Fig. 26.10 Pulsation artefact. MR knee coronal (**a**), axial (**b**) and both legs axial (**c**) showing pulsation artefacts

tells us whether fat is present or not. The disadvantage is in the frequency-encoding direction, it produces bands of increased and decreased signals. It can make one wall of a hollow organ or cyst look dark and thick and the wall opposite it, thin and isointense.

- Pulsation artefacts: These are seen both in T1 VIBE and spin echo sequences, but they are seen more in the SE sequence (Fig. 26.10). Solution: application of flow compensation, use of out-of-phase saturation pulses, increasing the number of acquired signals and switching the directions of the phase- and frequency-encoding gradients.
- Truncation artefact (Gibb's artefact): **Truncation artefacts** appear as alternating bands of light and dark shadows at boundaries where there is a high contrast difference between adjacent tissues (e.g. the interface between gray and white matter). These artefacts occur due to inadequate sampling of the data in the **phase-encoding direction**. This can happen if there is a reduced matrix size or insufficient number of phase-encoding steps. The artefact becomes more prominent when fewer phase-encoding lines are used to hasten the scan. It results in an underestimation of the sharp transitions between structures [12].
- Zipper artefact: This appears as a line of alternating light and dark signals, running across an image and is due to RF interference.
- Section overlap (crosstalk): This happens in multislab, multiangle sequences. The signal intensity due to the overlapping areas is heterogeneous.

26.12 MR Coils

In addition to the main superconductive coil in the MR system, there are other sets of coils used in MRI.

- Gradient coils: The gradient coils are located within the gantry in three planes: X, Y and Z. They create a secondary magnetic field that distorts the main magnetic field (B0), which makes the spins precess at different frequencies in all three planes. This variation in precession frequency allows spatial encoding of the MR signal along all three axes, thus enabling the localization of proton spins in three dimensions (X, Y, Z).
- RF coils [13]: These coils are located within the gantry and serve two main functions: transmitting RF pulses to excite protons in the body and receiving the MR signals emitted by the excited protons. After receiving the MR signal, the process of image formation involves a few steps. First, the received signals are amplified. Next, noise is filtered out, and the signals are converted from analogue to digital form. The **Fourier transformation** is then applied to the frequency-encoded data, allowing for the conversion of the signal from the time domain to the frequency domain. This final step enables the reconstruction of an image.
- Types of RF coils: They can be transmitted only, receive only or both transmit and receive types of coils. They can be rigid as well as flexible and are constructed in such a way that they can fit the geometry and size of the part under study. This close proximity of the coils to the body part improves the signal-to-noise ratio.
- Shim coils: These coils carry a small current that creates additional magnetic fields which compensate for the inhomogeneities of the main magnetic field (B0). The magnetic field is rendered uniform across the imaging area which results in improvement of the quality and accuracy of the MRI images.
- Body coils: These are large coils, made of multiple small coils and can be of various sizes. They are located within the gantry and are transmit/receive coils.
- Surface coils: Coils outside the gantry of the magnet are called the surface coils.
  (a) Surface coils: Surface coils, such as head coils and extremity coils, are generally used to **receive signals** [13]. Since these coils are positioned close to the body, they have a higher signal-to-noise ratio. Coils, such as **"birdcage" coils**, are commonly used for the head and extremities and can function as **transmit and/or receive coils**. Surface coils are removable and used when needed. They create a homogeneous RF excitation field across the region being imaged.
  (b) Phased array coils: These are collections of multiple small coils arranged in an array. They combine the benefits of both small coils (high signal-to-noise ratio for localized areas) and larger coils (coverage of a large imaging area), which improves spatial resolution and provide higher SNR across larger areas. Phased array coils can also hasten image acquisition and shorten scan times through the use of **parallel imaging techniques**, which reconstruct images by using data from multiple coils simultaneously. Parallel imaging techniques are known by various names, such as **SENSE** (Sensitivity Encoding), **GRAPPA** (Generalized Autocalibrating Partially Parallel Acquisitions) and **iPAT** (integrated Parallel Acquisition Techniques), depending on the vendor.
  (c) Advanced designs of receiver coils: These coils are designed to improve the uniformity of RF excitation across the region being examined, thereby enhancing the signal-to-noise ratio (SNR). They also support **multidirectional parallel imaging**, which reduces scan time using techniques like **integrated Parallel Acquisition Techniques (iPAT)**. Additionally, these coils help reduce susceptibility artefacts and anatomical distortions, leading to improved image quality. These advanced receiver coils can be used for imaging various parts, including the body, head and extremities.
  (d) Quadrature coil: This is an RF antenna designed to transmit and receive RF signals from multiple directions, thereby

producing high-quality images. It consists of two sets of coils positioned at right angles to each other, creating a **90-degree phase difference** between the two coils. This configuration improves signal reception and transmission efficiency, resulting in a higher signal-to-noise ratio (SNR) and better image quality.

(e) Endocavitary coils: These can be either endovaginal or endorectal. They improve the signal-to-noise ratio because of their close contact with the area under examination.

MR Spectroscopy: [14] (A, B) There are numerous protons (metabolites) in the body tissue. These Metabolites, that is, the protons keep precessing (revolving) in a magnetic field, at a certain frequency, called the precessional frequency which changes with the type of environment, the metabolite is in. This change in precessional frequency is called “chemical shift”, which forms the basis of MR spectroscopy. By using this difference in precessional frequency, the presence of various types of metabolites in a tissue, hence the nature of the tissue, can be determined. Therefore, this is a technique which enables visualization of the chemical composition of a mass.

For MRS, it is necessary to subdue water signals in the CNS and fat signals outside the CNS. This enables visualization of signals of the other metabolites which are present in much lower concentration, and whose signals are masked by the far larger signals of water and fat which are present in abundance in the body tissues.

The techniques can be single-voxel study (SVS) or chemical shift imaging (CSI) which is a multivoxel-based study. The aim of MRS is to detect the metabolic activity in that single or multivoxel region. SVS is used for focal or diffuse diseases while CSI is used for either larger irregularly outlined lesions or for comparing both sides.

To study MRS of tissues, a few methods are employed. These go by the acronyms of STEAM, PRESS, ISIS and CSI. The student can read more about them from books on MRI physics.

Spectroscopic images are displayed as parts per million. The study yields better results in a higher field strength magnet.

For MRS study, the SNR is improved by a longer TR. TE also plays an important role. Long TE (>135 ms) allows major brain metabolites to be visualized. These include choline, creatinine, NAA and lactate. On using shorter TEs (20–30 ms), metabolites which have a shorter T2 decay are visible. These are myoinositol, glutamine and glutamate.

Listed below are the commonly used metabolites and what they stand for:

Myoinositol (MI) is seen at 3.5 ppm, is a marker for astrocytic activity.

Choline (CHO) is seen at 3.2 ppm and is a marker of cell membrane turnover, such as in tumours.

Creatine (Cr) at 3.0 ppm is a marker for energy metabolism.

N acetyl aspartate (NAA) at 2.0 ppm is a marker of neuronal integrity.

Lactate peak set at 1.3 ppm is a marker for anaerobic activity.

Lipid Peak which is seen between 0.9 and 1.4 ppm is seen with necrosis.

Multislice Imaging. The time needed to excite and then encode a single slice is called a slice loop. In a given TR, the length of the TR divided by the slice loops determines the number of slices which can be acquired. If more slices are needed, it can be done by either increasing the TR, using faster gradients or applying multiple sets of repetitions.

Proton Density (PD) Sequence: This sequence is used predominantly in imaging the musculoskeletal system. It is based on the fact that all tissues have different proton densities (amount of hydrogen protons), hence they have different levels of magnetization. Water has more hydrogen protons and therefore will have a higher PD and appear brighter than those tissues which have lesser hydrogen protons. PD images are produced by increasing the TR and reducing the TE. The images look gray because the PD difference between tissues is small.

Pulse Sequences: These include spin echo (SE) sequences, gradient echo sequences (GRE), inversion recovery sequence (IR) and echoplanar imaging sequence (EPI).

Spin Echo Sequence: Two RF pulses applied at 90 and 180° are used to dephase and rephase the hydrogen protons, in order to produce images.

Gradient Echo Sequence (GRE): A **G**radient **E**cho **S**equence is a pulse sequence, which instead of using a 90- and 180-degree pulse sequence (spin echo sequence) uses gradient coils to rephase the transverse magnetization. The GRE sequences are faster because the flip angles are small. They are used for faster scanning.

Inversion Recovery Sequences (IR Sequences): These are sequences used to suppress either fluid signals (FLAIR sequence—fluid attenuating inversion recovery sequence or fat signals, STIR—short T1 inversion recovery sequence). A 180-degree pulse is applied first to flip the protons below the baseline. After a certain time called the inversion time TI, when the T1W of fat or fluid is zero in the Z-axis, a 90° pulse is applied. The signal generated is used to create the image. By varying the inversion time, signals from fat (which have a shorter inversion time than water) can be separated from water. Thus, fluid which appears bright can be distinguished from fat, which appears dark in the fat suppressed sequence.

A FLAIR sequence is an FSE sequence. The T1 value of the FLAIR sequence is long (1500–2500 ms). This allows suppression of the long T1 signals of CSF in the T2W brain imaging, thus highlighting bright signals associated with pathological lesions. FLAIR sequence can be both T1 and T2 FLAIR. The T1 FLAIR sequence is better than the conventional T1W sequence because it produces increased contrast differentiation between gray and white matter. It is a good technique for studying anatomical details and can also be used for contrast studies (Figs. 26.11 and 26.12).

There are other inversion recovery sequences. These are:

1. *MPRAGE* (Magnetization Prepared, Rapid Acquisition Gradient Echo sequence). In this sequence, the T1 is intermediate that is between 300 and 1200 ms and is used to produce T1-weighted images.
2. *SPIR*, which stands for Spectral Inversion Recovery pulse sequence. SPIR sequence is ideal for obtaining T1W FSE images.
3. *SPAIR* (Spectral Attenuated Inversion Recovery) sequence. This is also a fat suppressing sequence and ideal for T2W FSE sequence [5].
   (a) *Echoplanar Imaging (EPI)*: This is a single or multiple-shot GRE or SE rapid image acquisition sequence which col-

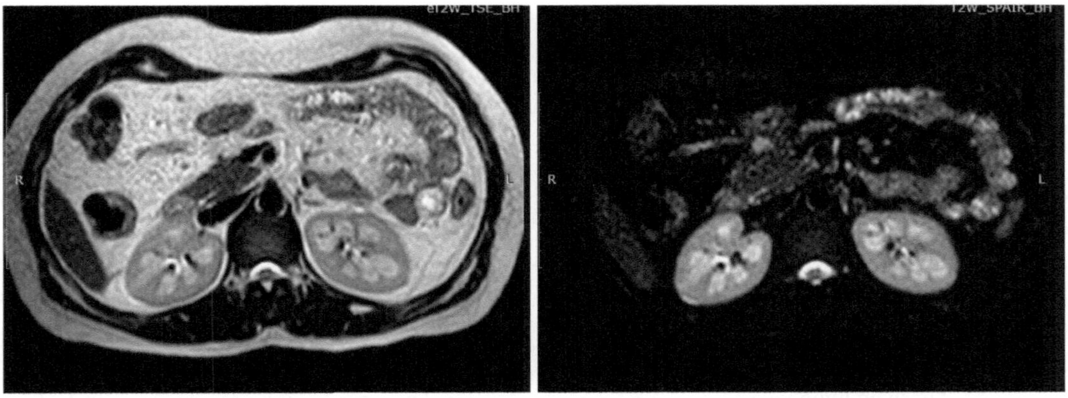

Fig. 26.11 T2 W sequence of the abdomen, without and with fat suppression

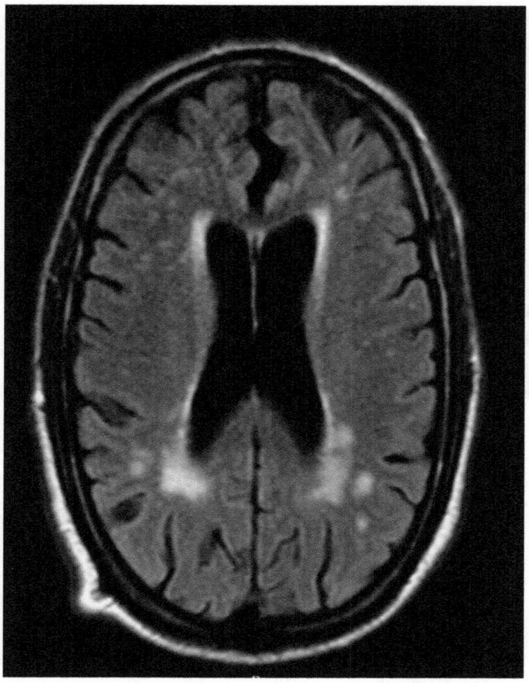

Fig. 26.12 Flair sequence: Note the CSF-containing spaces are dark as compared to the areas of abnormality which are bright. A longer TE eliminates signals from CSF. However, the brain parenchyma retains the same signal intensity as in an FSE or SE sequence

lects a complete range of signals within one TR and rapidly fills all the lines in a k-space, resulting in quick image formation. The images have low signal-to-noise ratio, low resolution and are affected by artefacts due to chemical shifts or susceptibility-related issues. This is because the horizontal filling of the k-space is quicker than the vertical filling. The problem can be solved by using quick multishot EPI. EPI is used in functional MRI studies.

(b) *Susceptibility-weighted sequences (SWI)* [15, 16]: SWI sequences are GRE sequences which utilize the T2* effect. The SWI sequences [15, 16] highlight veins carrying deoxygenated blood as dark tubular structures. The degree to which a substance is susceptible to becoming magnetized in the presence of an external magnetic field is known as its magnetic susceptibility. When tissues of different magnetic susceptibilities are in proximity in a magnetic field, there is distortion in the signals which result in signal loss. The tissues showing high magnetic susceptibility are referred to as **ferromagnetic**. Those with weak magnetic susceptibility are referred to as **paramagnetic** and those with little or no effect are referred to as **diamagnetic**. Examples are blood products, such as deoxyhaemoglobin and hemosiderin which are paramagnetic, calcium and bone minerals which are diamagnetic. Ferromagnetic and paramagnetic substances show a reduction in the MR signals and appear dark. Haemoglobin, when still containing oxygen, is diamagnetic because oxygen surrounds the iron in haemoglobin, thereby reducing the magnetic susceptibility. As the oxygen is used up and depletes, iron within haemoglobin is exposed becoming deoxyhaemoglobin and later on hemosiderin (paramagnetic, i.e. dark). Normal venous blood flow, air and metal also show signal loss and appear dark in the GRE sequence (T2* sequence). SWI sequence can detect subarachnoid haemorrhage (SAH), diffuse axonal injury, cavernous haemangiomas, intraventricular bleeding and bleeding within infarcts. A (minimum intensity projection image) MINIP sequence used with SWI further highlights the dark structures. The SWI sequence also enables differentiating between blood and calcium by using a phase mask and different T1 and T2 relaxation times (Fig. 26.13).

Paramagnetic Substances: These have unpaired electrons and are weakly attracted towards an external magnetic field. Examples of paramagnetic substances include oxygen, iron and rare earth elements such as Gadolinium.

Phase Encoding: Knowing a signal's anatomical location in relation to its surrounding tissues is crucial for creating an image. To do this and

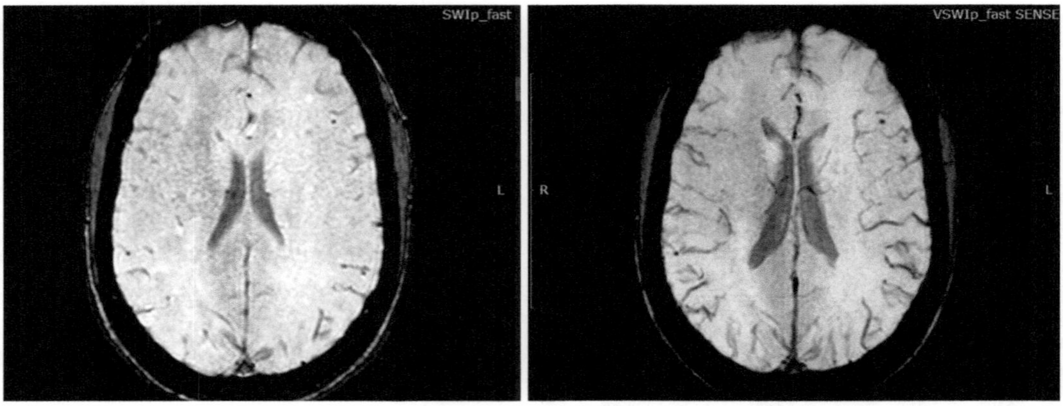

Fig. 26.13 SWIP (Susceptibility Weighted Image with Phase Enhancement) images developed by a certain vendor, with slice thickness of 2 and 10 mm. The latter image is a MINIP sequence, which highlights dark signals better by virtue of using thicker slices

make an image, three gradients, slice selecting, frequency-encoding and phase-encoding gradients are used. Having selected a slice along the Z-axis, a frequency-encoding gradient is applied along the X-axis and a phase-encoding gradient is applied in the "Y"-axis. Using the information obtained, the position of the hydrogen proton in a slice can be ascertained.

Pixel: The word stands for picture element. It is the smallest illuminated area in an image. Several pixels combine to form the final image. The higher the number of pixels, the better the displayed image.

PSIF Sequence: This is a preexcitation refocussed heavily T2 W sequence and is very sensitive to flow. Hence, it is used where CSF flow can disturb the anatomy. PSIF sequence is used to evaluate normal structures residing in the CP angle as well as to detect small lesions present in this area [17].

Quenching: MRI machines have a superconducting magnet which needs to be cooled to very low temperatures in order to produce a stable and strong magnetic field. This cooling is done by using Helium gas. If for some reason the temperature rises, Helium gas boils off and can damage the equipment as well as harm the patient. This is called "quenching". Quenching leads to loss of superconductivity of the magnet and will need refilling the lost Helium gas to cool down the magnet. It is a time-consuming as well as costly process.

Radiofrequency: This consists of waves, having a range of frequency within the electromagnetic spectrum, the range extending from 3 kHz to 300MHZ. It is used in MRI to alter the spinning of the hydrogen protons to produce an image. It is also used to heat and coagulate abnormal lesions in the body, particularly tumours in the liver, kidneys as well as in the treatment of bone lesions such as osteoid osteoma.

Ramping: Ramping is to change in the strength of a magnetic field.

Relaxation: This is a return of a spinning proton, excited by an RF pulse, to its original resting state. It also means that as the transverse magnetization decays the longitudinal magnetization is restored to its resting phase. The resting phase is reached when the spinning protons align in parallel to the main magnetic field "Z"-axis.

Resonance: This is a vibration which happens when the frequency of the RF pulse transmitted is equal to the frequency of the spinning hydrogen protons. The energy absorbed by the hydrogen protons in the slice is released and this energy is used to create an MR image.

RF Pulses: These are a bunch of radiofrequency (RF) energies, used to tilt the magnetic field of a hydrogen proton.

RF Shielding: This is done to prevent the extraneous RF pulses from interfering with the MRI system.

Saturation: This is a way of reducing unwanted signals, say from fat, background noise or blood flow, and is produced by repeatedly applying (saturating) RF pulse at Larmour frequency to the tissue whose signals are to be suppressed.

Shimming: The normal magnetic field is inhomogeneous, both due to the intrinsic make of the magnet as well as due to the outside magnetic fields which can stray into the MRI suite. This produces noise in the image. By using electric coils called shim coils, the noise is filtered out and the magnetic field is homogenized. This process is called active shimming. Passive shimming is also utilized by attaching pieces of ferromagnetic metal inside the bore of the scanner.

Signal-to-Noise Ratio: It is the ratio of MR signal to the background noise. It means that in order to produce a clear high-resolution image, the strength of a signal from an MR image section must be higher than the signals from the background noise. The signal-to-noise ratio can be increased by increasing the strength of the magnet, using surface coils or sampling a larger volume of the tissue.

Single-Shot Imaging: This means that by filling the entire K-space using a single excitation pulse, all the data necessary to form an image is acquired.

Slice Selection: Selection of a slice of tissue for studying is done by using a slice selective RF pulse along the "Z"-axis. Only the slice having the same frequency as the RF pulse of the slice selective gradient is chosen for display.

Spin Echo: This is an RF pulse sequence where initially a 90-degree excitation pulse is applied followed by a 180-degree pulse which refocuses the dephased spin. This results in production of an echo after a time "TE". By using the 180-degree RF pulse, there is removal of magnetic field inhomogeneities, improvement of image quality and mitigation of the effect of chemical shift which occurs between water and fat.

Spoiled Sequence: **Spoiler Gradient (Incoherent Gradient)**:

These are additional gradients which are used in gradient and FSE sequences in order to remove all the transverse magnetization at the end of each cycle, thereby minimizing artefacts which can result from the residual transverse magnetization. By removing the transverse magnetization and therefore the T2* effect, a T1 W image is obtained. The acronyms for spoiled sequences given by different vendors are T1 FFE, SPGR, LAVA, VIBE and THRIVE. FLASH is also a spoiled gradient fast sequence, which can also be modified to work as an unspoiled. GRE sequence. It is used where patient movement is an issue.

Steady-State Sequences (Coherent Sequence) [17]: These are gradient echo sequences in which the T2 signal is not suppressed or spoiled. In fact, the T2 signals get highlighted and fluid within any organ or blood vessel becomes easily visible. Depending upon what signals are sampled to create an image, the steady-state sequences can be:

(a) **Preexcitation refocused sequence**: which have acronyms given by different vendors such as steady-state free precession [SSFP, GE], PSIF [reversed FISP, Siemens] T2-FFE (Philips).
(b) **Post-excitation refocused sequences**: which are also known by acronyms, FFE, GRASS, FISP, etc.
(c) **Fully refocused sequences**: Gradients applied in all axes are balanced, and hence, these are called balanced steady-free precession sequences (balanced SSFP), with acronyms such as true FISP, FIESTA and BFFE.

Spatial Resolution: The smallest measurable distance between two points which allows clear separation is called "spatial resolution". In other words, the ease of separating two points is called spatial resolution.

Specific Absorption Rate (SAR): Is a measurement of the rate at which heat energy is deposited into one kg of tissue by an RF pulse. When the RF pulse is applied to generate a signal, it interacts with water molecules and by accelerating their motion, increases the kinetic energy which results in an increase in temperature in the body. Heat deposition in the body is regulated by an international standard and should not be more than 0.5° in the normal scanning mode. Heat deposition increases in obese patients. SAR can be reduced by reducing the flip angle of the refocusing pulse in the fast spin echo technique. Heat deposition can also be reduced by using parallel imaging and reducing the number of phase-encoding steps.

Steady-State Gradient Echo and Balanced Gradient Echo Sequence: In both steady-state gradient echo technique and balanced gradient echo, the transverse magnetization is allowed to remain along with the T1W contrast. In other words, they are predominantly T2W sequences. Balanced gradient echo sequences are called TrueFISP by Siemens, FIESTA by GE and bFFE by Philips and balanced steady-state sequence, b-SSFP sequence, by other vendors. The b-SSFP sequence provides a higher signal-to-noise ratio as compared to the balanced gradient sequences. Balanced sequences are used to study blood vessels, cardiac chambers, biliary system and CSF. All these structures appear bright in the balanced sequence. A modification of the steady-state sequence is called DESS (dual-echo steady-state) sequence which is a combination of T1-weighted spoiled gradient echo and a steady-state free precession T2* sequence. DESS is used predominantly in joints for examination of bone, cartilage and fluid.

Superconducting Magnet: A superconducting magnet uses a coil which is cooled to such a level that it does not offer resistance to the flow of electric current. This results in the production of a homogeneous and stable magnetic field. The superconducting material used in MRI is composed of niobium–titanium embedded inside a copper matrix.

Suppression: This technique enables suppression of signals from a particular constituent of an object under study. By minimizing the contribution of this component, the other constituents can be highlighted, as it happens in MRS.

T1 W Sequence: T1 stands for longitudinal relaxation time and is also called spin-lattice relaxation time. The RF pulse rotates the spinning proton from its relaxed state in the Z-axis (longitudinal axis of the main magnet) into the high energy state in the X/Y axis by tilting it 90° from the original state. When the RF pulse is switched off, the spins start losing their energy to the surrounding tissue latticework. There is recovery of the longitudinal magnetization. The longitudinal magnetization recovers from zero and grows up to 63% of its maximum value over a period of time T1. The faster the energy lost to make that recovery, the shorter the recovery time which is the T1 time and the brighter the signal is. (Fat, white matter, Gadolinium products, proteins and blood products (at a certain time interval of degradation of blood products) appear bright in T1W sequences). The longer it takes to relax (long T1) the darker the image is. Fluids such as CSF, urine and water appear dark in the T1W image. T1W sequence depends upon TR. A short TR and a short TE mean faster relaxation and lead to T1 shortening. When the TR is increased, the T1 effect is reduced. White matter in T1W sequence appears brighter than gray matter due to higher myelin and less water content than gray matter.

T2 W Sequence: This is called the spin-spin relaxation time. The application of RF pulse results in protons coming together and gradually spinning in phase, thereby attaining a magnetic moment (which is magnetic field strength and alignment in the xy direction) M_{xy}, which is equal to the resting phase magnetic moment M_Z. On switching off the RF pulse, the spins, by reacting with one another as well as with the local magnetic field inhomogeneities, start losing their magnetic moment M_{xy}, by dephasing and cancelling out each other's signals. The T2W symbol stands for the time taken for all of M_{XY} magnetizations to lose their energy/phase coherence and attain 37% of the magnetization at the start of the RF pulse. This sequence enables distinction between tissues based on their T2 values. The T2W sequence is produced by increasing the TR and TE. The TR should be 3 times the TR of T1W

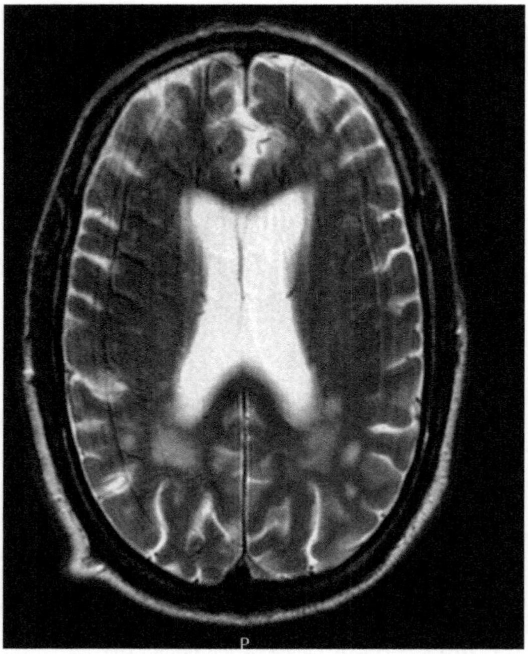

Fig. 26.14 T2W image: The TR is 4500 and the TE is 100. This is a longer sequence which shows artefacts produced by slight movement of the head. Note that in this T2W sequence, fluid in the CSF spaces (sulci, fissures and ventricles) is white

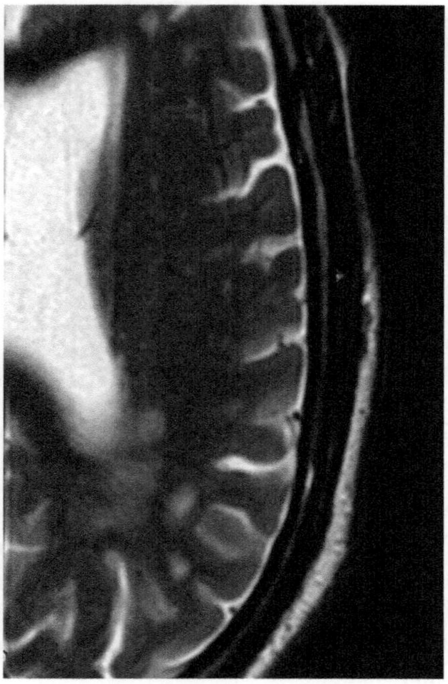

Fig. 26.15 Another T2W sequence: Note the difference between the gray and white matter. The gray matter is a few shades lighter as compared to the darker shade of the white matter. This is because there is more fat in the white matter myelin sheaths, as compared to water. And fat appears darker than water in the T2 W sequence

sequence, in order to reduce the T1 signal to <5%. TE of T2W sequence is longer than the TE of the T1W image so as to gather as much T2 effect as possible.

Spins which dephase quickly have short T2W, such as solids, proteins and blood products. Spins, which have a long T2W such as water, CSF, liquified abscesses, fluid-containing spaces and necrotic tumours, dephase slowly and appear bright. Slowly flowing or clotted blood may be bright in T2W sequence. Fat is bright in T1 FSE sequence. It will appear less bright in a T2W sequence. White matter appears darker in the T2W image as compared to gray matter, due to a higher myelin content within it (Figs. 26.14 and 26.15).

T2* Effect is the loss of phase coherence not only due to T2W effect but also due to inhomogeneities present in the local magnetic field. This effect is seen in susceptibility-weighted sequence.

TE: The echo time "TE", is the time between the application of the RF pulse and the arrival of the signal from the area of interest. The shorter the TE, the smaller the T2 signal. By varying the TE, the contrast of tissues, their appearance can be modified.

TR: This abbreviation, meaning "repetition time", stands for the time interval between two consecutive pulse signals applied to the same slice. The longer the TR, the longer the scan time and the greater the loss of T1 signal as the tissues have time to relax before the application of the next RF pulse.

Transverse Magnetization: When the spinning protons are tilted by 90°, from the main magnetic field (B_0), into the transverse plane (B_1), the magnetization converts from longitudinal to transverse magnetization. This is ultimately responsible for the generation of an MR signal.

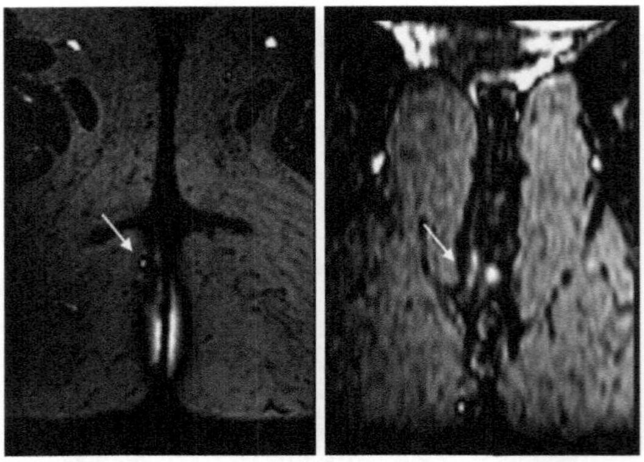

Fig. 26.16 Three-dimensional VISTA sequence using IV contrast used to demonstrate a fistula-in-ano (arrow)

Tesla (T): This is a measure of the magnetic field strength. Magnets come in various strengths from 0.2 to 7.0 Tesla. In practice, the strength of the magnet used commonly is up to 3 T at present.

Two-(2D) and Three-Dimensional (3D) Imaging. MR images can be acquired in 2D or 3D planes with T1, T2 or PD weighting. In a 2D sequence, a single slice is obtained while in a 3D sequence, a slab is obtained from which multiple slices can be elicited. The 3D sequence takes a longer time and can be affected by movement, resulting in the production of artefacts. SPACE/CUBE/VISTA sequences are the acronyms given by GE, Siemens and Philips, respectively, to the 3D sequences. Unlike 2D images, the 3D images are sharper because thinner slices can be selected from the data slab. Hence, 3D sequences are used in brain, inner ear, MRCP, fistulography and even in MSK studies (Fig. 26.16).

Voxel: A voxel stands for volume formed by a number of pixels. As the voxels increase, resolution of the image diminishes. There is more partial volume effect. However, the MR signals are brighter and the scanning time is reduced.

VIBE (Volume interpolated breathhold examination). This is a 3D GRE sequence, which is used with the administration of Gadolinium, in liver and abdominal imaging. It is a fast scan and yields excellent tissue contrast.

"W" stands for weighting or leaning towards a specific difference in the tissue contrast produced by the use of varying T1 or T2 parameters (Figs. 26.17 and 26.18).

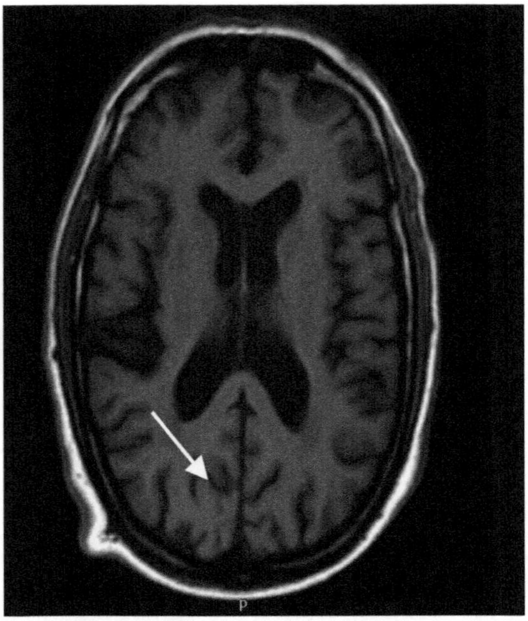

Fig. 26.17 T1W sequence of the brain: The TR is 571 and the TE 15. Note that fluid in the ventricles and sulci appears black

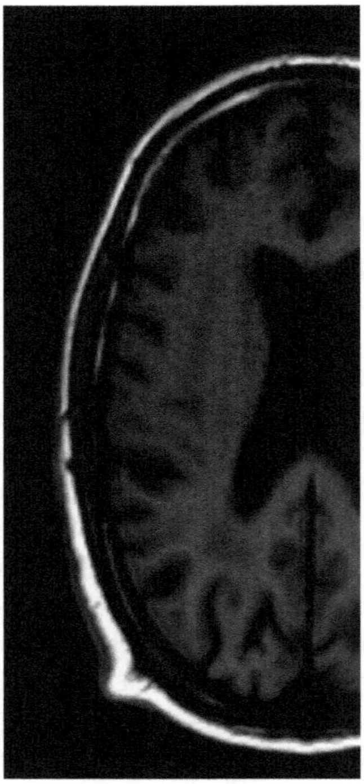

Fig. 26.18 Another T1W image: Note that the gray matter surrounding the sulci appears darker than the white matter. The gray matter contains more fluid, the white matter more myelin, hence the difference in their signal intensity

References

1. https://www.acr.org/-/media/ACR/Files/Radiology-Safety/MR-Safety/MRGlossary.pdf.
2. Jones J, Bell D, Murphy A, et al. B0. Reference article, Radiopaedia.org. Accessed 10 June 2024. https://doi.org/10.53347/rID-5854.
3. Weerakkody Y, Knipe H, Poirier-Quinot-, et al. MRI pulse sequence abbreviations. Reference article, Radiopaedia.org. Accessed 16 June 2024. https://doi.org/10.53347/rID-8073.
4. Yucel-Finn A, Mckiddie F, Prescott S, Griffiths R. Chapter 6. Magnetic resonance imaging. In: Farr's physics for medical imaging, 3rd ed. p. 135.
5. https://mriquestions.com/uploads/3/4/5/7/34572113/optimizing_spir_and_spair_fat_suppression.pdf.
6. Gallagher TA, Nemeth AJ, Hacein-Bey L. An introduction to the Fourier transform: relationship to MRI. Am J Roentgenol. 2008;190(5):1396–405.
7. Wymer DT, Patel KP, Burke WF III, Bhatia VK. Phase-contrast MRI: physics, techniques, and clinical applications. Radiographics. 2020;40(1):122–40.
8. Ballinger J, Bell D, Botz B, et al. Phase contrast imaging. Reference article, Radiopaedia.org. Accessed 14 June 2024. https://doi.org/10.53347/rID-22024.
9. Petrella JR, Provenzale JM. MR Perfusion imaging of the brain: techniques and applications. AJR Am J Roentgenol. 2000;175(1):207–19. https://ajronline.org/doi/full/10.2214/ajr.175.1.1750207.
10. Pusey E, Lufkin RB, Brown RK, Solomon MA, Stark DD, Tarr RW, Hanafee WN. Magnetic resonance imaging artifacts: mechanism and clinical significance. Radiographics. 1986;6(5):891–911.
11. https://sajr.org.za/index.php/sajr/article/download/127/139.
12. Noda C, Venkatesh BA, Wagner JD, Kato Y, Ortman JM, Lima JAC. Primer on commonly occurring MRI artifacts and how to overcome them. Radiographics. 2022;42(3):E102–3. https://doi.org/10.1148/rg.210021.pres.
13. Kwok WE. Basic principles of and practical guide to clinical MRI radiofrequency coils. Radiographics. 2022;42(3):898–918.
14. Danielson ER, Ross B. Magnetic resonance spectroscopy diagnosis of neurological diseases. New York: Marcel Dekker; 1999. p. 5–43.
15. Sven Haller E, Haacke M, Thurnher MM, Barkhof F. Susceptibility-weighted imaging: technical essentials and clinical neurologic applications. Radiology. 2021;299(1):3–26.
16. https://www.usa.philips.com/healthcare/product/HCNMRB460/swip-mr-clinical-application.
17. Chavhan GB, Babyn PS, Jankharia BG, et al. Steady-state MR imaging sequences: physics, classification, and clinical applications. Radiographics. 2008;28:1147–60.

Further Reading

Chavan GB. MRI made easy. 3rd ed. New Delhi: Jaypee Brothers Medical Publishers; 2022.

Runge VM, Nitz WR, Trelles M, Goerner FL. The physics of clinical MR taught through images. New York: Thieme Medical; 2014.

Commonly Used MRI Sequences 27

Abstract

Most MRI machines have preloaded vendor-driven protocols. These protocols are often adequate. However, the application specialist will tweak the protocols and add some additional sequences as per the need and preference of the MRI radiologist. The in-house technical team can also change the protocols whenever needed. The equipment allows such modifications.

Most MRI sequences are often similar across institutions. The vendor-specific abbreviations and acronyms may differ. Outlined in this chapter, are some of the commonly used sequences which are usually sufficient to provide the required information based on the clinical situation. The protocols are listed by anatomy as well as by clinical scenario.

Keywords

MRI · MRI protocols · Sequences

Some basic rules.

MRI is an investigation that takes time to complete. It has to be planned according to the clinical situation so that there is minimal need for repeating sequences. The scan should be evaluated by the on-duty radiologist and the experienced technologist to determine the adequacy of the study and whether additional sequences are needed. Every effort should be made to complete the entire study in one visit.

The image quality needs careful monitoring. All clinically relevant sequences must be obtained keeping in mind the clinical data. The studies can also be shortened ,especially in restless patients and children, once the clinical question appears to have been answered. This is also of particular relevance in "stroke" patients where it is essential to finish the studies so that the treatment can be started.

The examination must be performed with utmost care for the patient's safety.

Before commencing the examination, ensure all safety measures have been taken and the patient as well as the attendants are properly briefed abouted the study. Since the time taken to complete the study can be long, the patient should be stable enough to lie still while the examination is going on. Alternatively, the study can also be completed in parts. The urinary bladder should not be overdistended as the patient is likely to find it uncomfortable if the bladder overdistends and may move during the study. Also, bladder contractions may produce motion-related artefacts. Give the patient, earplugs to withstand the the noise within the gantry. Have an IV line ready, in case a contrast-enhanced scan needs to be performed. The image quality is likely to be degraded in small children, patients with tremors, and sick patients. The technician must know what to do in these situations.

R. Gothi, *Radiographic and Imaging Techniques for Radiology Residents and Technologists*, https://doi.org/10.1007/978-981-96-4816-0_27

Always perform those sequences first, which are likely to yield the most relevant diagnostic information. This is because the study may have to be abruptly terminated at any point in time due to various reasons.

Some patients may be claustrophobic despite the current MRI tunnels being shorter and wider than in the earlier types of equipment. These patients may need reassurance, sometimes sedatives and need to be scanned using a short protocol.

27.1 MR Sequences

These can be divided into the following groups:

1. Spin echo (SE) group.
2. Gradient echo (GRE) group.
3. Inversion recovery (IR) group (can be applied to both SE and GRE groups, but most often to SE group).
4. Echoplanar Imaging (EPI) group (can be used with SE and GRE groups but, unlike IR, it is most often applied to GRE group).

27.2 MR Sequences for the Brain: Some of the Core Sequences Will Be Discussed Here

Localizer: First perform a three-plane localizer. This is to ensure adequate coverage of the area under investigation, to obtain symmetry of the right and left structures of the brain parenchyma in the axial and coronal planes, and for proper midline sections in the sagittal plane (Fig. 27.1).

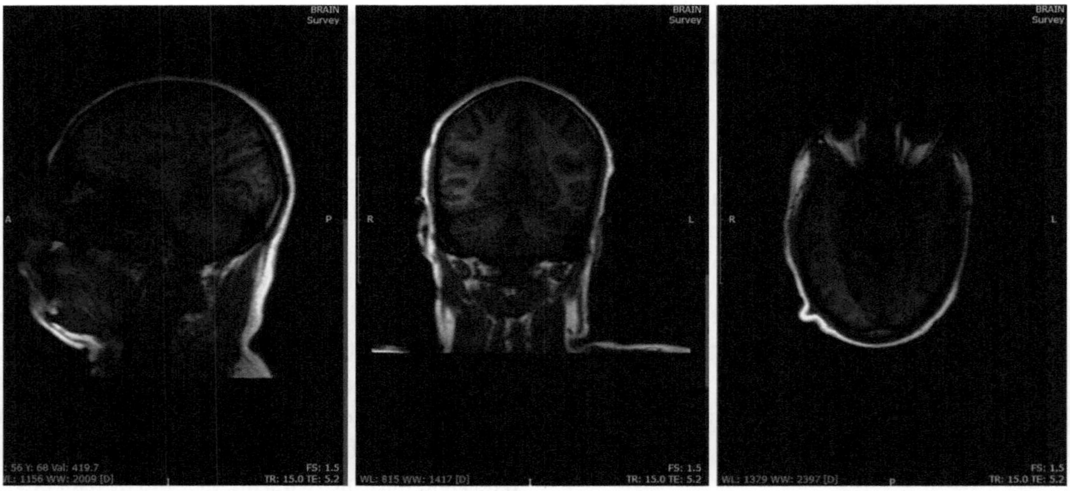

Fig. 27.1 Three-plane localizer: It can be either a T1W TSE (Turbo Spin echo) sequence or a T1 MPRAGE (gradient echo sequence) [1]

27.3 Non-Contrast Sequences

- **FLAIR sequence**: This is a T2W fluid attenuating inversion recovery sequence which lowers the T2 bright CSF signals, thereby enabling easy recognition of other bright signals originating from pathological lesions (Fig. 27.2).
- **T2W sequence**: The purpose of this sequence is to study anatomy and highlight pathological lesions in brain tissue which can either appear brighter or darker than CSF. Cerebral oedema appears bright. Some tumours appear isodense, clots appear bright and flowing blood appears dark (Figs. 27.3, 27.4, and 27.5).
- **DWI with ADC maps**: This sequence is used to detect lesions causing restricted diffusion. Lesions, which restrict the movement of water molecules, appear bright in the DWI sequence when higher gradient strengths are used and dark, in the ADC maps. This is called restricted diffusion and can be seen with infarcts, blood products, abscesses, solid and necrotic tumours (Figs. 27.6 and 27.7).
- **SWI sequences**: These are called susceptibility-weighted images. Ferromagnetic and paramagnetic substances including venous blood, clots and subacute blood appear dark in this sequence (Fig. 27.8).
- **T1 W sequence**. This is meant to study anatomy as well as detect lesions having a short T1W. The bright signals in this sequence are cast by fat, blood, proteinaceous material and contrast (Fig. 27.9).
- **TI Inversion recovery sequence:**

  This sequence provides improved SNR between gray and white matter [2] (Figs. 27.10 and 27.11).

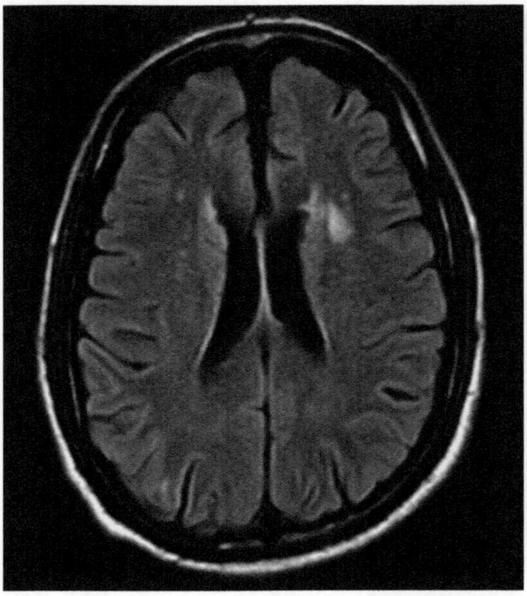

Fig. 27.2 FLAIR sequence. Note the difference between the attenuated T2W signals of the CSF present in the ventricles and sulcal spaces as compared to the bright signal produced by the lesion located close to the body of the left lateral ventricle

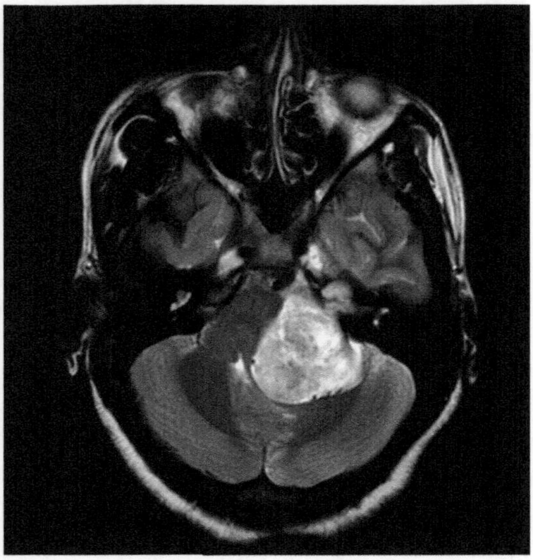

Fig. 27.3 T2W sequence showing a left CP angle tumour. Except for some tumours, most tumours generally appear bright on the T2 W sequence

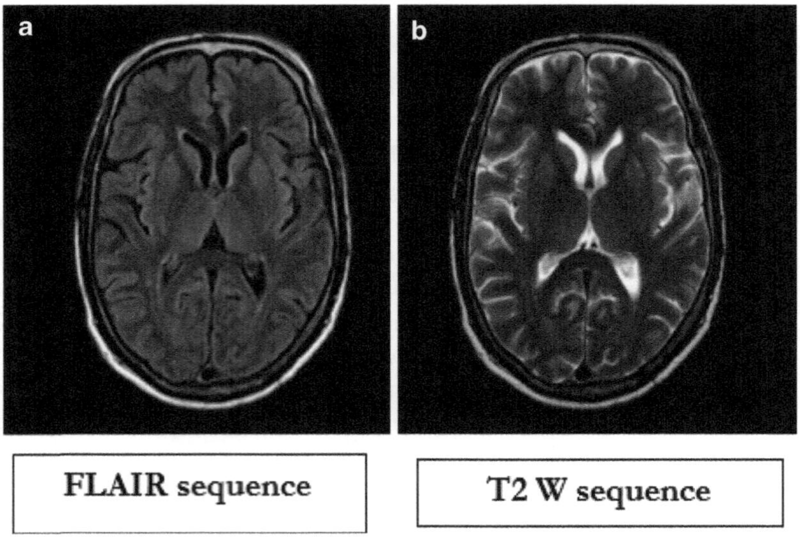

Fig. 27.4 (**a**, **b**) Comparison between FLAIR and T2W sequences (**a**): Note the dark signals of the CSF within the ventricles in the Flair sequence. (**b**) T2 W sequence: Note the bright signals of the lateral ventricles and CSF spaces

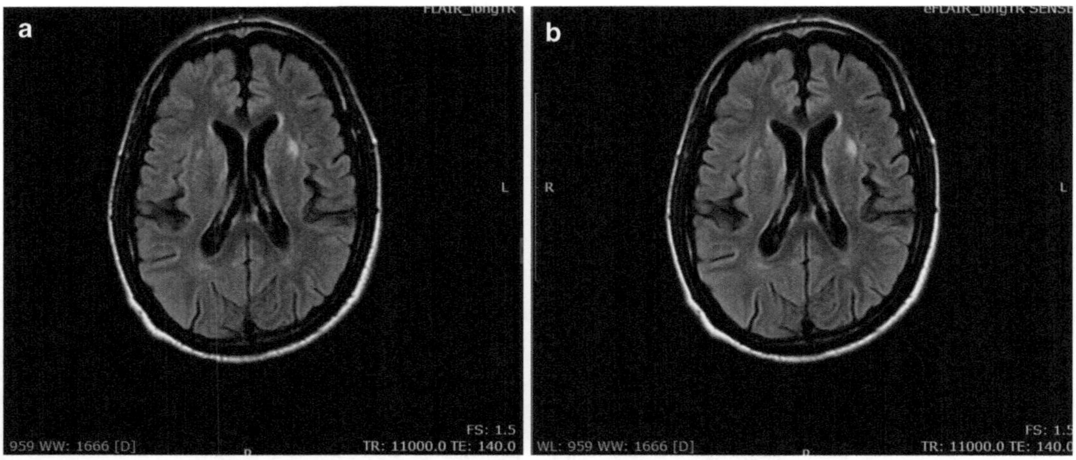

Fig. 27.5 (**a**, **b**) FLAIR sequences (**a**) normal and (**b**) using SENSE (parallel) imaging which reduces scan time. Note the long TR (11000) and long TE (140) used in the FLAIR sequence

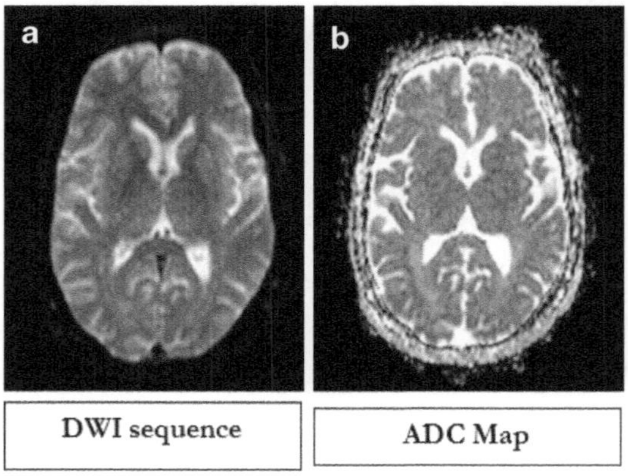

Fig. 27.6 (**a**, **b**) Normal Diffusion-Weighted images and corresponding ADC maps

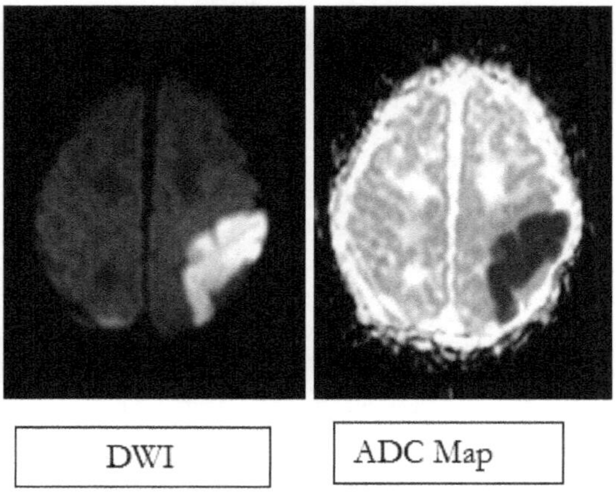

Fig. 27.7 DWI and corresponding ADC map, showing restricted diffusion in an area of infarction in the left parietal lobe. The infarcted area appears dark in the ADC map

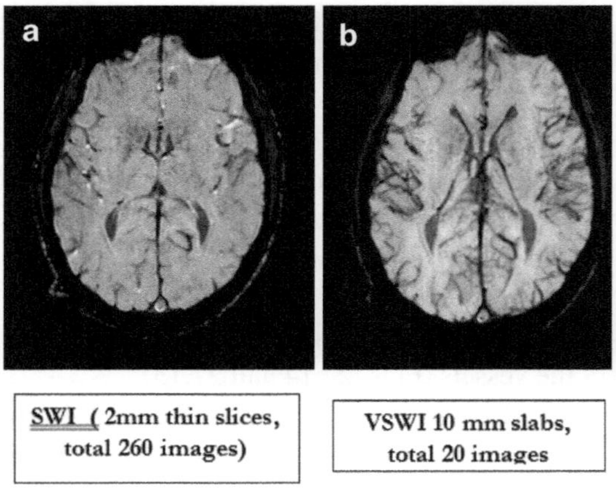

Fig. 27.8 (**a**, **b**) SWI images: These sequences are used to detect ferromagnetic, paramagnetic substances including intraparenchymal hematoma. The volume SWI (VSWI) image is a thick slab which averages the signals in that slab and gives a better idea of the venous blood flow in the brain parenchyma

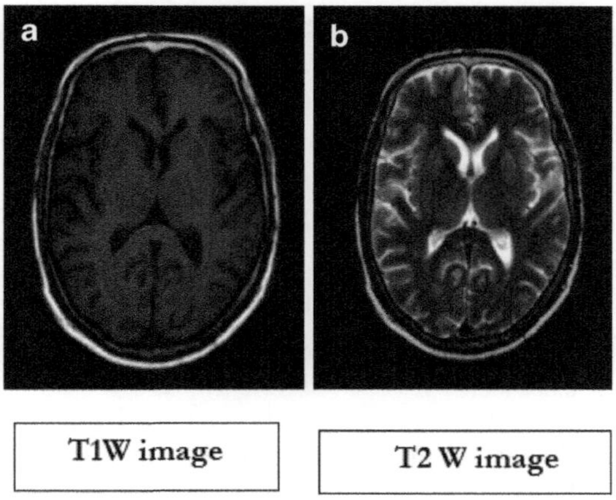

Fig. 27.9 (**a**, **b**) T1 (**a**) and T2 W (**b**) sequences. Note the appearance of CSF in the two images. Also, note that the white matter looks brighter than the gray matter in the T1W sequence and darker in the T2W sequence. This is because of the higher lipid content in abundant myelin sheaths of axons in the white matter as compared to the gray matter, which contains more water and less fat

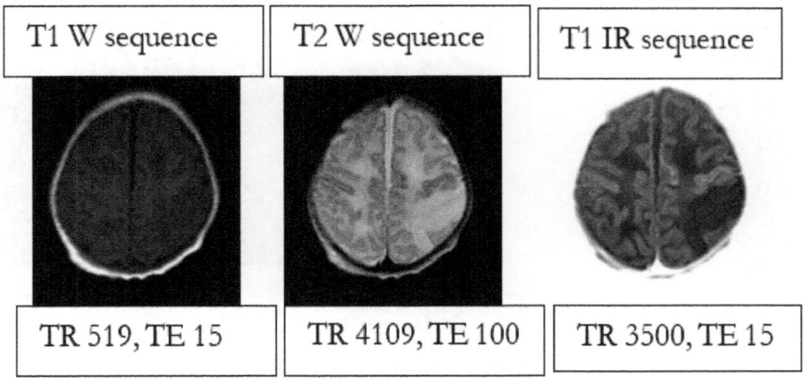

Fig. 27.10 Comparison of T1, T2 and T1 IR (inversion recovery) sequence. Note the improved gray-white differentiation in the T1 IR sequence as compared to the T1W sequence

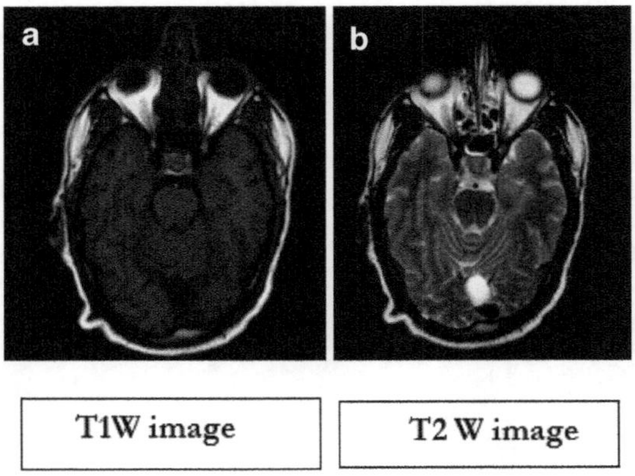

Fig. 27.11 (**a**, **b**) T1 W (**a**) and T2 W (**b**) sequences. Note the dark signal of flowing blood in the carotid siphon in both T1 and T2W sequences. When the blood clots, the T2 signals become bright

27.4 Vascular and Contrast-Enhanced Studies

- **Non-contrast MR angiograms (MRA)and venograms (MRV)** can be done using flow-sensitive time-of-flight (TOF) sequences or phase contrast sequences. MRA is performed using a 3D TOF sequence, while MRV is performed using a 2D TOF sequence. The drawback with these sequences is that since they are projection images and not contrast-enhanced studies, they suffer from artefactual distortions caused by turbulent blood flow, around areas of narrowing. Hence, they can overestimate the length of a stenotic segment (Figs. 27.12 and 27.13).

Contrast-enhanced MR angiography is performed using T1W 3D spoiled gradient echo sequences. If a contrast study is being performed, it must be clear whether it is for an angiogram, a venogram or a parenchymal study. This allows proper planning of the study. Angiographic and venographic studies are performed as soon as contrast is administered to capture densely opacified contrast flowing through these vessels. On the other hand, parenchymal studies can be performed after a few minutes delay in order to allow contrast to seep into the lesions through the break in the blood-brain barrier.

- **Contrast-Enhanced MRA:**

  A contrast-enhanced study is performed immediately after administering an IV Gadolinium-based contrast agent. A 3D GRE sequence is performed using short TR, TE (TR23 TE 6.5 for arterial phase and TR 15.0 and TE 6.6 for MRV sequence). A maximum intensity projection image (MIP) display is performed with these sequences to highlight the vessels (Figs. 27.14 and 27.15).
- **CEMRI**: This is a contrast-enhanced study for brain parenchymal lesions using a 3DT1 W sequence. It is timed differently as compared to an MRA or MRV sequence. The scan is usually carried out after an interval of 5–10 min post-IV contrast injection.

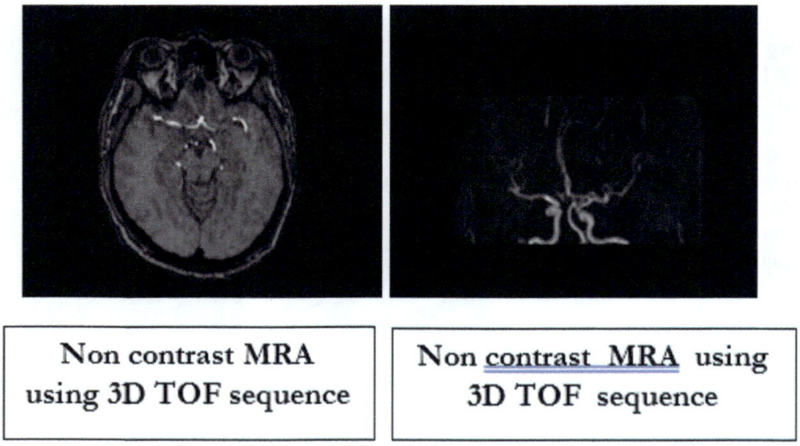

Fig. 27.12 Non-contrast Angiogram of the brain, using 3D TOF sequence

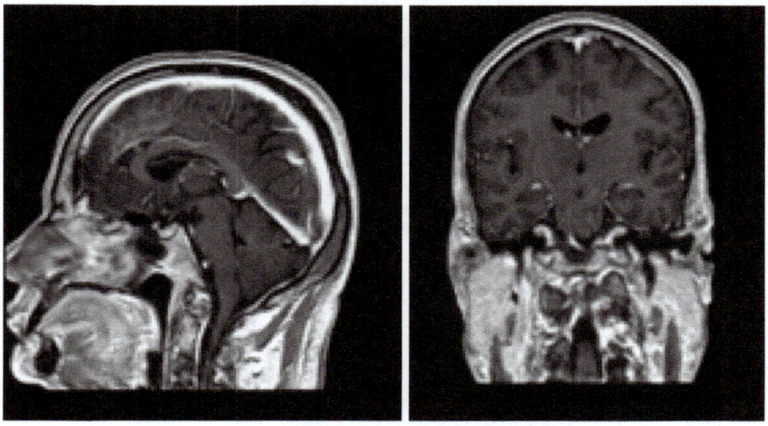

Fig. 27.13 Non-contrast MR Venography using 2D TOF sequence

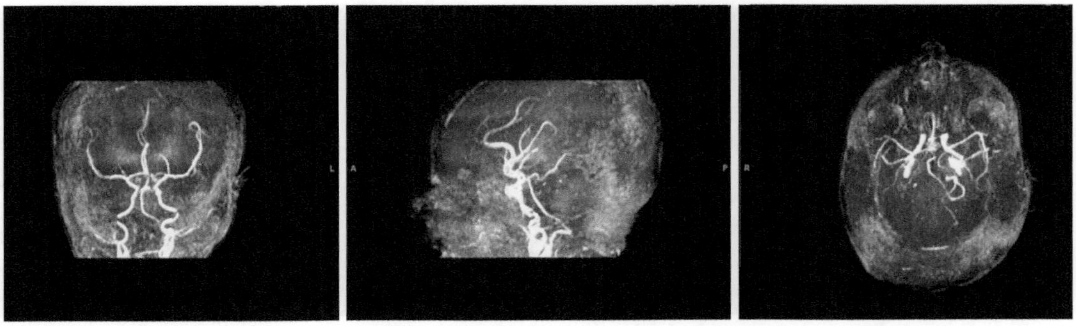

Fig. 27.14 Contrast-enhanced MIP, MRA sequence of the brain demonstrating the intracranial arteries

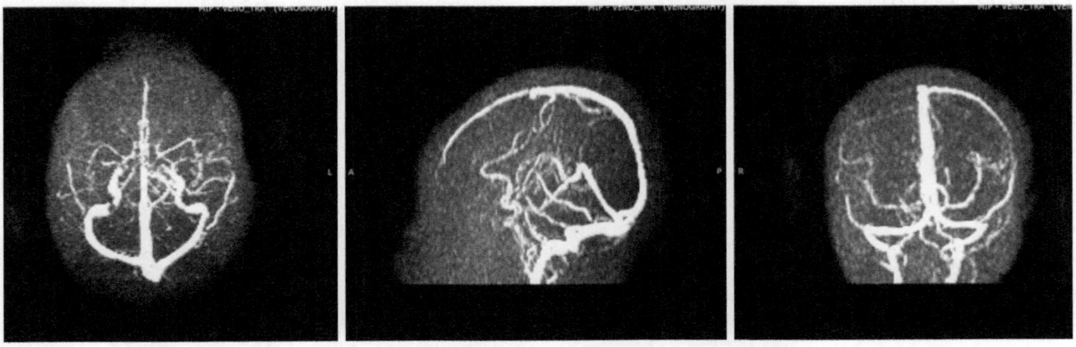

Fig. 27.15 Contrast-enhanced MIP, MRV sequence performed to demonstrate the dural venous sinuses

27.5 CSF Flow Study

- CSF flow studies require phase contrast imaging. CSF flows caudally during systole and cranially during diastole. Hence ECG gating is necessary. To assess CSF flow through the aqueduct, sagittal "in-plane" T2 W images and axial "through-plane", sections are obtained. Rapidly flowing CSF appears dark in this sequence. A magnitude and a phase image are also obtained, in addition to the T2W sequence, to map the CSF flow. The CSF flow is also shown in a graphic format with the cardiac cycle. The flow is below the baseline during systole and above it during diastole.
- **Study of Intracranial Nerves** [3]:
  These include 3DFLAIR, 3DT1, 3DT2, 3D contrast-enhanced sequences, Steady-State Free Precession (SSFP) sequence and DWI sequences. A T2 DRIVE, which is a fast T2W sequence, in which the TR is shorter compared to the conventional T2 W sequence, is particularly useful for studying the CSF-containing regions such as in the internal auditory canal [3], around the brainstem and spinal cord. The CSF looks brighter, and the nerves as well as the cord stand out as dark structures against the white CSF background (Figs. 27.16 and 27.17).

MR Spectroscopy: The sequences used for MRS are tailored to detect metabolites having different resonant frequencies. These sequences can be single voxel or multivoxel sequences. Since the resonant frequencies of metabolites are very close to one another, they need to be spread apart on the baseline to distinguish them from each other. This is done by using short TE or long TE sequences. Short TE sequences use a TE of 25–30 ms while long TE ranges between 135 and 144 ms.

How to view the MR images: Pair them with one another or place them in sets (Fig. 27.18).

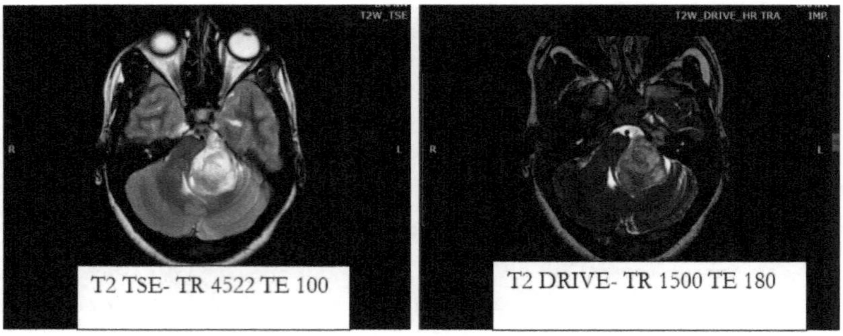

Fig. 27.16 Comparison between T2 TSE and T2 DRIVE. Note the shorter TR in the DRIVE sequence and the brightness of the CSF surrounding the left CP angle mass

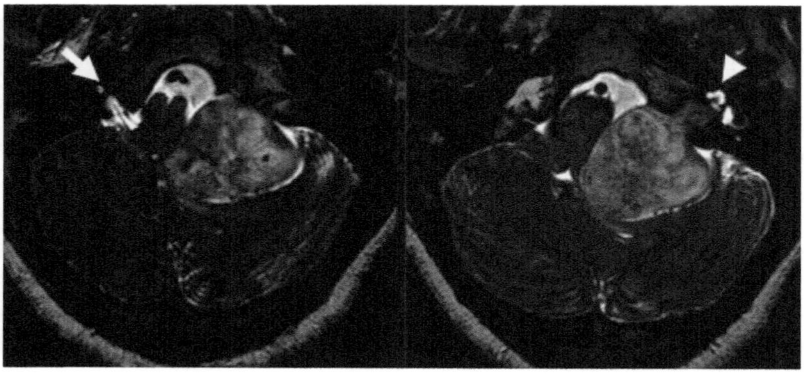

Fig. 27.17 T2 DRIVE sequence. Note the structures in the internal auditory canal (arrow) as the inner ear structures (arrowhead)

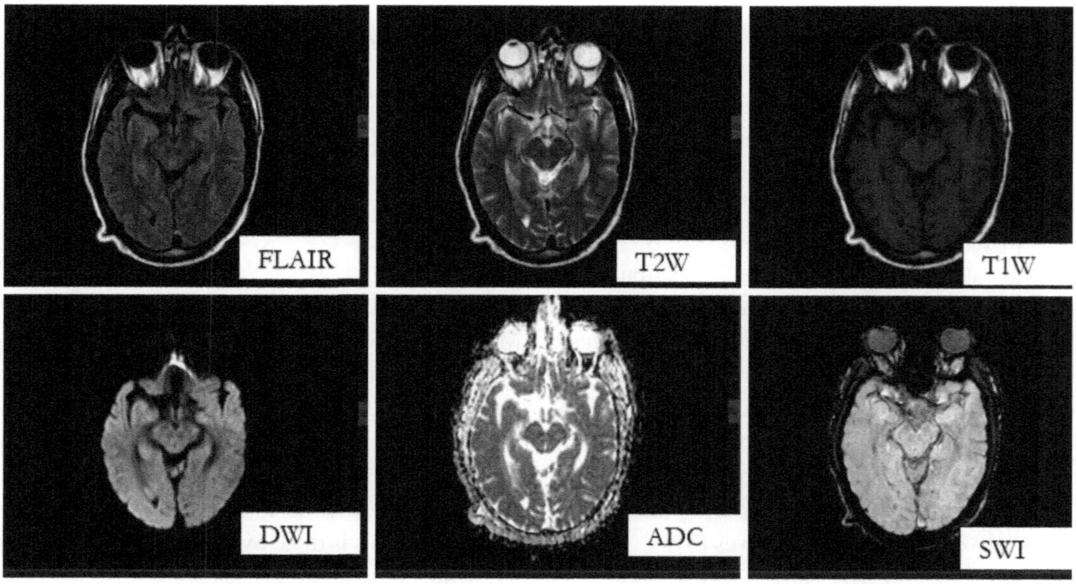

Fig. 27.18 Set of images stacked for viewing. It is good to arrange images as a set of different sequences. In this way, the appearance of the pathological lesion in various phases can be easily compared and studied

27.6 MRI Sequences for Body Imaging (Abdomen and Pelvis)

There are several techniques available for performing body MRI. Most of these techniques incorporate certain basic sequences which will be discussed here.

- **Localizer**: Obtain a 3-plane single breathhold, end-expiratory, localizer with a large field of view. The localizer could be a T1 W fast spin echo sequence, an SSFSE (HASTE) or a balanced gradient echo sequence. The SSFSE and balanced sequence often provide clinically relevant information, such as the presence of calculi in a distended gall bladder and CBD. The balanced GRE sequence can be distinguished from the SSFSE sequence, by the bright signals of blood flow it shows in comparison to the dark signals of flowing blood seen in the SSFSE sequence. A T2W spin echo sequence is not used as a localizer, because of the long time it takes to complete (Fig. 27.19).
- **T2W sequence**: This sequence provides information about cystic lesions, bowel loops, the urinary tract, the biliary system and iron deposition (which appears dark on the T2W sequence). To acquire T2W images, fast spin echo or turbo spin echo sequences (FSE or TSE, F standing for fast, T stands for turbo), SSFSE and sometimes balanced steady-state sequences are used. The advantage of the SSFSE and balanced steady-state sequence is that, since these sequences are very fast and require breathhold for a few seconds only, Also, if for some reason the study has to be discontinued, the information gained from fluid-filled structures may be sufficient to arrive at a preliminary diagnosis. Non-fluid-containing areas appear too dark in these heavily T2W sequences for a meaningful interpretation, hence a conventional T2W sequence (with and without fat suppression) is always needed. In patients where respiratory motion-related artefacts are anticipated, respiratory gating can be applied to get a respiratory blur-minimized image. The images of the abdomen in the T2W sequence are obtained in axial and coronal planes. In the 2D SSFSE sequence, images are acquired in coronal and in the 3D sequence, in orthogonal (multiple) planes. The FOV in the SSFSE sequence is limited to the area under investigation. To minimize blurring in the T2 W sequence, fast scanning using parallel imaging (SENSE) can also be applied. The SSFSE sequences can be replaced by steady-state sequences which also provide T2 weighting at a fast speed. One of the advantages of steady-state sequence over SSFSE sequence is that blood appears brighter in this sequence, a phenomenon called flow-related enhancement. It happens because the background signals are suppressed by repeated application of RF pulses, but the continuously

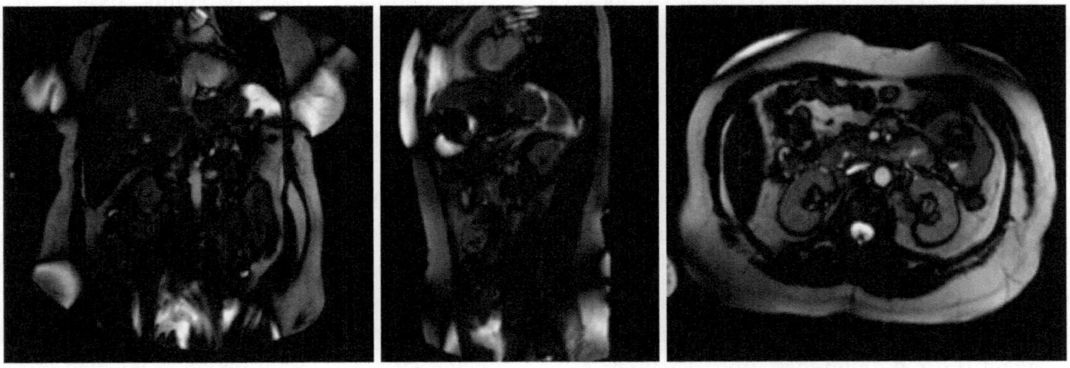

Fig. 27.19 A 3-plane balanced steady-state sequence used as a localizer. Note the bright signals in the aorta

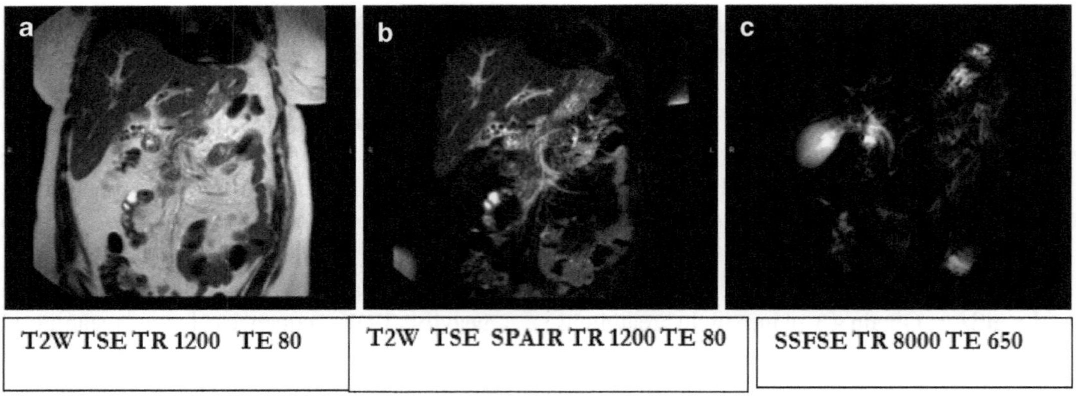

Fig. 27.20 (a–c) T2W TSE, T2 TSE SPAIR (fat suppressing inversion recovery sequence used with T2 weighting sequence) and SSFSE sequences

inflowing blood does not stay for too long in the slice to get saturated and therefore appears bright. This enables the detection of intravascular clots which appear dark in the bright signal-intensity flowing blood. The signal-to-noise ratio is higher in the SSFSE (MRCP) sequence as compared to the balanced sequence; hence, it is preferred for performing MRCP studies (Fig. 27.20).

The T2W sequences can be performed immediately after a localizer scan, especially if IV Gadolinium contrast is to be administered. This is because IV Gadolinium contrast may alter the signals of the tissues surrounding the fluid-containing structures and affect the interpretation of the T2 W images. The same principle applies to contrast-enhanced MR urography. The T2 W sequence must be performed first and then Gadolinium be administered.

T2W 3D sequences: These are sequences which produce images of excellent resolution and are used for prostate imaging, female pelvis imaging and oblique views of the rectum. They are known by acronyms CUBE (GE), SPACE (Siemens) and VISTA (Philips). These are single acquisition sequences with a shorter scan time capable of multiplanar reconstructions.

- **T1 W sequences**: These sequences are used primarily before Gadolinium-based contrast agent (GBCA) administration. They are also markers of protein contents in the body. That is why the normal liver, pancreas, blood clots, necrotic lesions and melanin appear bright in the T1W sequence. T1 W gradient echo sequence as well as in- and opposed-phase sequences are used for the detection of fat and iron. Fat signals are dropped in the opposed-phase sequence, while iron signals are dropped in the in-phase sequence. Presently, the 4-point Dixon technique is used instead of in- and opposed-phase sequences, as it provides images of in and opposed phases as well as fat-only and water-only sequences (Fig. 27.21).
- **T1 Contrast Sequences**: T1W sequences are performed with IV contrast administration. These T1 W sequences are spoiled gradient echo 3D sequences with fat suppression, in which the transverse magnetization is spoiled. This suppresses bright signals from the adjoining stationary fluid-containing tissues and highlights T1 short lesions and Gadolinium-related contrast enhancement. They require a few short and successive breathholds. They are commonly used for liver imaging and are known by acronyms such as VIBE, THRIVE and LAVA (as per vendor's nomenclature). They are fast scans with short acquisition time (approximately 15–20 s breathhold). Parallel imaging is also applied to these sequences. The contrast-enhanced study is performed using IV Gadolinium which is injected intra-

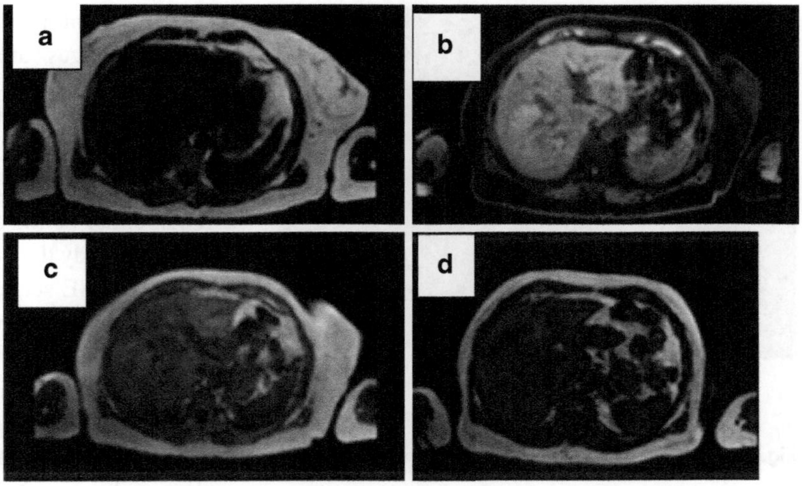

Fig. 27.21 A four-point Dixon technique, showing (**a**) fat-only, (**b**) water-only, (**c**) in- and (**d**)opposed-phase images

venously in a dose of 0.1–0.2 mL/kg body weight, with a slow injection given at the rate of 1–2 mL/s. Delayed arterial at 35 s, and venous phases at 70 s are routinely obtained. The late phase at 7–10 min post-injection may also be obtained to understand how contrast is distributed in lesions such as haemangiomas. An even further delay of up to 155 min may be needed in patients with tumours containing a high level of desmoplastic tissue, which enhances slowly.

- **Diffusion-Weighted Imaging (DWI) and ADC Maps**: These sequences are performed using T2 gradient echoplanar imaging. Tumours, especially solid and metastatic tumours, abscesses and lymph nodes, particularly necrotic, appear bright and are well delineated by DWI sequence. The "b" value (which depends on gradient strength and its duration of application) should be kept a 1000 or higher. A "b0" gradient strength is like a T2W image. The higher the b value, the greater the suppression of Brownian motion in liquid-containing areas resulting in diffusion restriction. At higher b values, only abnormal tissue will show diffusion restriction, that is they will appear bright in the DWI sequence and dark in the ADC map. The DWI sequence can be performed after IV contrast administration.

27.7 Additional Sequences

- *MRCP Sequence*: This is an optional sequence and is always used when evaluation of the biliary tract is the primary objective. It is a heavily T2W, SSFSE sequence using a high TE to suppress the background signals including signals of flowing blood and highlight signals of fluid-filled structures such as the biliary system. Both 2D and 3D sequences are obtained. The former can be done without respiratory gating while the latter needs respiratory gating. The images are obtained in the coronal plane (2D) as well as in the orthogonal plane (3D sequence) (Fig. 27.22).
- *Forced Recovery (Driven) Fast Spin Echo Sequence*: This sequence is also known as "Driven Equilibrium Fourier Transformation" (DEFT) sequence. In this sequence, another 180° refocusing pulse followed by a 90° RF pulse, to quickly drive the magnetization back to the "Z"-axis, is applied. This hastens recovery of longitudinal magnetization, which means that tissues having a long T1 relaxation time, such as water/CSF, can be visualized using a short TR. The sequence provides, both, a good T2 contrast density as well a fast speed. Its TR and TE are between those of T2W TSE and SSFSE sequences.

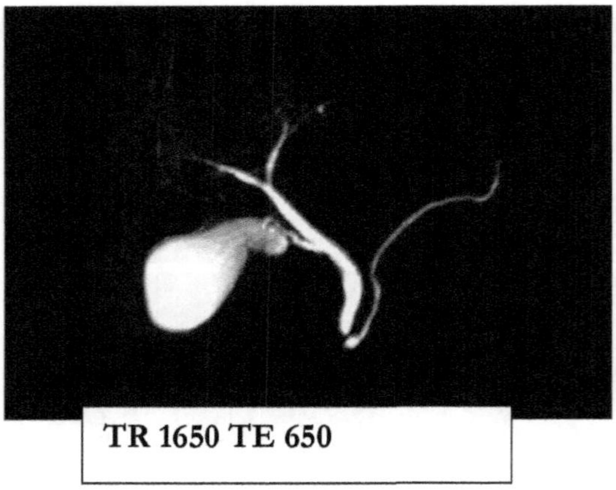

Fig. 27.22 Heavily T2 W, SSFSE MRCP sequence

- *Parallel Imaging*: This is a technique which can be applied to any sequence to reduce scan time (speed up the scanning). It is done using a phased array (multi-element) surface coil.

27.8 Patient Preparation and Planning for Abdominal and Pelvic MRI

- **MRI of the Abdomen**: The patient should be fasting for 4 h. There is no restriction on medication and water, except when MRCP is being performed. The urinary bladder should be partially filled. Since the procedure may get prolonged, a patient with a full bladder might get uncomfortable and may move during scanning, hence the precaution. Make sure to check all records before commencing the procedure. The patient should wear loose clothes and leave valuables outside the gantry room in a locker or with an attendant.
- **MRI of the Pelvis**: The urinary bladder should be partially filled. Plan the study along the orientation of the uterus, so that coronal, axial and sagittal scan images are obtained along the length and true axial planes of the endometrium. T2TSE sequence in axial, coronal and sagittal planes with and without fat suppression and T1 TSE with and without fat suppression are obtained. A 2D T1-SPGR sequence with fat suppression is also obtained when IV contrast is administrated. Diffusion weight images are obtained especially in tumour evaluation.
- **MRI in Ob-Gyn**: The patient is imaged in the supine position using a phased array coil. The area covered depends on the clinical scenario. It can either be the entire abdomen or just the pelvis to study the uterus and adnexa. A multiplanar SSFSE sequence is used. Axial, coronal and sagittal views are obtained based on the clinical question. In case where a foetus/foetal organ/anatomy is to be evaluated, planning is modified accordingly. The scan is mainly focused on the fetal anatomy where an abnormality is suspected or has been detected by prior ultrasound examination. A T1 SPGR sequence can be added to look for any intracranial bleeding. DWI sequence is included in the protocol, as it helps determine placental infiltration into the myometrium, especially in cases of placenta accreta syndrome. IV contrast is avoided during pregnancy.
- **MR enterography**. The patient should be on a liquid/semisolid diet for 2 days, to clear the bowel of any solid contents. Then, on the day of scanning, about 1.2–1.5 L of mannitol, 2.5% is given, which is to be had within 45 min. This contrast has a biphasic effect, in that it appears dark on T1 and bright on T2 sequences. The T2 W sequences used are SSFSE and balanced gradient echo sequences, with and without fat suppression, with images obtained in coronal and axial planes. In the balanced sequence, the intraluminal contrast as well as the mesenteric vessels are better seen. The SSFSE sequence with fat suppression shows mucosal oedema more clearly. The T1W study is a 2D and 3D sequence both without and with fat suppression (fat suppression is needed if administration of IV Gadolinium is contemplated). Before starting this sequence, an antiperistaltic agent is administered to reduce bowel movement. The imagies are acquired in coronal and axial planes. IV contrast images should be obtained during delayed arterial and delayed venous and parenchymal phases. This is because some of the lesions show delayed contrast enhancement, especially if there is

fibrosis in the bowel wall. A DWI sequence can also be added to detect bowel wall oedema as well as the presence of mesenteric nodes. DWI sequence is also useful in the detection of tumours, especially residual, following adequate surgical/ medical treatment. The slice thickness should be between 3 and 5 mm, and scans should be performed using breathhold or respiratory gating, to minimize motion-related artefacts.

- **MR Urography**: The patient should be fasting for 4 h. Before beginning the study, ensure that the patient is well hydrated, for good hydration helps in distending the renal outflow tract. Hydration should be through the intravenous and not oral route or else fluid in the stomach and bowel loops might overly the urinary tract and obscure abnormality, if any. The urinary bladder should not be overdistended. Coronal T2W sequence using SSFSE is used to evaluate the entire urinary tract. In order not to miss any small lesion, the pelvic region can be evaluated separately, in the axial plane. The use of intravenous contrast is indicated when a tumour is being studied, otherwise it is not necessary and should be avoided, especially in a case of chronic kidney disease or acute renal failure [4]. Intravenous injection of Gadolinium 0.1 mL/kg body weight diluted with an equal volume of normal saline or distilled water is injected at 2 mL/s. A T1W spoiled gradient recalled echo (SPGR) sequence is performed in coronal and sagittal planes. Fat-suppressed 3D T1 W SPGR sequence is also run. This sequence is performed using a large flip angle, for better suppression of background noise. In and opposed sequences are also performed to detect fat within renal masses. The slice thickness is kept at 3 mm. The study can also be performed using a diuretic, such as Lasix (Furosemide). When administered with intravenous fluids, it leads to increased production of urine and distension of the urinary outflow tract.
- **MR Fistulography**: The study can be performed without preparation and breathhold. After obtaining a 3-plane localizer of the pelvis, scanning is performed in axial and coronal planes, by applying T2 FS or STIR sequences and using a small field of view (FOV). Axial and coronal T1 W sequences are also obtained with and without fat saturation, to evaluate the anorectal region and ischiorectal fossa area for any abnormality in the surrounding fat planes, the presence of a fistulous tract which appears dark due to fibrosis should be looked for, in this non fat suppressed T1W sequence. A contrast-enhanced T1 W sequence may also be obtained to look for any active disease in this region. Abscesses will be visible in a T1FS sequence as a hyperintense collection. A DWI image may also be added to highlight active lesions, such as abscesses, which will appear bright in this sequence and dark in the ADC map. The study should cover the pelvis from the sacrum to the anal verge and the slice thickness to be used should be 3 mm.
- **MRI for Pelvis Floor** (MR defecography). Axial images are obtained using T1TSE and T2TSE sequences in planes parallel to the anorectum. Sagittal T1 and T2 W images are also obtained. The scans are performed both in the resting phase and while performing the act of defecation. The defecating phase is the dynamic component of the study and needs fast scanning using multiple images. This is done by using a balanced steady-state free precession sequence. For this sequence, the anorectal region is first distended with ultrasound gel which is introduced per-rectally. The patient is asked to squeeze, hold and then relax. This manoeuvre should be rehearsed at least 3–4 times, before the final performance. In this way, the pelvic floor descent, hence incompetence, can be visualized.
- **MRI for Rectal Cancer**: In this study, T1TSE and T2 TSE weighted sequences **without fat saturation** are obtained. Fat saturation can mask tumour infiltration and peritoneal reflections. Scanning is performed in axial, coronal and sagittal planes. The axial plane should be at right angles to the rectal mass. The sagittal plane should align with the anorectum while the coronal plane should be parallel to the length of the tumour. Fat suppressed contrast-enhanced and DWI sequences are used following surgery or chemotherapy to look for

residual tumours or local recurrence. These post-operative studies should be performed after at least 6–8 weeks interval [5]. The slice thickness, as for the other regions, should be 3 mm. Spasmolytics may be needed where there is excessive bowel movement, which can be judged from the localizer images.

Note: There is no restriction on medications, especially in hypertensive and diabetic patients for any of the above studies.

- **MRI of the Prostate**: A phased array pelvic coil is used. An endorectal coil if available gives a better resolution of the prostate. However, if a 3 T instead of a 1.5 T magnet is used, the resolution is excellent in most cases the endorectal coil may not be needed. The sequences used are multiplanar T2 W TSE sequence, DWI sequence and dynamic contrast-enhanced (DCE) sequences. The field of view should be small (between 12 and 20 cm), and the echo-train length of the T2 W TSE sequence should be short because a long echo-train length causes blurring of images. The DCE sequence should preferably be a 3D sequence. The scan plane should be aligned with the prostate in all sequences [6, 7].
- **MR Angiography**: This can be performed with or without using IV contrast. When performing scans with contrast, obtain a precontract 3D T1 SPGR sequence. Then depending upon whether the thoracic aorta or abdominal vessels are being evaluated, use ECG or respiratory gating. The thoracic aorta is evaluated at the end of diastole when the cardiac motion is at its minimum. Evaluation of extremity vessels is done in multiple steps of table movement to cover the entire area., Atleast two phases, early and late arterial should be acquired. Thereafter, subtraction of the pre- from the post-contrast scan yields only an enhanced image of the vessels and their branches without any other background shadow.

  Contrast-enhanced time-resolved MRA can also be performed to ascertain the rate and direction of contrast flow through an image. In these sequences, multiple images are acquired from a vessel every 1–3 s. This enables visualization of the rate of blood flow from the artery to the veins.

  A non-contrast MRA can also be performed using a 3D steady-state free precession (balanced steady-state sequences). These sequences are better than TOF sequences because the latter have a longer scan time and also are affected by the tortuosity of vessels, where there can be signal loss. The steady-state sequences need ECG gating for the thoracic vessels. In the abdomen and pelvis, there is a need for background suppression which can be done by adding an inversion pulse sequence. Subtraction is also possible in this sequence. Images are obtained in both systole and diastole. There is suppression of only arterial signals in systole while both arteries and veins are visible in diastole. Thus on subtracting the systolic image from the diastolic images, only arteries are imaged.

  To study the velocity of blood flow, phase contrast MRI can be used. Using the VENC (velocity encoding) sequence, the velocity of blood flow can be assessed. VENC values in cm/s are chosen according to which vessel, a vein or an artery, is being examined. For veins and CSF flow, a low VENC is chosen while for arteries, a higher VENC is applied.

  Phase contrast MRI can either be a 2D acquisition to evaluate intracardiac velocities or a 3D acquisition, to evaluate velocities in all directions. The intracardiac velocity is obtained by combining the velocity encoding sequence obtained in the X, Y and Z axes with time-resolved data. This becomes a 4D acquisition.

  In addition to the above sequences, vessel wall imaging, using dark blood 2D or 3D TSE sequence can also be performed to evaluate vessel wall diseases. These include the study of atherosclerosis, vasculitis, presence of haemorrhage or fat in the vessel walls. The stiffness of vessel walls can also be estimated using MR elastography.
- **MR Sequences for Musculoskeletal Imaging** Before commencing the study, it is good practice to look at all previous records. Plain films

of the affected area must be reviewed. A detailed history and physical evaluation always help.

- The following sequences are applied:
  - Fluid-sensitive sequence, both with and without fat suppression is used. It is T2 TSE with FS. A STIR sequence can also be used. In these sequences, muscles, tendons, nerves and cartilages such as menisci appear dark.
  - Hydrogen-rich sequences such as proton density sequences are preferred by many because compared to the T2 W sequence, the images are less dark (greyish) and allow adequate tissue differentiation.
  - T1 TSE sequence is used to study bones, fat, muscles and masses, if any. In a T1W, fractures are seen as dark lines traversing the bones.
  - If IV Gd is likely to be administered, T1 TSE with fat saturation should be used. A STIR sequence will obscure everything capable of T1 shortening, including the signals of IV contrast.
  - A 3D fat-suppressed T1 SPGR sequence may be used to study the physes in children.
  - A dual-echo steady-state (DESS) sequence is used for cartilage evaluation.
  - The images acquired by fluid-sensitive T2 W sequence and PD sequence should be in axial, coronal, oblique and sagittal planes, relative to the bone and joint under examination. The T1 W scan should be sagittal and coronal relative to the bones and joints.

MR of the Chest in Children and Adults: Most small children will need sedation. Older children and adults will need to be explained the study in detail and made comfortable. They wilol need earplugs and some other distracting device which will let them stay still during the examination. They may have respiratory distress, hence scanning should be quick and tailored to acquire relevant data quickly. A surface coil, meant to receive signals, should be closely fitting for a better signal-to-noise ratio. Fast sequences such as T2TSE, SSFSE and GRE sequences should be used. The T2W, fat-suppressed sequences are used to show fluid-containing parenchymal lesions, such as consolidation, necrotic masses, acute interstitial lung diseases and vascular lesions. These sequences are obtained in coronal and axial planes. The GRE sequences such as SPGR and balanced steady-state sequences are used for imaging blood vessels, airspaces and airways. Vessels and airways appear dark in the spoiled gradient echo sequences. In the balanced sequence, vessels appear bright. The airways can be dynamically studied using a narrow 3D SGPR sequence with images obtained during various phases of free breathing, especially to assess the presence or absence of tracheobronchomalacia. The lung parenchyma can also be assessed by the 3D GRE sequence to look for any evidence of parenchymal bleeding, bronchiectasis with retained secretions, bronchial asthma with mucus plugs or mass with mixed attenuation values. This can be followed by a contrast-enhanced 3D SPGR sequence with fat suppression, especially for evaluation of any lung or pleural mass. The same sequences can be used to evaluate the mediastinum in coronal and axial planes. Fat suppression may be needed to rule in rule out fat-containing lesions.

MRI of Heart and Great Vessels: This region is studied using fast T1 and T2 W spin echo and gradient echo sequences such as SPGR and SSFP sequences to produce dark and bright blood images. The images are obtained in all three axes both with and without fat suppression. Breathholding is not needed. For children, a body-hugging receiver coil is preferred to achieve a better signal-to-noise ratio. A delayed contrast-enhanced dark blood sequence is also obtained to look for any enhancing endocardial/myocardial lesion. Steady-state sequences can also be used to produce cine images of the cardiac shadow.

MR Neurography: This technique is used to study peripheral nerves, brachial and lumbosacral plexus. A 3 T MR is preferred over a 1.5 T unit. Following a multiplanar localizer, scanning is performed along the direction of the nerves and plexus in all planes. Both T1 and T2 TSE sequences are acquired. This enables the study of muscles which can atrophy and show fat replacement., following nerve damage. Additional images are obtained using STIR sequences to improve nerve-to-muscle contrast [8] and adequately suppress fat signals [9]. However, the STIR sequence suffers from noise and image degradation. Hence, a T2 SPAIR sequence is preferred. Sometimes signals from surrounding vessels, fat, muscles and bones interfere with the MR signals of nerves These signals can be suppressed using Gadolinium-enhanced 3D FSE, and STIR sequences [9, 10]. Besides all these sequences, conventional MR images with a large field of view should also be obtained. A dual-echo steady-state (DESS) sequence may be considered especially for the evaluation of facial nerve [11].

Flexible surface coils, which fit well in the area under investigation, should be used. For MR neurography. Respiratory gating may be needed to obtain movement-free images of the brachial plexus.

In conclusion, these are some of the MR protocols, which are used in routine practice. They are often modified and remodified as per institutional preferences and with evolving expertise.

References

1. Di Muzio B, Murphy A, Lecyk J, et al. Brain screen protocol (MRI). Radiopaedia.org. Accessed 18 June 2024. https://doi.org/10.53347/rID-37784.
2. Shawky M, Habib R, Elsawaf A. T1 inversion recovery pulse sequence: could it replace T1 spin echo sequence in neuroimaging by improving tissue contrast? Egypt J Radiol Nucl Med. 2019;50:26. https://doi.org/10.1186/s43055-019-0028-5.
3. Romano N, Federici M, Castaldi A. Imaging of cranial nerves: a pictorial overview. Insights Imaging. 2019;10:33. https://doi.org/10.1186/s13244-019-0719-5.
4. Weinreb JC, Rodby RA, Yee J, Wang CL, Fine D, McDonald RJ, Perazella MA, Dillman JR, Davenport MS. Use of intravenous gadolinium-based contrast media in patients with kidney disease: consensus statements from the American College of Radiology and the National Kidney Foundation. Kidney Med. 2020;3(1):142–50. https://doi.org/10.1016/j.xkme.2020.10.001. PMID: 33604544; PMCID: PMC7873723.
5. Seo N, Kim H, Cho MS, Lim JS. Response assessment with MRI after chemoradiotherapy in rectal cancer: current evidences. Korean J Radiol. 2019;20(7):1003–18. https://doi.org/10.3348/kjr.2018.0611. PMID: 31270972; PMCID: PMC6609432.
6. Papoutsaki MV, Allen C, Giganti F, et al. Standardisation of prostate multiparametric MRI across a hospital network: a London experience. Insights Imaging. 2021;12:52. https://doi.org/10.1186/s13244-021-00990-y.
7. Yuan Q. Prostate MRI protocols. PhD Department of Radiology UT Southwestern Medical Center Dallas, Texas. AAPM; 2021. http://amos3.aapm.org/abstracts/pdf/166-57948-15651646-171901-482520230.pdf.
8. Sneag DB, Daniels SP, Geannette C, Queler SC, Lin BQ, de Silva C, et al. Post-contrast 3D inversion recovery magnetic resonance neurography for evaluation of branch nerves of the brachial plexus. Eur J Radiol. 2020;132:109304.
9. Jung JY, Lin Y, Carrino JA. An updated review of magnetic resonance neurography for plexus imaging. Korean J Radiol. 2023;24(11):1114–30. https://doi.org/10.3348/kjr.2023.0150. PMID: 37899521; PMCID: PMC10613850.
10. Zhang Y, Kong X, Zhao Q, Liu X, Gu Y, Xu L. Enhanced MR neurography of the lumbosacral plexus with robust vascular suppression and improved delineation of its small branches. Eur J Radiol. 2020;129:109128.
11. Kwon D, Lee C, Chae Y, Kwon IJ, Kim SM, Lee JH. Clinical validation of the 3-dimensional double-echo steady-state with water excitation sequence of MR neurography for preoperative facial and lingual nerve identification. Imaging Sci Dent. 2022;52(3):259–66. https://doi.org/10.5624/isd.20220035. Epub 2022 May 13. PMID: 36238701; PMCID: PMC9530289.

Contrast Studies in CT and MRI

28

Abstract

Oral and Intravenous contrast is often needed in both MRI and CT scans to evaluate anatomical and pathological processes involving the gut, blood vessels, in the evaluation of vascular lesions and for vascular mapping in transplant patients. It is also needed in trauma patients, in studying response to treatment and in patients having active and profuse bleeding from any where in the body.

Therefore, it is essential to know about contrast medium which are used in imaging studies.

The CT contrast is iodine based while MR contrast is gadolinium based. While both contrasts have clinical uses, it must also be remembered that they can have side effects ranging from minor to very severe side effects. In this chapter, we will briefly view the various types of contrasts used in daily clinical practice.

Keywords

CT contrast · MR contrast · Iodinated contrast Gadolinium-based contrast · Side effects

CT Contrast: Contrast medium used in CT scans can be divided into oral, rectal, intravenous, intracavitary and intrathecal.

- **Oral contrast medium** [1–4]: The primary aim of oral contrast is to delineate the lumen of the stomach and small loops which gives an idea of luminal and mural pathology. Contrasts medium can be positive (iodinated, such as Gastrografin) or neutral (such as water, mannitol 2.5%, Volumen 0.1%, polyethylene glycol, milk and low-density barium). Negative (air) contrast, already present in the gastrointestinal tract, is also useful in evaluating both luminal and mural-based abnormalities. Oral positive contrasts are administered to evaluate perforations, post-operative anastomotic leaks and distinguishing peritoneal lesions and lymph nodes from bowel shadows. The drawback of oral positive contrast is that it obscures the intravenous contrast enhancement of bowel walls. It is akin to performing a conventional barium study which is purely an luminal study. Orally administered contrast is often unable to distend small bowel loops uniformly either due to reduced or rapid peristaltic activity. This leaves some of the small bowel loops in a contracted state even in an enteroclysis.

  There are several situations where routine administration of oral contrast of any type is unnecessary. These include patients with acute or chronic small bowel obstruction (particularly in those cases where plain films show air-fluid levels), cases of peritonitis, trauma,

R. Gothi, *Radiographic and Imaging Techniques for Radiology Residents and Technologists*,
https://doi.org/10.1007/978-981-96-4816-0_28

calculus disease of the urinary tract and gastrointestinal bleeding. Many patients are unable to drink the requisite amount of oral contrast due to nausea, vomiting or sheer dislike of the taste of contrast. The gut has a typical anatomy and disposition in the abdomen. Pathological bowel loops are often dilated or constricted. They can be thick-walled and maybe mass-forming. They may also be malpositioned, clumped, displaced or fixed in position (which might be seen in biphasic or delayed studies) hence, they can be distinguished from non-pathological loops. In such cases, giving IV contrast is sufficient because the intravenous contrast enhancement, if any, of the mucosa and bowel walls can be easily identified. With a little experience, bowel loops can also be easily distinguished from adjoining nodes or peritoneal lesions. Giving oral contrast routinely, delays scanning till the patient has consumed all the oral contrast. In patients who are likely to undergo conservative management, oral positive contrast can be administered and followed up with X-rays rather than a CT scan. The use of oral contrast is a debatable topic and often depends upon the institutional and radiologist's preference.

- **Rectal Contrast**: Air, water and positive iodinated contrast (20 mL iodine 300 mg/mL diluted in a litre of water) can be introduced rectally as an enema. The volume of contrast administered depends upon the patient's tolerance and capacity to retain it for the period of the study. Once contrast has been administered, if possible, the patient should be asked to roll over 360° on the couch, to allow proper dispersal of contrast in the left and right colon.
- **Intravenous Contrast**: Non-ionic iodinated contrast is used. The strength of iodine varies from 300 mg/mL for parenchymal study to 350–370 mg/mL for vascular study.
- **Intracavitary Studies**: These studies include CT cystogram, hysterogram, sinogram and contrast administration through colostomy to evaluate the distal colonic tract. An infant feeding tube or a cannula can be used to introduce contrast (usually iodine 300 mg/mL). The quantity of contrast needed depends upon the examination being conducted.
- **Intrathecal Contrast**: About 10–20 mL iodinated non-ionic contrast (Omnipaque 300 mg/mL) is injected under fluoroscopic guidance through a lumbar puncture. The patient is then turned prone with the chin flexed. The table is tilted by 45° and the patient is kept in the Trendelenburg position for approximately 2–5 min after contrast administration [5]. This allows the contrast to enter the basal intracranial CSF cisterns. Scanning of the paranasal sinuses, which includes the skull base, is performed in the supine position [6]. The scan sections are obtained from the top of the frontal sinuses till below the level of the maxillary sinuses. The images are displayed in both soft tissue and bone windows. The soft tissue windows are meant to see the density of fluid in the sinonasal area. High density of the fluid is consistent with leaked contrast enhanced CSF. Bone window images help delineate the integrity of the bony structures from where CSF leak can occur. This study is performed to determine the site of the leak in a case of CSF rhinorrhea. It is always wise to obtain a pre-contrast CT of the paranasal sinus. This helps in distinguishing high-density CSF from other causes of fluid collection in the paranasal sinuses.

28.1 MR Contrast: Gadolinium-Based Contrast Agents (GBCA)

Gadolinium (Gd)-based contrast is used to detect the contrast uptake in non-vascular structures as well as for the performance of angiography. Gadolinium is a paramagnetic substance from the Lanthanide group of heavy metals. Compared to CT contrast, it is relatively safer. However, it can also cause hypersensitivity reactions. Nephrogenic system fibrosis can occur in patients with severe renal impairment. It can also affect the pancreas, causing pancreatitis [7], deposit in the brain and affect nerve conduction and muscle contraction [8].

To ensure quick exit from the body and to avoid or minimize toxicity, Gd is chelated to a molecule which forms a complex that remains stable, till the time of its excretion from the body. The half-life of most gadolinium-based contrast agents (GBCA) is between 30 min and 2 hrs [9]. However, Gd can still deposit in bones [9] as well as in the brain [10], especially if it is injected multiple times. These molecules (or ligands) are either ring-shaped (macrocyclic) or open-chained (linear). The GB contrast agents can also be broken down into ionic and anionic / non ionic categories. The FDA has classified GBCAs into groups 1–3, based on their linear or macro-molecular structure and whether it is non-ionic or ionic. Groups 2 and 3 macromolecules and linear ionic contrasts dissociate less in the body as compared to group 1. Hence they are safer than the other GBCAs.

Most GBCAs are excreted through the urinary tract. Some GBCA can be excreted through both the urinary tract as well as through the biliary system. These are called hepatobiliary agents and can be used to study liver lesions as well as the biliary systems.

Some of the commonly used contrasts are:

- Gadopentetate dimeglumine (Magnevist) which is a linear ionic contrast group 1 contrast with a 2% dissociation.
- Gadobenate dimeglumine (Multihance) which is a linear ionic group 2 contrasts with a 2% dissociation. It can be used both for the study of vessels and vascularity of lesions as well as for hepatobiliary imaging.
- Gadoxetate disodium (Eovist) which is a linear ionic group 3 contrasts with a 1.1% dissociation rate. It is also used for hepatobiliary imaging.
- Among the macrocyclic non-ionic group 2 contrast with dissociation rate < 0.1% are Gadobutrol (Gadovist), Gadoteridol (Prohance) and Gadoterate meglumine (Dotarem).

It is safer to use group 2 contrast medium as per ACR guidelines. The macrocyclic grade 2 agents have a negligible effect on the brain and various other organs including the kidneys.

References

1. Heimer MM, Sun Y, Bonitatibus PJ, Yeh BM. Oral CT contrast agents: what's new and why, from the *AJR* special series on contrast media. AJR Am J Roentgenol. 2024;223:e2329970. https://doi.org/10.2214/AJR.23.29970. Epub ahead of print. PMID: 37877595.
2. Callahan MJ, Talmadge JM, MacDougall R, Buonomo C, Taylor GA. The use of enteric contrast media for diagnostic CT, MRI, and ultrasound in infants and children: a practical approach. Am J Roentgenol. 2016;206(5):973–9.
3. An C, Obmann MM, Sun Y, Wang ZJ, Sugi MD, Behr SC, Zagoria RJ, Woolen SA, Yeh BM. Positive versus neutral oral contrast material for detection of malignant deposits in intraabdominal nonsolid organs on CT. Am J Roentgenol. 2022;219(2):233–43.
4. Buturović-Ponikvar J, Višnar-Perovič A. Ultrasonography in chronic renal failure. Eur J Radiol. 2003;46(2):115–22. https://doi.org/10.1016/S0720-048X(03)00073-1.
5. Steele JR, Hoffman JC. Brainstem evaluation with CT cisternography. AJR Am J Roentgenol. 1981;136(2):287–92.
6. Hablas LT, Ammar AM, Elnagar RM. CSF rhinorrhea: non-contrast CT, contrast-enhanced CT cisternography or combined? Egypt J Radiol Nucl Med. 2022;53:201. https://doi.org/10.1186/s43055-022-00889-8.
7. Blasco-Perrin H, Glaser B, Pienkowski M, Peron JM, Payen JL. Gadolinium induced recurrent acute pancreatitis. Pancreatology. 2013;13(1):88–9. https://doi.org/10.1016/j.pan.2012.12.002. Epub 2012 Dec 10. PMID: 23395575.
8. Fraum TJ, Ludwig DR, Bashir MR, Fowler KJ. Gadolinium-based contrast agents: a comprehensive risk assessment. J Magn Reson Imaging. 2017;46(2):338–53. https://doi.org/10.1002/jmri.25625. Epub 2017 Jan 13. PMID: 28083913.
9. Darrah TH, Prutsman-Pfeiffer JJ, Poreda RJ, Ellen Campbell M, Hauschka PV, Hannigan RE. Incorporation of excess gadolinium into human bone from medical contrast agents. Metallomics. 2009;1(6):479–88. https://doi.org/10.1039/b905145g. Epub 2009 Sep 16. PMID: 21305156.
10. Kanda T, Fukusato T, Matsuda M, Toyoda K, Oba H, Kotoku J, Haruyama T, Kitajima K, Furui S. Gadolinium-based contrast agent accumulates in the brain even in subjects without severe renal dysfunction: evaluation of autopsy brain specimens with inductively coupled plasma mass spectroscopy. Radiology. 2015;276(1):228–32. https://doi.org/10.1148/radiol.2015142690. Epub 2015 May 5. PMID: 25942417.

29 Image Gently: Patient Safety in the Radiology Department

Abstract

X-rays, CT and MRI often are among some of the investigations used frequently in the management of patients. These investigations require radiation exposure, IV contrast administration and use of strong magnetic fields which can have adverse side effects, especially in the vulnerable population. The foetus in a pregnant woman, children and young persons must be specially cared for and imaged gently. Wherever possible non-radiation and non-contrast studies should be used. The harmful effect of MRI is lesser than X-rays and CT scans. Hence ultrasonography and MRI should be substituted, wherever possible. However, if it is a matter of choosing the most appropriate investigation in a given situation, there should be no hesitation in using X-rays and CT scans. The radiation and contrast-related risk may be much less than the lifesaving advantage, these investigations can offer.

Keywords

Safety · Harmful effect x-rays · CT · MRI risk benefit · Radiation · Contrast · Magnetic effect

The use of imaging modalities such as X-rays, CT and MRI is increasing exponentially. IV contrast is often needed in all modalities. X-rays and CT also suffer from the adverse risk of radiation to the patient while MR can cause potential harm through its powerful magnet and the use of IV GBCA, though this effect has reduced significantly with the availability of safer macrocyclic ionic (group 2) Gadolinium based contrast agents.

Keeping in mind the side effects, there is a need to reduce repeat scans and use appropriate doses of IV contrast and low radiation dose.

The term "image gently" was introduced to sensitize radiation technologists, radiologists and especially colleagues from the clinical disciplines to the harmful effects of several reimaging techniques and how best to lower their risk to the patient.

29.1 Some of the Steps that Can Be Taken to Safeguard Patients Are Described Herewith

X-rays

- Always enquire about any previous records. Old records are a great help in deciding whether the currently requested investigation is necessary or some other investigation should be substituted. Sometimes diseases have been present for a along time and without the benefit of previous records, they can be mistaken for a new development.

R. Gothi, *Radiographic and Imaging Techniques for Radiology Residents and Technologists*, https://doi.org/10.1007/978-981-96-4816-0_29

- The equipment should be adequately maintained and calibrated so that no untoward accident or abnormally high radiation exposure is given to the patient.
- While performing X-rays, try to obtain the most informative film on the first go.
- Collimate the X-ray beam to include only the part being investigated and avoid radiating the rest of the body.
- For small patients or while examining extremities, one can obtain a good film without the use of a bucky.
- Do not use fluoroscopy unnecessarily, especially to position the patient.
- Do not keep the fluoroscopy on for a prolonged period.
- The image intensifier should be close to the table, while the X-ray tube should be no less than 40 cm from the patient.
- Shield the gonads, breasts and thyroid if possible.
- The "10-day" rule should be applied to females coming for X-rays. The 10 days begin following the onset of menstruation [1].
- Technologists and radiologists should use lead aprons and thyroid shields while performing image-guided procedures.
- Hands should also be kept outside the radiation field while performing fluoroscopic procedures.

CT Scans

- Always check for previous records.
- Always consider whether the risk from pathology is more than the risk from scanning [2].
- If a child or a young adult is sent for scanning, discuss with the clinician, suggest alternative investigation and tailor the study to limit the radiation dose.
- Be careful when using IV contrast. The patient could have a severe reaction. Have emergency drugs on standby and provide continuous training to the personnel in the CT department, in managing a crisis. The personnel on the ground will form the first line of defence for the patient.
- The intravenous contrast medium dose should not exceed the dose beyond what is enough to provide diagnostic-quality images.
- Use an extension tube while injecting contrast.
- Keep the contrast at room temperature.
- Kidney function tests (KFT) are mandatory in all hospitalized patients unless time is the constraint. Patients with diabetes mellitus and acute or chronic renal failure need special consideration and deliberation with the treating doctor.
- IV contrast should be avoided if eGFR is less than 30 mL/min/1.73 m^2.
- In emergencies such as trauma, stroke, shock or suspected vascular catastrophe, one can go ahead with a contrast CT scan rather than waiting for reports of KFT.
- Scans of the thorax and extremities can be performed in pregnant patients.
- Avoid iodinated contrast agents during pregnancy, as they can cross the placental barrier [3].
- Routine use of shielding is not necessary as most dose to the foetus comes from the internal scatter [4].

MRI [5, 6]

- Always check the current and previous records.
- Be prepared for all types of complications and side effects while doing the MRI.
- The patient may get claustrophobic when inside the bore of the MRI. To avert this, prepare the patient and if need be arranged for sedation.
- Check renal functions, if IV Gadolinium is likely to be used.
- Patients who have been exposed to iodinated contrast medium and GBCA in the past are more likely to have adverse contrast reactions.
- Do not allow unauthorized entry into the gantry room.
- Remove all ferromagnetic substances from the patient's person as well as from the vicinity of the MRI room.

- Even a non-ferromagnetic material such as aluminium may feel the power of the magnetic field, pushing it back.
- Be careful about foreign bodies and implants. Despite having undergone MRI safely, on some other machine, the implant may prove unsafe in a different MRI machine.
- Provide earplugs to prevent temporary hearing loss.
- Patients may have seizures due to the rapid pulsed gradient sequences. Hence, monitor the patient continuously.
- Ensure that the patient's body is not touching the innermost part of the MRI bore. This can lead to local heating and burns.
- Wires, leads, tattoos and wet diapers can get heated and cause local burns.
- Pacemaker leads are not contraindications, but some patients may have adverse effects, and hence, a careful watch is needed in these patients.
- Do not let any patient or personnel stay inside the gantry room in case of helium leakage or during quenching. The patient may asphyxiate or get a frostbite on encountering helium.

Summing up, despite the rare chance of an untoward side effect of these imaging techniques, the radiation technologist and radiologist must always be on guard, while performing any of these investigations.

References

1. https://www.iaea.org/resources/rpop/health-professionals/radiology/pregnant-women.
2. Wiles R, Hankinson B, Benbow E, Sharp A. Making decisions about radiological imaging in pregnancy. BMJ. 2022;377:e070486. https://doi.org/10.1136/bmj-2022-070486.
3. Singh V, Sandean DP. CT patient safety and care. [Updated 2023 Jan 2]. In: StatPearls [internet]. Treasure Island: StatPearls Publishing; 2024. https://www.ncbi.nlm.nih.gov/books/NBK567800/.
4. Tirada N, Dreizin D, Khati NJ, Akin EA, Zeman RK. Imaging pregnant and lactating patients. Radiographics. 2015;35:1751–65. https://doi.org/10.1148/rg.2015150031. PMID: 26466183.
5. Shah A, Aran S. A review of magnetic resonance (MR) safety: the essentials to patient safety. Cureus. 2023;15(10):e47345. https://doi.org/10.7759/cureus.47345. PMID: 38021512; PMCID: PMC10657250.
6. Kanal E, Borgstede JP, James Barkovich A, Bell C, Bradley WG, Felmlee JP, Froelich JW, Kaminski EM, Keeler EK, Lester JW, Scoumis EA, Zaremba LA, Zinninger MD. American College of Radiology white paper on MR safety. Am J Roentgenol. 2002;178(6):1335–47.

Part IV

PET Scans

Introduction to PET Scan

30

Abstract

Positron Emission Tomography (PET) is a nuclear medicine imaging technique in which a radiopharmaceutical or radiotracer, bound to a radioactive material is injected intravenously. This is taken up by many normal and abnormal tissues with ongoing metabolic activity. In other words, it is a functional study. Metabolic activity is high in many normal body tissues. It increases in muscles, especially following physical activity. Tumours and inflammatory lesions also show increased uptake. These lesions, therefore, stand out in the PET scan and can be easily identified. PET scans are coupled with CT or MRI scans. Hence, they can be either PET-CT or PET-MRI scans.

Keywords

PET scan · PET-CT · PET-MRI
Radiopharmaceutical · Radioactive material

There are several instances where pathological lesions are not easily detectable by conventional CT or MRI. There are also occasions where the number of lesions, their location and their state of activity are not apparent by the usual imaging modalities. A PET scan helps locate such lesions by demonstrating their metabolic activity.

The most common radiopharmaceutical or radiotracer used in practice is FDG (Fluorodeoxyglucose), a glucose analogue. This is tagged to a radionuclide F-18. Other radionuclides include Carbon-11 and Oxygen-16 [1]. FDG, which contains fluoride, is a glucose analogue and is taken up by lesions having high metabolic activity. Pathological lesions, such as tumours and infective/inflammatory processes, have a high metabolic activity. The FDG gets trapped in these tissues as it cannot undergo any further change beyond the phosphorylation stage. The scintillation detectors (made of Bismuth germinate, Cerium-doped lutetium oxyorthosilicate (LSO), or Cerium-doped gadolinium silicate (GSO) detectors) convert the gamma rays emitted by F-18-FDG avid lesions into a bright signal which is detected by photomultiplier tubes connected to the detectors within the PET scanner. In this way, lesions showing avid metabolic activity are detected by the PET scanner. However, the images of a PET scanner are not able to convey the exact location and relationship of PET avid lesions with respect to other organs in the body. For this reason, PET scanners are linked to either a CT or an MRI scanner. Thus, the final product is a PET-CT or a PET-MRI.

Indications of PET-CT: The scanner is used for the detection of tumours, the cause of fever of unknown origin and determination of disease activity. It is also used for identifying an easily accessible lesion amongst multiple lesions for a biopsy and in the follow-up of cancer patients after treatment.

R. Gothi, *Radiographic and Imaging Techniques for Radiology Residents and Technologists*,
https://doi.org/10.1007/978-981-96-4816-0_30

Preparation of patient: The protocol includes:

- Informing the patient that PET-CT is a lengthy examination and may take 2 h or more from end to end.
- Fasting for 4–6 h is required.
- Blood sugar levels should be under control, if possible.
- Blood sugar level should be obtained before commencing the study. This will help in interpreting the PET studies.
- The patient should not do exercises before scanning as this increases uptake by muscles and cardiac shadow.
- The urinary bladder should be empty. The patient should not be incontinent, as the diaper will be soaked with radioactive material.
- The patient must relax and avoid talking for several minutes before the scanning. This is to avoid uptake by active muscles of speech.
- Oral positive contrast is given to patients of malignancy as it helps distinguish bowel loops from adjacent structures.
- Both NCCT and CECT can be performed in PET-CT.
- Imaging commences after an hour from the injection time. The CT scan takes a few seconds to minutes, depending upon the type of scanner and the need for any IV contrast injection. The PET scan takes half an hour to 40 min.
- It is recommended to avoid contact with the patient following injection of the isotope [2].

30.1 Scanning Technique

- The PET scanning gantry looks like a CT or MRI gantry. The CT scanner is in front, and the PET scanner is lined behind it within the same housing. (Both units are separate and can also be used as individual units). The alignment of the CT and PET scanner is such that there should be no mismatch between the CT and PET images. The lesion seen in the PET scan must correspond with the lesion identified in the CT scan (Fig. 30.1).

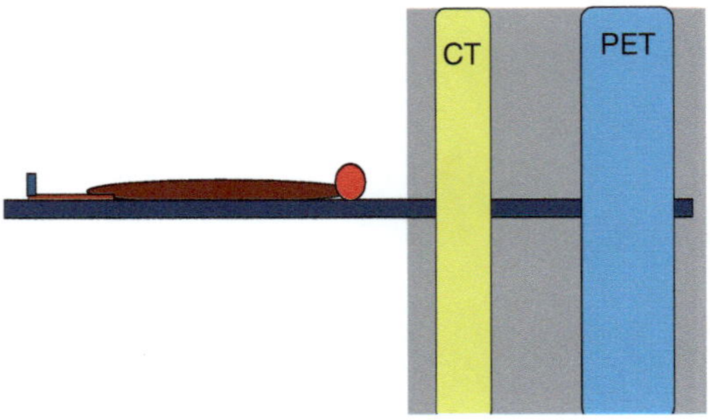

Fig. 30.1 CT PET Gantry. The CT scanner is in front of the PET scanner within the same gantry housing

- A CT scan is performed first. A non-contrast CT is adequate, especially if a recent contrast enhanced study is available. It saves the risk of contrast reaction, movement or vomiting when inside the gantry. However, by taking special precautions and using remote-controlled injectors, IV and oral contrast studies can also be performed. The scan covers the head, neck, chest, abdomen and pelvis.
- Then, without disturbing the patient, by sliding the couch inside the gantry, PET scanning is performed.
- The images obtained are PET tracer uptake images (black and white), CT images and combined PET-CT images which are colour-coded. However, it is possible to acquire only PET, only CT or combined PET-CT images (Fig. 30.2).
- The images can be interpreted visually. Areas of high uptake appear bright yellow as compared to areas showing normal uptake.
- The quantity of metabolite taken up can also be assessed and is given a value, called "standardized uptake value" (SUV). This value does not indicate the nature of the disease. Both inflammatory and malignant diseases can have high SUV values. Higher SUV values mean that the disease has higher metabolically activity.

FDG Uptake by Normal Tissues [3]: FDG uptake is typically seen in the normal liver, spleen, bowel loops, anorectal region, urinary tract (including kidneys, ureters and bladder), myocardium, salivary glands and muscles.

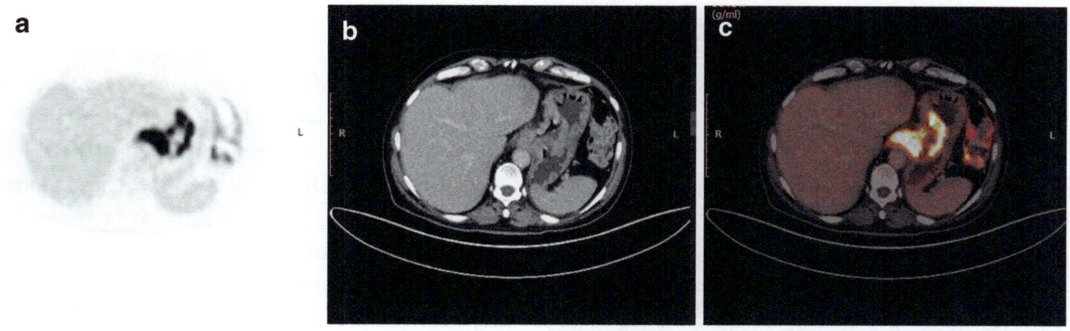

Fig. 30.2 (**a–c**) PET scan of a patient showing tracer uptake image (**a**), CT image (**b**) and PET-CT hybrid image (**c**)

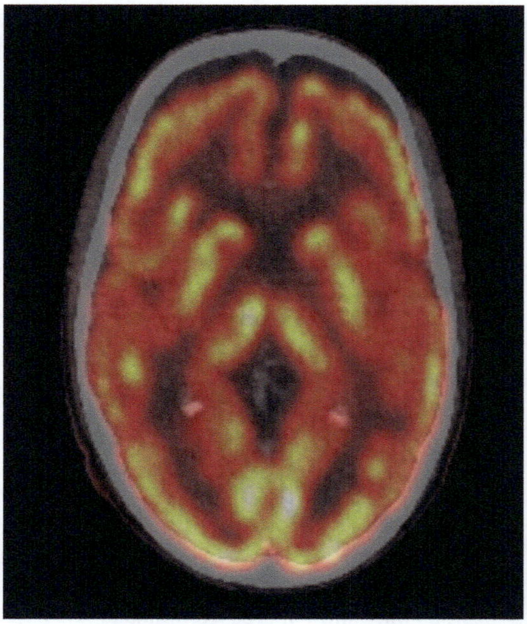

Fig. 30.3 Normal uptake in the brain

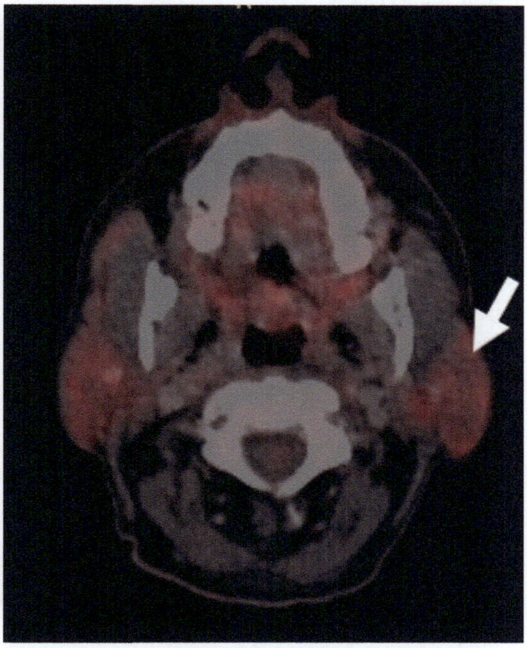

Fig. 30.4 Uptake by normal parotid salivary gland (arrow)

The uptake depends upon the ongoing metabolic activity in these areas and the time elapsed after the injection [4]. These activities can be peristaltic activity, anal sphincteric contraction, excretion in the urinary tract and menstrual activity involving the endometrium and ovaries. Vigorous activity, before scanning, can increase FDG uptake in muscles (Figs. 30.3, 30.4, 30.5, 30.6, and 30.7).

FDG Uptake due to Motion: Cardiac and respiratory activity and Gastroesophageal reflux during scanning can induce an artefact. Similarly, increased uptake may be seen with peristaltic activity in the bowel loops. If the patient moves during scanning, movement artefacts can be produced, which result in blurring of the images and misalignment between the CT and PET images. This misregistration affects ascertaining the amount of FDG uptake by a lesion [5]. Patients should, therefore, be cautioned not to move while the scanning is on [1].

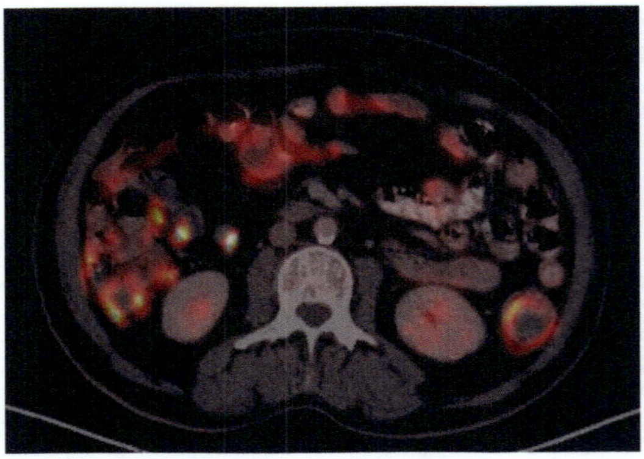

Fig. 30.5 Normal uptake by small and large bowel loops as well as the kidneys

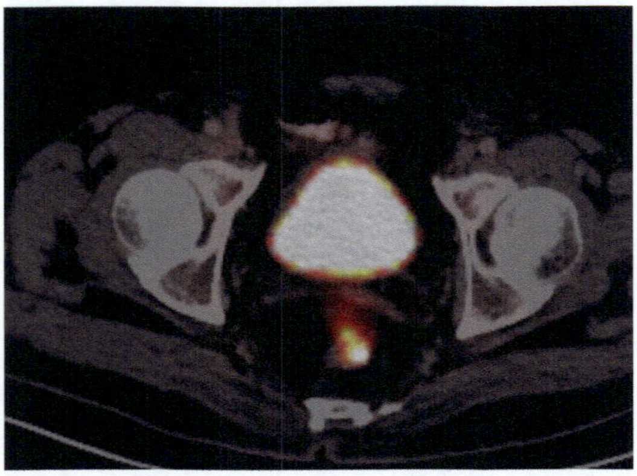

Fig. 30.6 Normal appearance of the urinary bladder filled with F-18 FDG labelled urine. Also, note increased activity in the anorectal region due to sphincteric activity

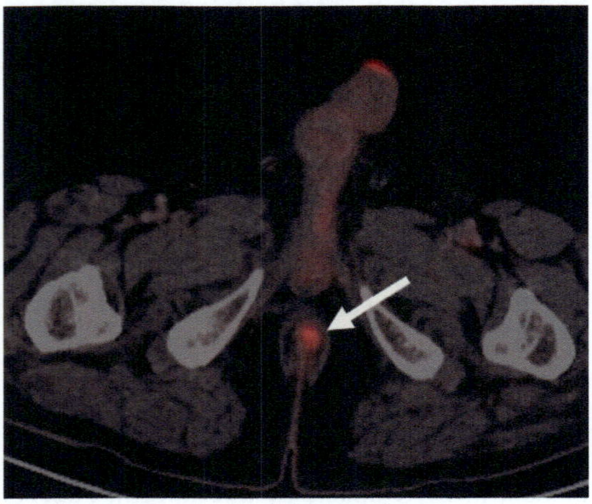

Fig. 30.7 Physiological uptake by anal sphincter

FDG Uptake in the Presence of Prosthesis: Metal implants in the body produce streak artefacts, which can affect the images [5]. Stents in the bile ducts may artifactually increase the FDG uptake which may result in misdiagnosis [6].

PET-CT in Obese Patients: These large patients can suffer from a mismatch between the imaging field obtained by a CT scan as compared to the field acquired by the PET scan. This discrepancy between the two fields of view (FOV) results in truncation artefacts if the PET scanning extends beyond the field of view of the CT scan. This will lead to an underestimation of the concentration of activity in an FDG-avid lesion and needs to be kept in mind and suitably corrected.

30.2 A Few Other Pitfalls Which Also Need to Be Remembered

These include:

- Increased uptake by the cirrhotic liver and in chronic hepatitis. This increase in uptake should not be mistaken for liver malignancy.
- High blood sugar levels in diabetic patients, by interfering with FDG transportation and metabolism, may affect the uptake in all parts of the body. Early pancreatic malignancies may be missed [7, 8].
- Both acute pancreatitis and benign pancreatic lesions may show increased uptake.
- Some tumours such as minimally invasive lung cancers and signet cell carcinoma of the stomach may not show avid FDG uptake. Physiological activity of the stomach, acute gastritis and lymphomas may show increased uptake [6].
- Brown fat deposited in the neck may show avid FDG uptake.
- Many benign bony lesions, including osteophytes and degenerative disc diseases, may show high FDG uptake and be mistaken for malignancies. Therefore, comparing the PET images with CT images will help in minimizing this pitfall [9].

- Fractures may mimic metastatic deposits. The colour-coded images may mask the underlying bony architecture. Here, examining the CT images and evaluating the SUV values is important. The SUV values will generally be higher in malignancies, as compared to fractures. The SUV values of fractures will also decrease with healing.
- Immediate/recent post-operative scans show increased FDG uptake. PET scans do not give a histopathological diagnosis of a lesion. The uptake is dependent on the metabolic activity and may be high even in benign, especially inflammatory diseases. It should not be used to make a histopathological diagnosis.

30.3 Role of PET-CT in Current Practice

PET-CT is used in

- Oncology, to detect lesions (Fig. 30.8).
- Patients having fever of unknown origin, to detect the source of infection (Figs. 30.9 and 30.10).
- Guiding biopsy. Demonstrating the active and most accessible lesion helps plan the biopsy.

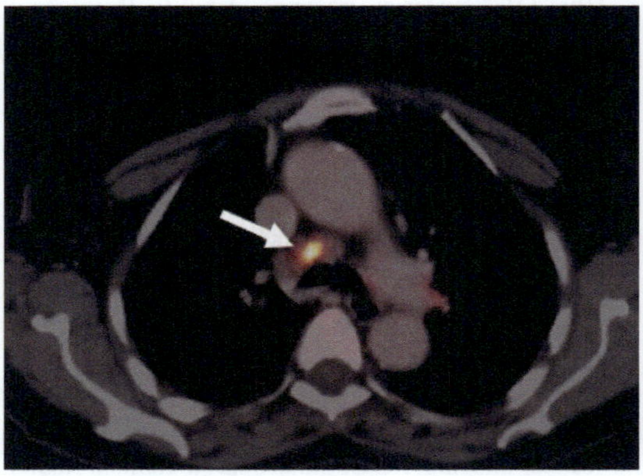

Fig. 30.8 FDG uptake in a small right paratracheal node (arrows). The uptake suggests active disease, suitable for transbronchial biopsy

- Evaluation of disease activity. For example, it is used in Sarcoidosis to identify disease activity.
- Follow-up of patients undergoing treatment for malignancies, infections and inflammatory disorders.

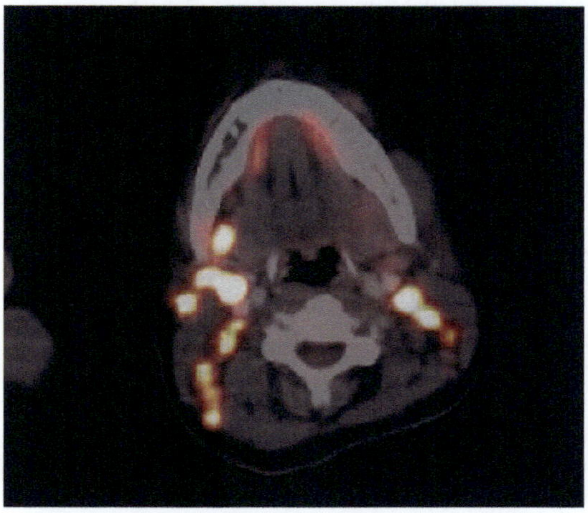

Fig. 30.9 Multiple FDG avid nodes in the neck in a case of fever of unknown origin. The biopsy revealed a granulomatous disease

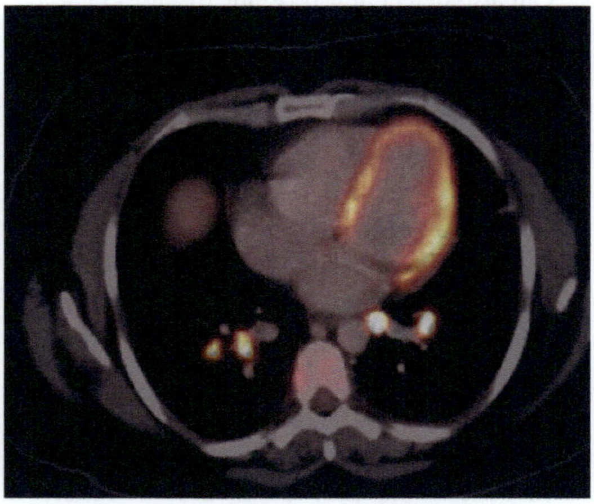

Fig. 30.10 A case of Sarcoidosis showing bilateral intrathoracic nodes. The myocardial uptake is normal and shows normal PET avidity

30.4 Advances in PET Scan

- Fibroblast activation protein is expressed by tumours with strong fibroblastic reaction. Fibroblastic activity in the lungs, liver and kidneys as well as in inflammatory disorders such as Crohn's disease, pulmonary thrombosis, myocardial ischemia and wound healing suggests the presence of ongoing disease.

  Gallium 68 FAPI PET scan is a new tracer which has shown promise in the detection of many cancers and their distant metastasis as well as in the study of many other non-cancerous diseases [10, 11].
- Prostate-specific membrane antigen (PSMA) is a test which measures prostate-specific membrane antigen, a glycoprotein produced by the prostate cells, both normal and tumour cells. This antigen is overexpressed by cancer cells. The study of the spread of cancer of the prostate has brought to the fore PSMA PET scanning which is used to detect nodal and skeletal metastasis as well as biochemical recurrence of prostatic cancers after curative surgery. It is more sensitive than bone scans and CT scans. However, its specificity in detecting prostatic cancers has been called into question because it can also detect non-prostatic diseases [12].

30.5 A Word About PET-MRI

PET-MRI combines the MRI images with the PET scan images. MRI images have better soft tissue contrast details due to their multiple sequences and do not require radiation [13]. However, it takes a longer time to complete an MRI and it is more costly than PET-CT. Its precise role in clinical practice is still evolving.

In conclusion, PET-CT is used routinely in oncologic practice and many other situations. It is a hybrid technique where both imaging as well as nuclear medicine collaborate. Radiologists are often called upon by clinicians to interpret PET scan images. This brief introduction is provided to enable radiology technologists and physicians to approach this modality with a basic understanding.

References

1. Kapoor V, McCook BM, Torok FS. An introduction to PET-CT imaging. Radiographics. 2004;24(2):523–43.
2. Benamor M, Ollivier L, Brisse H, Moulin-Romsee G, Servois V, Neuenschwander S. PET/CT imaging: what radiologists need to know. Cancer Imaging. 2007;7 Spec No A(Special issue A):S95–9. https://doi.org/10.1102/1470-7330.2007.9012. PMID: 17921089; PMCID: PMC2727970.
3. Vangu MDT, Momodu JI. F-18 FDG PET/CT imaging in normal variants, pitfalls and artifacts in the abdomen and pelvis. Front Nucl Med. 2022;1:826109. https://doi.org/10.3389/fnume.2021.826109.
4. Shreve PD, Anzai Y, Wahl RL. Pitfalls in oncologic diagnosis with FDG PET imaging: physiologic and benign variants. Radiographics. 1999;19(1):61–77.
5. Corrigan AJG, Schleyer PJ, Cook GJ. Pitfalls and artifacts in the use of PET/CT in oncology imaging. Semin Nucl Med. 2015;45:481–99. https://doi.org/10.1053/j.semnuclmed.2015.02.006.
6. Lin E, Alavi A. PET and PET/CT—A clinical guide. 3rd ed. New York: Thieme; 2019.
7. Hamidian Jahromi A, Fallahzadeh MK, Takalkar A, Sheng J, Zibar G, Shokouh Amiri H. Impact of plasma glucose level at the time of flurodeoxyglucose administration on the accuracy of FDG-PET/CTin the diagnosis of pancreatic lesions. Int J Endocrinol Metab. 2014;12:e16429. https://doi.org/10.5812/ijem.16429.
8. Diederichs CG, Staib I, Glatting G, Berger HG, Reske SN. FDG PET: elevated plasma glucose reduces both uptake and detection rate of pancreatic malignancies. J Nucl Med. 1998;39:1030–3.
9. Costelloe CM, Murphy WA Jr, Chasen BA. Musculoskeletal pitfalls in ^{18}F-FDG PET/CT: pictorial review. Am J Roentgenol. 2009;193(3_supplement):WS1–WS13.
10. Mori Y, Dendl K, Cardinale J, Kratochwil C, Giesel FL, Haberkorn U. FAPI PET: fibroblast activation protein inhibitor use in oncologic and nononcologic disease. Radiology. 2023;306:e220749.
11. Mori Y, Novruzov E, Schmitt D, et al. Clinical applications of fibroblast activation protein inhibitor positron emission tomography (FAPI-PET). npj Imaging. 2024;2:48. https://doi.org/10.1038/s44303-024-00053-z.
12. Sivathapandi T, Gunasekaran G. Role of Ga68 prostate-specific membrane antigen positron emission tomography-computed tomography in prostate cancer imaging. J Gastrointestinal Abdominal Radiol. 2024;7:121–47.
13. Ehman EC, Johnson GB, Villanueva-Meyer JE, Cha S, Leynes AP, Larson PEZ, Hope TA. PET/MRI: where might it replace PET/CT? J Magn Reson Imaging. 2017;46(5):1247–62. https://doi.org/10.1002/jmri.25711. Epub 2017 Mar 30. PMID: 28370695; PMCID: PMC5623147.

GPSR Compliance

The European Union's (EU) General Product Safety Regulation (GPSR) is a set of rules that requires consumer products to be safe and our obligations to ensure this.

If you have any concerns about our products, you can contact us on ProductSafety@springernature.com

In case Publisher is established outside the EU, the EU authorized representative is:

Springer Nature Customer Service Center GmbH
Europaplatz 3
69115 Heidelberg, Germany

Batch number: 09403631

Printed by Printforce, the Netherlands